Administration In Nursir

Administration In Nursing

Mary D. Shanks, Ed.D.

Caroline F. Rupert Professor of Nursing
and Director of the School of Nursing
Illinois Wesleyan University, Bloomington
Commander, U.S. Navy Nurse Corps Reserve

Dorothy A. Kennedy, M.A.

Coordinator and Major Professor
Undergraduate and Graduate Program
Maternal and Child Nursing
College of Nursing
University of Delaware

Second Edition

McGraw-Hill Book Company
A Blakiston Publication

New York St. Louis San Francisco Düsseldorf
London Mexico Panama Sydney Toronto

Administration In Nursing

Library of Congress Catalog Card Number 79-126180

56405

Foreword

The authors of this text present three basic concepts: (1) nursing will improve as the individual in nursing improves, (2) nursing will improve as the individual nurse improves her own practice of nursing, and (3) the nurse must complement and facilitate the practice of all other persons who are engaged in nursing.

With these three concepts in mind, the authors define the kind of person needed to do the job, the kind of place where much of the job is done, and the process through which the job is successfully accomplished. Finally, by means of case studies, the reader is challenged to think about the principles and the components of the administrative process in carrying out nursing activity.

New to nursing texts is the *administrative blueprint,* presented in Chapter 11; it is a design for *doing* the job. The authors state that the process involves components that are not sequential; that the components are concomitant and interdependent, and that each component must be applied to the performance of each administrative function. Each activity, they insist, is an *intellectual* activity. Their proposal that the administrative process be implemented by the principles inherent in the blueprint is based on the premise that thinking in preparation for doing is a rewarding and exciting experience.

With this in mind, it is easy to see why they have devoted so much space to the person, the individual. They believe that philosophy, religion, and the arts are vital influences from which the individual can develop and nurture desirable characteristics that will enable him to enrich his personal life as well as to improve his professional performance.

This text is not one that can be scanned lightly. The thoughtful reader, for instance, may find that Parts II and III may be reread as independent units without repeated reference to Parts IV and V. All readers will not agree with this presentation, but all should find it interesting and provocative.

The book can be recommended to three distinct groups.

1. The students who are still involved in the formal learning process.

2. The beginning practitioners who need expert on-the-job help to develop to the highest degree the application of the "administrative

process." This text could well be used for Nursing Management Courses intended for the Assistant Head Nurse level.

3. The long-time practitioners who have learned, as many of us have, by doing, and who, with thoughtful study of the text, will recognize the *process* which has so often been neglected in favor of intuition.

Unlike most books, this one can be used equally well by the beginning practitioner and the skilled administrator. It is also extremely valuable for the graduate student and for on-the-job training programs. It can be used in part, or as a whole; as a classroom text, or as a reference volume. Some readers will be interested in researching the hypothesis and investigating in selected settings whether this guide really details a "scientific process."

Last, but not least, the case studies are developed in such a way that they can be used readily by the individual reader or by a group. The cases are carefully selected and are meaningful. The case notes are helpful. The case discussions, while detailed, leave room for much discussion and perhaps even disagreement by the reader. It certainly induces the reader to participate actively.

However the book is used, the reader will not be indifferent to it.

Evelyn M. Hamil, R.N.
Director, Nursing Services and Education,
Los Angeles County
University of Southern
California Medical Center

Preface

The theory of administration and the educated practice of administration are excitingly scientific. Theory formulation is new to nursing administration, but it undoubtedly plays a valuable role in the quest for new administrative knowledge based on fact and scientific inquiry.

This book proposes the theory that *the administrative process is a scientific process.* From this theory, it can be anticipated that testable hypotheses may be derived and subjected to the rigors of the scientific method by the many practitioners of nursing administration who, in fact, are students of administration. In this way the theory will be substantiated or refuted and supplanted by an alternate proposal, thus adding to the now scant body of knowledge of administration in nursing.

The assumption upon which this theory is based is that prescribed techniques for doing are no longer sufficient to the complicated administrative tasks at hand. Recognizing that the scientific exploration of the proposed theory will take time, we offer an *administrative blueprint* as a source of assistance to nurses who, in the absence of immediately available administrative knowledge, perform administrative functions. The blueprint is a design for doing the job and has been found to be effective by those who have followed it in the performance of the job.

The subject of administration concerns itself, however, not only with the process, or with the job to be done, but also with the person who is doing the job and the place in which the job is done. And there are some provocative theories relating to both of these aspects of administration being proposed by scholars in other disciplines. For example: "Personality is the major consideration in the establishment of an organizational structure." This and several other theories are explored in terms of their relevance to nursing administration.

Theories, however, ultimately are valued directly in proportion to the degree to which they improve practice. Throughout this book suggestions for improvements are identified extensively, through guided opportunities to experience the practice of nursing administration in a controlled environment, by means of the comprehensive case studies documented herein.

This book has been written for all professional nurses. Daily, nurses are called upon to perform one or several functions that are administrative in nature. This is not a temporary situation due to what is frequently termed the transitional stage through which nursing is presently passing. Rather, administrative performance is an integral component of nursing—nursing at any functional level from general duty nursing to directing a nursing service, in any setting—such as a hospital, public health agency, or industry. For example, because the concept of team nursing is spreading from the hospital to long-term care institutions and home care programs, professional nurses will have to exert considerable administrative leadership in planning and organizing the care given these patients.

The responsibility is not new. Through the years all nurses have been evaluated in terms of ability to plan and organize their own work and the work of others, and to direct the activities of others—patients and coworkers. Evaluated, yes; prepared, not always. Time must be made available for the teaching of administration in basic educational programs.

But what of the practitioner of nursing who has not had this preparation, as well as the future student and teacher of nursing? It is with these persons in mind that this book has been designed to bring together in one readily available source much of the existing knowledge and to present some new knowledge pertaining to administration in nursing.

The present revision reflects the usual updating of content, bibliographical references, and the like, but also reflects a somewhat unusual steadfast commitment to the original concepts, principles, and philosophy of administration—the very nature of which has dictated a change of title. If, indeed, the proposition that "administration and the administrative process occur in substantially the same generalized form in the industrial, commercial, civil, educational, military, and hospital organization" is accepted and supported throughout the text, then the title *The Theory and Practice of Nursing Service Administration* was misleading and far too delimiting. If every function of the nurse has administrative components, and nurses are functioning *every place,* then surely we need to broaden the perspective—hence, *Administration in Nursing.*

Mary D. Shanks
Dorothy A. Kennedy

Contents

Administration In Nursing

part 1
Introduction

1

Administration in Nursing Practice

The fundamental goal of the nursing profession is to provide patients with the best possible nursing care. Throughout the history of their profession nurses have strived to attain this goal while confronted by vast technologic, economic, and sociologic changes that have exerted a challenging impact on the nature of the health services provided. Nursing has responded to the demands imposed by these changes and will continue to respond in order to accomplish the goals of the profession. As health services increase, the need for nursing services increases, and more and more persons become involved in providing these services. The role of the professional nurse now ranges from the giving of care to the direction and supervision of other persons who give care to patients. Administrative skill has become indispensable in providing creative, need-fulfilling patient care within this many-faceted and multidisciplinary approach to the giving of nursing care.

Administration is that organization through which persons in a given social setting achieve a desired and defined goal. This definition of administration embodies the concept that the components of the system are persons, purpose, place, and process. It implies a personal element, in that individuals participate in and direct the necessary activities. It includes a sociologic element, in that participants should understand and appreciate the setting for the activities. It prescribes a philosophical approach, in that a goal must be both desired and defined. Inherent in this definition, also, is the concept that the person, the purpose, the place, and the process contribute equally to the performance of administrative functions in any setting, be it a business, educational, industrial, military, governmental, hospital, or health agency.

Administration of professional nursing practice is that organization through which nurses in a hospital or another type of health agency are able to provide the best possible nursing care for patients in the hospital or under the jurisdiction of another type of health agency.

The administrative process is a series or cycle of actions that leads to the accomplishment of a defined goal. The administrative process is utilized whenever an individual nurse gives care to an individual patient. The elements of the process are used in planning the patient's care, in directing the care, in arranging and controlling the setting, and in facilitating the accomplishment of the care.

An administrator is a person who guides others toward the accomplishment of an objective by coordinating their activities. Throughout this text the term *administrator* refers to all nurses—staff nurse, supervisor, or director of nursing—who perform functions that are essentially administrative. In nursing this term is traditionally associated with the positions of director and assistant director of nursing service, nursing service supervisor, and head nurse. It is the thesis of this text, however, that the staff nurse in any employment setting also is a nurse administrator.

What then, is the administrative role of the staff nurse? What are her responsibilities, her functions? The American Nurses' Association defines the general duty (staff) nurse as follows: ". . . a registered professional nurse, employed by a hospital or an institution, who is responsible for the direct and/or indirect total nursing care of the patient."[1] The Association adds that general duty nurses are aware that they must be given the opportunity to participate in the development of administrative policy if they are to function effectively in work situations. The preparation, administration, and supervision of a patient care plan certainly have administrative implications.

Another major function for the general duty (staff) nurse is specified as participation in the administration of nursing service in a general or special hospital or other health agency. The components of that participation are listed as follows:[2]

A. Interprets philosophy, aims, and policies of hospital administration to:
   1. Patients and family
   2. Hospital personnel
   3. Allied health groups
   4. Community

B. Participates in intra- and interdepartmental activities designed to assist the hospital and nursing administration in improving the service of the hospital.

C. Establishes and maintains good interpersonal relationships.

[1] *Functions, Standards, and Qualification for Practice of the General Duty Nurse,* American Nurses' Association, New York, 1956, p. 1.

[2] *Op. cit.*, p. 2.

D. Coordinates the objectives and aims of nursing service.
E. Assumes responsibility for contributing to the educational program of any student who is having clinical experience under the nurse's guidance.
F. Contributes to the improvement of nursing care.

Since it is from the staff nurse position that professional nurses advance to greater degrees of involvement in the administrative process, more attention must be paid to the beginner if there is to be any hope for advancement of administration in nursing.

The literature is replete with references to the changing role of the staff nurse and the dichotomy between the educational preparation of the nurse for practice and the expectations of the employing agencies for the functions of the staff nurse. Much of this literature calls attention to the staff nurse's desire to return to the bedside of the patient and recommends that she be allowed to do so. Too many persons insist, however, that in returning to the bedside the nurse would have to discard all administrative responsibility—responsibility so frequently regarded as "unwanted" and "inflicted" upon staff nurses by the present organization of health agencies. Administration is conceived of in this text as being as integral a part of patient care as so-called true bedside nursing. Without administrative functions true bedside nursing does not exist.

Writers in the professional nursing journals, physicians, sociologists, other interested and concerned professionals, and writers of lay literature decry the present state of affairs in which the true nurse has been displaced by the "paperwork" nurse. No one will argue with this. Many of the management functions of the staff nurse could be delegated to others. Esther Lucile Brown expressed the belief that nursing and nurses must be ". . . the major agent for maintaining a socially therapeutic environment in those parts of the hospital where patients spend most of their time." [3] This cannot be accomplished without the administrative process, and in this effort the staff nurse has a role as important as that of other nurse administrators. There is a need for a more creative approach, at all levels, to the administration of nursing services. This concept must be instilled in the minds of nursing students, staff nurses, and other nurse administrators. Every nurse must be encouraged to approach her role in a dynamic manner and toward an optimal approach to nursing service administration.

[3] Esther Lucile Brown, *Newer Dimensions of Patient Care*, part I, Russell Sage Foundation, New York, 1961, p. 117.

THE PURPOSE OF THIS BOOK

The task set for this book is to present some theories of administration, to relate these theories to the administration of professional nursing practice, and to offer guidance to nurses about to assume staff positions and to nurses already engaged in the practice of their profession. The primary focus of this approach to administration is on nursing practice in hospitals, only because hospitals employ almost two-thirds (62 per cent) of the professional nurses engaged in active practice.[4] It may be assumed that the administrative principles and techniques essential for the provision of nursing services in the hospital are equally applicable to the provision of nursing services to patients in any social setting.

BASIC BELIEFS ABOUT ADMINISTRATION

There are, of course, many ways to approach a discussion of administration in nursing. Profound beliefs about the process of administration and the role of the nurse as an administrator have guided the authors in the practice of administration and in formulating the plan for this book. The presentation in this book has evolved from these beliefs, as stated below:

1. The goal of administration in any setting is service; the service activities are carried out by persons, through persons, for other persons.

2. The primary role of the administrator is to coordinate whatever is necessary so that everyone else can accomplish his job.

3. The degree to which the administrative process is effective in the achievement of a goal depends upon:

a. The extent to which all persons involved subscribe to the defined goal.

b. The extent to which all persons work together toward the goal.

c. The extent to which the elements of the process are used by all persons involved.

d. The extent to which the persons involved know, understand, and appreciate the social structure of the setting.

e. The characteristics of the person occupying the administrative position.

4. The administrative process in hospitals and in other health agencies is the same as in business, educational, industrial, military, or governmental organizations.

5. Administrative functions have greater importance than in the past as

[4] American Nurses' Association, *Facts About Nursing,* New York, 1968, p. 12.

a result of today's broader concept of health and nursing and the increasing complexity of health agencies.

6. It is essential that every nurse have an understanding of the theory and practice of administration, for the administrative process is involved whenever an individual nurse gives care to an individual patient.

THE DESIGN OF THIS BOOK

This book is presented in five parts. Part I introduces the reader to the scope of nursing administration and to the formulation of theories of administration. If advances are to be made in nursing administration and if the profession is to meet the increasing demands for nursing care, nursing must devote time to the development of theories of nursing administration and to the testing of these theories.

Part II describes some of the desirable characteristics of *the person* in administration—the administrator. Because the administrative process is utilized whenever an individual nurse gives care to an individual patient, the characteristics desirable in the administrator are, in reality, the characteristics desirable in all nurses.

What are the characteristics, tangible and intangible, that identify the administrator and are essential for leadership in the provision of nursing care for people? Can these be uncovered and developed in the nurse? Chapter 3 describes some of the desirable characteristics of the administrator as they have been manifested by successful administrators in nursing and in allied professions. These descriptions may motivate nurses, whether they be students of nursing, staff nurses, head nurses, supervisors, educators, or directors of nursing, to pause, to reflect, and to evaluate themselves in relation to the desirable characteristics of the administrator.

Because of our deep faith in the contribution that the liberal arts can make to nursing, to nursing education, and to the personality of the individual nurse, we asked colleagues from the academic world to present their views on the influence of philosophy, religion, and the arts on an individual. In Chapter 4, Dr. John VanderWaal, a teacher, philosopher, and minister delineates the contribution the study of philosophy, particularly the art and practice of thinking, can make to an individual.

Dr. Richard Stegner, a teacher and minister, discusses in Chapter 5 the influence of religion in enhancing the characteristics of the person. He describes the ways in which religion "shapes what a person is and does" and examines questions relating to the meaning of "vocation," the nature of man, and the ethics of man's relationship with others. In essence, he is not seeking to proselytize, but rather to encourage the reader to define for himself an ethical approach to the practice of his profession.

Ethical and spiritual values have been mentioned in the past in reference to the nurse and to nursing, but seldom does one find any consideration of the contribution that the fine arts can make to nursing and to the nurse. In Chapter 6 Rupert Kilgore, a teacher and painter, lifts the reader from a mundane, merely practical outlook on life to the realm of inspiration to be derived from an esthetic response to life and to the influence this attitude can have on the characteristics desirable in the nurse. In Chapter 7 Dr. Marie Robinson, a teacher and public speaker, emphasizes the ideas the artist, the musician, the writer, and the dramatist can communicate to an individual.

A thorough knowledge and understanding of the setting is essential to effective administration. What is the *place* in which this person, the administrator, functions? Is a health agency unlike other kinds of institutions? What influence does the setting have on the person and the administrative process? An understanding of a major health agency, specifically, the hospital, is presented in Part III by Dr. D. Paul Miller, a sociologist interested in and familiar with hospitals but not emotionally involved in medicine or nursing. Thus he is not compelled to preserve the myth that the hospital is an enigma which can be understood only by those within. He discusses the hospital as the place in which the administrator functions, the community in which the hospital is an integral part, and the effect the modern world has on the nature of the hospital. He also explores the factors that make the hospital unique among social institutions—the dichotomous chain of command and the service to persons who are ill—with the intent of contributing to the knowledge needed by the nurse.

The *process* of administration in nursing is presented in Part IV. Theories of the administrative process are presented in Chapter 9. These theories have yet to be tested, even though they appear to be substantiated by the experiences of persons in administrative positions in nursing as well as in other fields.

So much has been written about the "changing role of nurses" that nurses, colleagues, and the public are confused about what to anticipate from the profession. For this reason, the expectations of nurses themselves regarding administrative functions are explored. Chapter 10 is devoted to an examination of the statements of functions, standards, and qualifications nurses have established through their professional organization, the American Nurses' Association. Particular emphasis is given to the functions professional nurses describe as administrative in nature and to the differences in degree of involvement required of the general duty nurse, the head nurse, the supervisor, and the director of nursing service.

From personal experiences and the experiences of others in administrative settings the authors have drafted an *administrative blueprint* which can be used in the performance of administrative functions. Chapter 11 presents this approach to the administration of care—an approach that has proved effective in a variety of settings. As an example of the theoretical application of the design, the blueprint is applied in Chapter 12 to the staffing function—one of the broad functions of administration for nursing service.

Part V provides comprehensive experiences in the administrative process within a realistic setting—the hospital—within patient-nurse situations. Given a specific incident, how can the nurse administrator approach it, analyze it, change it, resolve it? What action should she take? What knowledge is necessary for a relevant decision? As a prelude to the presentation and discussion of actual incidents in nursing service, the process of case analysis is explored in Chapter 13. Suggestions are presented to help the reader view each case as a learning situation, not simply as an account of a past happening. To provide a degree of anonymity for the settings of the incidents described, actual cases have been altered only to adapt them to one fictional setting, a hypothetical hospital which is a composite of several hospitals and one which has all the elements found to a greater or lesser degree in any hospital. The Charles Evans Memorial Hospital, the composite setting, is described in Chapter 14.

The case incidents illustrated in Part V are intended to encourage the reader to reflect, to evaluate, to draw principles from the discussions, and to foresee ways of applying these principles to other situations. The primary person involved in several of the incidents described is the staff nurse, the general duty nurse. This selection is deliberate, because administrative responsibility is first assumed at this level of practice and because it is from the staff nurse position that the nurse advances to positions of supervision over a greater number of persons and thus to broader administrative responsibility.

The closing chapter of this text is an attempt to prophesy some of the contributions that nursing can and should make to the field of nursing administration and therefore to the science of administration.

2

Theory Formulation

Of the many theories of administration that have been proposed, none of them originated with nursing. This fact, however, does not make them less interesting and appropriate to nursing, nor less deserving of attention. A theory, by dictionary definition, is "a proposed explanation or hypothesis designed to account for any phenomenon." But this definition does not include several other qualifications that have become attached to the term. In the interest of fostering a scientific approach to theorizing, Herbert Feigel proposed that theory be defined as "a set of assumptions from which can be derived by purely logico-mathematical procedures a larger set of empirical laws." [1]

If one admits that a theory is essentially a set of assumptions, it follows that a theory cannot be substantiated or verified by experiment. Herein lies the real value of theory; from stated assumptions testable hypotheses can be derived. It is generally agreed that the study of administration has infrequently included the application of the rigors of the scientific method, but that theory formulation, with its resulting hypotheses, makes it possible to utilize this method. The focus is redirected from technique, long the method used in nursing, to processes and relationships.

Another qualification of the definition of theory is that it must describe the phenomenon. The three theories of leadership proposed by Ross and Henday are (1) leadership as traits within the individual leader, (2) leadership as a function of the group, and (3) leadership as a function of the situation.[2] Each statement attempts to define leadership. That the three statements are incompatible points up another value of theorizing—hypotheses that have been tested and refuted generate new theories.

Who may theorize? The opportunity is open to anyone who has a recog-

[1] Herbert Feigel, "Principles and Problems of Theory Construction in Psychology," *Current Trends in Psychological Theory,* Pittsburgh University Press, 1951, p. 82.

[2] Murray G. Ross and Charles Henday, *New Understanding of Leadership,* Association Press, New York, 1957, pp. 17–31.

nized thought in the form of an assumption. The practicing nurse, for example, is in an enviable position to observe administrative phenomena and to state them in the form of assumptions that may make it possible to formulate theories and concepts of administration that can be tested by the scientific method.

Rather than recount the efforts of the many theorists, the work of the two authorities whose theories have had the greatest influence on the development of the thesis of this text will be presented in some detail. In this chapter Edward H. Litchfield's administrative propositions will be discussed, and in Chapter 9 Griffith's theory pertaining primarily to the administrative process will be explored.

Litchfield made the following criticisms of existing administrative thought and theory: [3]

1. We are unable to speak precisely excepting in our own immediate circles where we have developed ephemeral professional dialects.
2. Present thought has failed to achieve a level of generalization enabling it to systematize and explain administrative phenomena which occur in related fields. We appear to maintain that there is not a generic administrative process but only a series of isolated types of administration.
3. We have failed to accord a broad role to the variables in the administrative process.
4. We do not understand the attributes and characteristics of administration as a totality.
5. We urgently need our thought set forth in straightforward propositions which we may then establish, modify, or destroy as research or more careful analysis may dictate.

He then enumerated a series of working hypotheses or propositions that may eventually lead to a broadly conceived theory of administration:

First Major Proposition. The administrative process is a cycle of action which includes the following specific activities:

A. Decision-making
B. Programming
C. Communicating
D. Controlling
E. Reappraising

Minor Proposition. Decision-making may be rational, deliberative, discretionary, purposive, or it may be irrational, habitual, obligatory, random,

[3] Edward H. Litchfield, "Notes on a General Theory of Administration," *Administrative Science Quarterly*, vol. 1, pp. 3–29, June, 1956. (*By permission.*)

or any combination thereof. In its rational, deliberative, discretionary, and purposive form, it is performed by means of the following subactivities:

a. Definition of the issue
b. Analysis of the existing situation
c. Calculation and delineation of alternatives
d. Deliberation
e. Choice

Minor Proposition. Decisions become guides to action after they have been interpreted in the form of specific programs.

Minor Proposition. The effectiveness of a programmed decision will vary with the extent to which it is communicated to those of whom action is required.

Minor Proposition. Action required by a programmed and communicated decision is more nearly assured if standards of performance are established and enforced.

Minor Proposition. Decisions are based on facts, assumptions, and values which are subject to change. To retain their validity, decisions must therefore be reviewed and revised as rapidly as change occurs.

Second Major Proposition. The administrative process functions in the areas of:

a. Policy
b. Resources
c. Execution

Minor Proposition. Action in each functional area is accomplished by means of the action cycle previously described.

Minor Proposition. Each function seeks a value which when realized is its contribution to the administrative process.

Minor Proposition. Each function has distinctive characteristics which govern the application of the cycle to it.

Minor Proposition. The functional areas of administration are integrally related to one another.

Third Major Proposition. The administrative process is carried on in the context of a larger action system, the dimensions of which are:

a. The administrative process
b. The individual performing the administrative process
c. The total enterprise within which the individual and the enterprise function.
d. The ecology within which the individual and the enterprise function.

Minor Proposition. While constant in basic structure, the administrative process will vary in important aspects, depending upon the personality of the person performing it.

Minor Proposition. While constant in basic structure, the administrative process will vary in important respects, depending upon the character of the total enterprise within which it is performed.

Minor Proposition. While constant in basic structure, the administrative process will vary in important respects, depending upon the environment in which the individual and total enterprise function.

Minor Proposition. The types of relationships existing among the three dimensions other than the administrative have an effect upon the administrative process.

Fourth Major Proposition. Administration is the performance of the administrative process by an individual or a group in the context of an enterprise functioning in its environment.

Minor Proposition. Administration as a totality has definable attributes. They are:

a. It seeks to perpetuate itself.
b. It seeks to preserve its internal well-being.
c. It seeks to preserve itself vis-a-vis others.
d. It seeks growth.

Minor Proposition. The attributes to the totality of administration have significant effects upon administrative behavior.

Fifth Major Proposition. Administration and the administrative process occur in substantially the same generalized form in industrial, commercial, civil, educational, military, and hospital organization.

This obviously is a comprehensive view of administration. Although Litchfield never stated a theory of administration, he implied the concept succinctly, and in a form that makes each proposition amenable to scientific treatment. Knowing that the aim of science is to describe, explain, and predict, the thought that eventually each one of these propositions will be fully described and explained is an exciting prospect. But of even more practical value will be the forecasts that can be made.

The above propositions will be considered throughout this text as the person, the purpose, the place, and the process are discussed.

part 2

The Person

3

Administrative Theory in Relation to the Characteristics of the Person

The process of administration as it is *commonly* conceived of in nursing encompasses the theory and practice of nursing service administration. But to discuss the process without first considering the person in administration and the place in which he performs his role is to view administration narrowly and to lose sight of the human element in administration. The minor proposition that identifies the significance of the effect of the personality of the administrator on the outcome of the administrative endeavor was stated by Litchfield as "While constant in basic structure, the administrative process will vary in important aspects, depending upon the personality of the person performing it." [1]

Which of the important aspects of the administrative process will vary, depending upon the personality of the administrator? Is an administrative personality identifiable? Is it possible to predict an individual's success in the performance of the administrative process? Simply stated, Litchfield's minor proposition suggests that the personality of the administrator is extremely important to the successful performance of the job. The quantity of research that has been done by other disciplines in efforts to identify the administrative personality attests to this fact. Studies in which the personality of the administrator has been considered a significant variable have been classified according to a number of current concepts relevant to the dynamic attributes of personality—attitude, values, adjustment, and motivation—as well as to cognitive abilities. The progress made in these research efforts toward defining the desirable administrative personality has been stated best by Hemphill et al. in a study of the principal of a simulated elementary school.[2]

[1] Edward H. Litchfield, "Notes on a General Theory of Administration," *Administrative Science Quarterly,* vol. 1, p. 24, June, 1956.

[2] John K. Hemphill, Daniel E. Griffiths, and Norman Frederiksen, *Administrative Performance and Personality,* Bureau of Publications, Teachers College, Columbia University, New York, 1962, p. 7.

At the outset, the researchers agreed that the science of administration was immature to the degree that "no known theory of administration was substantial enough to support the study." Consequently, they decided that their primary concern should be with "making observations of administrative behavior—observations which are the prerequisite of theory building." The approach we use in delineating the personality of the person in nursing administration is precisely the same as that used by Hemphill et al. For the most part, what is known about the nurse administrator is empirical. Thus, the characteristics that have been found to be desirable in the person can be described only in terms of gross observations. Our commitment to the theory that the personality of the person in administration is important allows the inclusion of somewhat nonscientific data simply because it represents the best knowledge available.

Griffiths et al. have said, "It is probably as sound to pick key individuals and build the organization around them as it is to establish the administrative structure and then seek to fill the key posts." [3] This is a forceful testimonial in support of the importance of the person to the job. But how does one recognize this individual? Is there an identifiable administrative personality? In the belief that there is, and that it is most immediately apparent to the possessor, we conducted an informal opinion poll over a five-year-period. A large number of persons in diversified occupations were queried. The only criterion for qualification was that the subject be in a position that was obviously administrative in nature—a nursing service administrator, a dean of a school of nursing, a *maître d'hôtel,* a newspaper editor, etc. Each person was asked, "When did you first know you had administrative ability?" Without exception, the answer was "Always." When asked, "What do you think are your characteristics of personality that are unique to an individual with administrative ability?," they could not answer as readily. This is where one is forced to describe empirically the characteristics that are common to persons who successfully occupy positions of administration.

If any one characteristic can be deemed to be more important than any other one, then surely this can be said of the characteristic *respect. Respect for the individual*—recognition of the inherent dignity and worth of man, is a primary condition of this characteristic. The two distinct but inseparable components of this characteristic are (1) respect for self and (2)

[3] Daniel E. Griffiths and others, *Organizing Schools for Effective Education,* Interstate Printers and Publishers, Danville, Ill., 1962, p. 51.

respect for others. They are named in this order inasmuch as the conviction is held that respect for others develops simultaneously with respect for self.

Inherent in the respect for self is the need to know the self. The process of learning about the self is never-ending. It entails an interest in and a willingness to continuously evaluate what one thinks and does. Has thought always preceded action? Of both can one be proud? If an individual eventually can identify himself as a person with a degree of wisdom and a strong sense of worth he acquires a belief in himself and a philosophy that is workable and sustaining throughout life. The development of self-respect is contingent upon the threefold process of (1) critical examination of the self, (2) self-improvement as a result of what one has learned about himself, and (3) acceptance of the self.

It is a sad event, for example, for a nurse to learn that she does not really like people. They do not respond favorably to her, and she devises ways of avoiding contact with them. It is sad to learn this, but it is a greater misfortune not to know it when it is true. Having identified a facet of her personality that is objectionable to herself and to others, she is now in a position to initiate corrective measures. The greatest hurdle is in recognizing the shortcoming. The ensuing self-analysis, with or without assistance, may disclose the course of action that may bring about self-improvement.

Having learned to know and respect oneself as a changing, improving person allows one to accept others on the same terms and to respect them as individuals in the state in which he finds them. This is a right of every person with whom the nurse is in contact, and the numbers are many: patients, their families, coworkers (including peers), physicians, nursing personnel with less preparation, and the personnel of other departments in the hospital. Each of these persons can expect from the nurse a genuine interest in him as an individual as well as an ability to listen and to "hear" what he is unable to say. A concern on the part of the nurse for everything that is of concern to the individual—concern evidenced not only by verbal but also by empathic response—tells a person that he is important as an individual.

A second aspect of this characteristic, which seems to be common to persons who have successfully occupied administrative positions, is *respect for the place*—the place meaning both the employing institution and the community in which the institution is located. To respect is to hold in esteem, and this is possible only if one is thoroughly familiar with the setting, has appraised it, and is in accord with its philosophy and purposes. It is at this point that respect for the place is recognized, and the recognition imposes the obligation to support and further the efforts of both. Respect is never a passive activity. If a community is to continue to grow and to maintain respect, participation in the activities of the community is required. In the past too many nurses have shunned community responsibility, possibly attributable in part to having to live in hospital housing. A great number of nurses now are property owners or at least live out in the community, and they are assuming a more active role in fundamental civic affairs; in politics, in religion, and in community planning and development.

Within the agency proper this respect is even more readily observable. The nurse who respects an institution is interested in its physical plant and will neither abuse nor allow abuse of the facilities. She will direct her efforts toward improving the general tone of the institution—the morale, attitudes, friendliness, cohesiveness, and unity of purpose—elements that are elusive but contribute remarkably to the success of the institutional endeavor.

The third and last aspect of this characteristic is *respect for the job.* Traditionally nurses have respected nursing. Within the last decade, however, the job has changed and many nurses are having considerable difficulty in accepting the new job and in giving it the respect it deserves. When nurses learn all that can be learned about their role, they proudly recognize the contributions they can make to the care patients require. They also give their best talents to performing their roles, and they regain respect for their profession. The nurse who has accepted that nursing is administrative in nature and that the role of the nurse is to give care, in part, through other individuals, finds her job a challenging and inspiring one. Respect is a healthy, vigorous factor which motivates the very best in human beings—both donors and recipients. The present concern, however, is not with belaboring the value nor the desirability of the aforementioned characteristics but with how to promote the acquisition of desirable characteristics by all nurses. This is especially important, at least, until the administrative personality is defined scientifically.

Our firm commitment to the value of a liberal education compels the belief that assistance in the acquisition of known desirable characteristics is forthcoming from the areas of philosophy, religion, and the fine arts. The following four chapters will describe the influence philosophy, religion, and the fine arts can have on the administrative personality of the nurse.

4

The Influence of Philosophy

by John A. VanderWaal

A discussion of the influence of philosophy seems particularly appropriate in the effort to describe the characteristics of the administrative personality. Philosophy, according to the historical definition of the term, is the love of wisdom. But the love of wisdom, as Plato points out, implies its absence rather than its possession. Philosophy bids one beware of the person who is no longer searching after wisdom but claims to be already wise. He is either an imposter or a fool.

Wisdom, then, is the perennial goal of philosophy and is as relevant today as ever before. A glance beyond the smoke of one's own chimneys reveals that in spite of the enormous accumulations of knowledge, wisdom is badly needed in the conduct of the affairs of mankind. The persistent search after wisdom, however, encourages us to believe that it is to be found and that the search is not destined to end in utter futility. Granted that wisdom is one of the most elusive and intangible of realities and eludes the grasp of most, it does come to some, who are enlightened thereby. Wisdom is its own justification for being.

Ultimately, philosophy may lead not only to wisdom, but also to clear thinking and orderly intellectual processes. Philosophy is the enemy of merely impulsive behavior, although, alas, many persons still exist according to the dictates of the impulse. Sometime ago, in Paris, at the Louvre Museum, a man stood in front of da Vinci's *Mona Lisa.* He had a stone in his pocket and on impulse, according to his confession, he decided to throw it at the portrait. The stone chipped the left elbow of the masterpiece, and a restorer had to spend fourteen hours in repairing it. Contrast this impulsive action with the attitude of Colonel John Glenn while he waited for his first space flight to take place. There was delay after delay, and the public marveled at his calm. When questioned about it, Colonel Glenn replied that he had learned early in flight-test training that one has to control his emotions. The astronaut refused to allow the delay to affect his ability to perform his mission. Although Colonel Glenn makes no pretense of being a philosopher, his clear thinking while under strain is worthy of emulation. Whenever there is reason in action, calm under stress, deliberation before decision, and order where there could be chaos, philosophy's fruits are present, whether openly recognized or not. They may be present in the surgeon's knowing when to operate, in the nurse's refusal to omit the most tedious task when it is tempting to do so, or in the administrator's submitting of the new budget to the hospital board.

A dominant characteristic of the person enhanced by philosophy is a broad intellectual horizon. Plato, in his famous "Myth of the Cave," *Republic VII,* illustrates this point. According to this myth, man is a prisoner shackled by fetters of ignorance, and until he is brought out of his cave into the sunlight of knowledge and truth, he does not even realize that an intellectual world exists. Education liberates man, but until man is educated his ability to perceive reality is limited. One needs to see from many perspectives, and philosophy is able to come to his rescue. An untraveled world lies just beyond, although it is not uncharted. Philosophy has been there before him. The matter can be summed up by stating that the person who has dipped into the wide realm of philosophy will possess greater intellectual comprehension than the person who has not. In this one world of time and space he will discover many worlds.

Such broadening helps to offset the ever-increasing specialization of this era. In a highly technical society it is inevitable that many persons be specialists. Knowledge in many areas has advanced in geometric progression, and it has become impossible for one person to master all knowledge. Specialization is the order of the day and society is the richer, and the poorer, for it. The inevitable result of specialization is that the individual knows more and more about less and less. The doctor is no longer a general practitioner of medicine; he is a heart doctor, or a lung specialist, or a psychiatrist, etc. There is much justification, then, for seeking the broadening influences of philosophy. Plato regarded the philosopher as the spectator of all time and existence, and he believed deeply in the capacity of philosophy to bring together what appears to be apart. Plato's vision concerning the function of philosophy has as much value today as it had centuries ago. Philosophy helps one to see facts in their relationships; it helps him to relate different fields of knowledge; it aids him in making value judgments; it teaches him to think; it liberates him from the tyranny of prejudice and dogmatism; it stimulates his mind into initiating thought about the most complicated problems of reality; it opens to him new vistas of time and space. The most decisive cure for narrowness of outlook and a cramped view of the world is a healthy dose of philosophy. It is not without reason that William James used to maintain that the most important question that could be asked of a young person is: "Hast thee any philosophy?"

Philosophy enhances the personality further by satisfying a person's intellectual curiosity about the character of the world in which he lives and moves and has his being. This kind of curiosity seems to be universal. It is one of the fundamental prerequisites for intellectual development The ancient Greeks were more curious than their neighbors, and philosophy arose among them. They had a passion for asking useless questions about their natural and social environments. Philosophy still glories in this unpragmatic approach. Philosophy is valued for its own sake, not necessarily for the uses to which it can be put. Philosophy ministers to the irrepressible metaphysical curiosity of man. What reality is like in itself, beyond and behind sense appearances, without subjective distortion, and free from all anthropomorphic ways of thinking, philosophy can help us to determine.

For an introduction to the most influential ideas of the world's great thinkers, past and present, East and West, one must go to philosophy. These ideas have shaped the course of civilization and have sometimes toppled kings from their thrones. For the person whose appetite has been whetted, it is not difficult to enjoy a sumptuous banquet at the feast of ideas. Philosophy confronts him with innumerable choices. The growth and free play of ideas is of the essence. Plato's dialogues represent one of the finest arrays of ideas ever presented to the mind of man, and we have every reason to believe that Plato enjoyed turning ideas loose just to see what would happen to them. What a spectacle emerged—of creative encounter, of dramatic conflict, and of minds in juxtaposition.

Perhaps the outstanding feature of the ideas of philosophy is their sheer diversity. They come in all shapes, sizes, and colors. There is something in philosophy to suit every taste. Depending upon one's point of view, some ideas of the philosophers are judged to be safe and sane; others are classified as radical and subversive. Some are in harmony with what seems to be common sense; others lead to the most baffling paradoxes. Some defend the status quo; others would overturn it at once. Some exalt man as the most lustrous gem of a wondrous world; others contend that man is an accidental offshoot of a fortuitous concourse of atoms. Some assert the existence of a Supreme Being who guides and guards the destinies of men and nations; others maintain that such a notion is a crutch that was useful, even necessary, during the childhood of mankind; but now that man has reached maturity the crutch may be discarded. At any rate, there are no sacred cows in philosophy. Nothing is off limits. Nothing is protected from analysis, exposure, or even ridicule. The searchlight of philosophy probes into the darkest corners and the most unlikely places.

When all is said and done, the individual is the final judge of the dazzling and bewildering array of ideas. Philosophy exercises no coercion over the mind, nor does it wish to. Ideas may be true or false, meaningful or meaningless, relevant or irrelevant, profound, commonplace, or ludicrous. Much depends upon how the individual and his cultural heritage assess the ideas. If philosophy has any eternal truths, it is still up to the individual to acknowledge them to be such. And a profound philosophy may be profoundly true or profoundly false. One of the proudest aspects of the heritage of philosophy is that she wishes to set the mind free from all intellectual shackles, unfounded dogmas, and petty prejudices. If philosophy has a faith, it is that truth will emerge in the marketplace of the free play of ideas and that the individual is under the moral obligation to follow only that which he sees with the eye of the mind to be truth for him. Truth alone has coercive influence over the intellect.

To broaden intellectual horizons, to satisfy intellectual curiosity, and to explore the dynamic ideas of the civilizations of the past and the present are worthwhile endeavors, but philosophy purports to enable one to do more than this. The study of philosophy aids one in developing a world-view, or philosophy, of life. This is not to affirm that everyone who has touched the hem of the garment of Dame Philosophy has a neatly organized and systematic world-view of his own. It is to affirm, rather, that each person must somehow come to terms with reality and make his own private assessment of its character. A person may come to optimistic, pessimistic, or indifferent conclusions about the ultimate nature of reality; provisional conclusions may differ from ultimate conclusions. But some conclusion each individual must deliberately or unconsciously reach. Philosophy helps a person to develop a satisfactory world-view which, at least in everyday experience, makes some sense.

Philosophers differ radically among themselves as to the ultimate character of the world. Some argue that it is of the nature of the mind and consciousness. Others insist that only matter and its configurations count in the long run and that the mind does not have metaphysical status. Some even pronounce reality as irrational and not to be grasped by the human intellect. Whatever the belief about the character of the world as a whole and man's place in it in particular, philosophy does stimulate the individual, at the least, to examine reality for himself. This is the perennial invitation and challenge of philosophy.

An absolutely satisfactory philosophy of life is always in the making, and never made, for many individuals. Philosophy's chief concern is that a person develop a view of life and the world that to him makes philosophical sense. Although philosophy does not provide a faith and does not necessarily replace existing faiths, it is nonetheless the case that achieving a satisfactory world-view entails a philosophy which renders meaningful and constructive experiences and does not ignore distinctions of value. Who needs this kind of outlook more than a person engaged in health services? He is constantly in touch with patients whose needs are personal, psychologic, emotional, physiologic, and medical. The particular outlook on life held by a nurse or a doctor may be as influential in bringing about the patient's recovery as the formal therapeutic measures used. A renowned psychiatrist has stated that the main problem he encountered in persons near the middle years of their lives was that of finding a satisfactory philosophy of life. How frequently these days does one not hear words to this effect? It may well be that the kindness and encouragement of the nurse in the hospital room does as much as anything else, in a particular case, to promote recovery, kindle the desire to get well, and provide the incentive to the patient to resume his normal place in society. On the other hand, it is entirely possible that the nurse with a dour disposition and a pessimistic temperament may be an inhibiting factor in the course of the patient's recovery. Surely a dour personality on the part of a person engaged in humanitarian services is deplorable and is itself symptomatic of failure to achieve a satisfactory interpretation of experience. Before this person can contribute to the healing process, she needs to be healed. The deleterious effects she may have on the person in the sick room are forbidding.

Another characteristic of the personality enhanced by the influence of philosophy is a higher-than-average capacity to think. Philosophy teaches one how to think, and to know how to think is commonly and correctly regarded as a rare virtue. Most of us admire the person who thinks. The conception of *thinker* has a number of overtones, most of them favorable. It connotes the image of a person with a peculiar toughness of mind and the ability to bring to a subject concentrated mental energy. These qualities are thought to be the prerogatives of the gifted few, not of the unthinking many. To know how to think implies the attainment of a philosophical perspective upon life. The possession of philosophical perspective is conducive to employing thought before action, to careful deliberation before making decisions. The person with such perspective is characterized by calmness of attitude and a determined refusal to be carried away by emotion. There is a stability in his outlook on life as a whole. Both in everyday living and during the crises of human existence such a person lives intelligently, conducts his affairs without worry, and anticipates the future without fear. This is an idealized picture of what human existence can be like, of course. It can nonetheless be cherished as a goal that is realizable to a considerable extent. If such qualities of personality are within the reach of those who know how to think, it is at once obvious that to gain this knowledge is a matter of importance, even of urgency.

Unfortunately, no simple definition or foolproof formula for thinking can be submitted. Thinking is not just one thing to the exclusion of all others. Thinking may be construed as an art and a science, with much overlapping between the two. As an art, thinking is above the law, so to speak, and is subject to no rigorous norms. As a science, thinking is subject to established techniques. Sometimes thinking is spontaneous and creative; at other times it is sustained and technical. If thinking is indeed the ambiguous process it seems to be, small wonder that to define it accurately is next to impossible. Suffice it to state that to think means "to employ the powers of the mind in deliberate reflection with the objective of arriving at reliable conclusions."

Numerous obstacles stand in the way of one's efforts to realize his own capacity to think. Much of the time we are under the tyranny of our emotions, prejudices, and feelings. We are human beings, after all, not simply mathematical formulas. For better or for worse, we are endowed with emotional biases which, time and again, tend to preclude clear thinking. Reenforcing these natural biases is natural mental inertia, resulting in mental sluggishness and just plain laziness. These weaknesses exist in varying degrees in all of us and are formidable enemies. Battles have to be waged with them constantly. Even in the most energetic of individuals these weaknesses are never routed completely. Who knows what potentials of thought are never realized, due to the antagonism of natural mental inertia. Even when one applies himself fairly conscientiously, most of what he learns is soon forgotten. Memories are faulty instruments. One usually recalls only that which he has heard or seen frequently and recently. He excuses himself for not remembering more details of what he has learned by stating that the educated man is one who knows where to look for the facts, not one who is a walking encyclopedia. He exercises remarkable ingenuity in excusing his failure to expend mental effort. Experience has been the best teacher in demonstrating that thinking always requires effort and expenditure of energy, that it rarely becomes habitual.

Although no infallible method of clear thinking can be set forth, one should, as a minimum, be aware of the distinction between deductive and inductive reasoning. These two forms of reasoning can be distinguished in theory; but in practice frequently they are inextricably related. In deductive reasoning statements entail other statements, premises entail conclusions. They do so in the sense that the conclusion states explicitly what is contained implicitly in the premises. Thus the conclusion is a kind of unfolding of what is implicit in the premises. If one begins with the premise that all men are mortal, for example, and if it is known that Socrates is a man, then it follows necessarily that Socrates is a mortal. Or, if one begins with the premise that all roses are red, and if he knows that the object in hand is a rose, then it follows necessarily that the rose is red. The reasoning is valid. There is no doubt whatever that the conclusions in these two examples follow from the the given premises. This kind of reasoning is called *deductive reasoning.*

Not all deductive reasoning is as easy to follow as the foregoing examples would lead one to believe. Suppose the premise is that "All men are able to reason." Let this be followed by the premise, "Some machines are able to reason." What deductive conclusion could be drawn from these two premises? It is tempting to conclude that "Some men are machines," but this would not be a valid inference. Nor is the inference that "Some machines are men" valid. In fact, no valid conclusion can be drawn from the given premises because of the technical factor classical logic calls the "undistributed middle term." It is beyond the purpose of this essay to elaborate upon the formal rules of syllogistic argument. What has been given is sufficient to show that one must be on guard when he employs so seemingly innocent a device as deductive reasoning.

Sometimes conclusions arrived at by means of valid deductive reasoning from given premises are later discovered to be unreliable conclusions. A conclusion is reliable only when it is known to be true, and the reliability of the conclusion depends upon the reliability of the premises from which the conclusion is drawn. It is often exceedingly difficult to achieve premises that are absolutely reliable. To be absolutely reliable means to be certainly true, and to be certainly true means to be true without exception. An absolutely reliable premise is more difficult to achieve than a valid conclusion. After all, the validity of our reasoning depends upon formal considerations that can be mastered. On the other hand, reliability pertains to content. It is here that inductive reasoning makes its appearance.

Inductive reasoning involves more than one simple operation. Basically, *inductive reasoning* means "to reason from particular instances to a general conclusion." In many cases the conclusion requires a "leap" which may or may not be warranted from the instances examined. The leap from particulars to the general is called *inductive inference*. For example, suppose one knows that Smith is a medical doctor. The temptation may be to assume that because Smith is an accredited medical doctor he is also a member of the American Medical Association (AMA). Many doctors are members of the AMA. It could be the case now that there is a mistake in this belief about Smith. He may not be a member of the AMA, although he is a doctor. In the assumption about Smith, the fallacy of hasty generalization has been committed. This is a common fallacy and its source is faulty inductive reasoning. One should be exceedingly cautious in making generalizations that admit of no exceptions. More often than not, one should say "some" instead of "all," "seldom" instead of "never," "sometimes" instead of "always." Generalizations should be tentative rather than sweeping. Only in cases in which all instances or possibilities have been enumerated is it possible to make generalizations of an absolute nature. Most of the time we have to be content with varying degrees of probability instead of with absolute certainty.

Some individuals apparently are unable to think because they do not possess a systematic technique for coping with problems. They simply do not know how to think. To such persons it is happily possible to suggest a very practical method of inquiry that may prove to be helpful. First of all, thinking, which is different from undirected mental rambling or daydreaming, should commence with a problem to be solved, i.e., a problem situation. At times the problem situation is not of one's own making. It is foisted upon him by the circumstances of his life or of his work, over which he may have little or no control. Sometime ago in a hospital in a large American city, a number of infants died from a seemingly mysterious cause. This situation was alarming and it demanded immediate inquiry by the finest medical minds. Experts at once went to work on the case and, although they were baffled for a while, they came forth with the answer. The cause of the mysterious deaths was finally discovered to be the catastrophically high salt level in their bodies. An accident had occurred. A practical nurse had filled the canister in the formula room with salt instead of with sugar.

The problem situation with which thinking commences is not always, of course, foisted upon the individual by some external circumstance. The situation may be of his own devising. He may deliberately employ his power of thought to conceive a problem situation which, in turn, requires for its solution the most patient and painstaking inquiry. The graduate student, for example, as he approaches the climax of his studies, will be required to embark upon a program of research leading to the writing of a dissertation. The nature of the research itself will be determined by the kind of problem to be investigated. Thought comes into play at the outset of the process. In consultation with his major advisers and others, and after preliminary research, the graduate student will engage in careful deliberation, the outcome of which is the setting up of a problem to be investigated through well-tested methods of research. Occasionally, as in the careful and accurate observation of some external phenomenon, the individual is merely a passive spectator of what forces itself upon his attention. For the most part, to think implies active and deliberate inquiry.

From all that the foregoing suggests, it should be clear that reflective thinking involves encounter with a particular problem situation. If the problem is to be resolved satisfactorily, it is desirable to achieve a clear formulation of the problem. This formulation should be followed by the accumulation and classification of relevant factual data and the eventual formulation of proposed solutions or hypotheses to the problem. The hypotheses then must be tested for confirmation, modification, or rejection, as the case may be. The process of testing the adequacy of a hypothesis is called *verification.* An adequate hypothesis explains the factual data relevant to the problem situation.

Often, more than one hypothesis can be advanced as a plausible solution to a problem. The selection of the most adequate hypothesis may result from the progressive elimination of each of the other hypotheses. This can be accomplished at times through mental processes, i.e., through trial and error thinking. At other times it may involve the setting up of an experiment. At times all hypotheses prove to be false and force one to rethink the entire situation; at other times one of the hypotheses may prove to be on the right track but stand in need of revision. The step to take at this point is to revise the hypothesis and test the revised hypothesis for its adequacy. No rule of thumb can serve as the clue to the formulation of an adequate hypothesis. Much depends upon the background, maturity, and experience, or perhaps the particular mental ability or state, of the person doing the thinking. When an adequate hypothesis is discovered, the original problem may be said to be settled and the act of reflective thought, for the moment, consummated. Thought is at rest. This particular inquiry is finished. The temporary cessation of thought does not rule out the possibility that the solution may serve to stimulate further reflection and continuing inquiry.

The above discussion gives the essence of what is usually called the scientific method of acquiring truth or knowledge. The scientific method is not different in kind from reflective thinking. What the natural sciences have, and everyday thinking does not have, is an array of precision instruments that help to refine their measurements. The scientific method as a whole is simply an extension of reflective thinking. T. H. Huxley was fond of saying years ago that we are all scientists, whether we know it or not, whenever we bend our minds to the solution of a particular problem.

How does one go about improving the quality of his thinking? That thinking can be improved is one of the axioms of a basic faith in human intelligence. The individual is not condemned by nature to live out his span of years on the level of instinct, habit, and tradition. Many persons can improve the quality of their thinking by first cultivating the practice of occasional solitude. The pressures of modern life do not permit much time for concentration and studied thought, and he who would think through his problems must isolate himself now and then. Everyone reaches a point, occasionally, at which he complains that he cannot call even his soul his own. He grows weary of the demands of life and the sameness of everyday routine. To collect his thoughts in private and to win back his self may be just what he needs.

All solitude need not be of the exterior variety. Interior solitude, through mental concentration, is also a definite possibility. Who has not known a person who seems to be capable of concentrating in a crowd and whose thoughts seem to be his very own, although he is surrounded by people? Others never seem to be able to concentrate, and their disordered minds are the fruits of their failure. To concentrate means "to focus the mind intently upon one thing at a time." Such concentration is necessary to clear thinking and is not likely to be present when factors favorable to its development are absent. Nervousness and fatigue are certainly not conducive to concentration. Excessive eating and sleeping are no help either. Anxiety and worry conspire further to prevent concentration. In order to improve the quality of one's thinking through concentration, it will be necessary to practice a stillness of mind by eliminating distractions.

To improve the caliber of thought, it will be helpful to develop a cautious attitude toward so-called obvious truths. Much of what has seemed obviously true to mankind in his relatively brief history has turned out to be false. It was once obviously true that the earth was flat, that the sun revolved around the earth, and that witches existed and had to be burned at the stake. These beliefs, and innumerable others, were surrendered as man's knowledge and understanding of his world increased. Some beliefs that are obviously true are actually accepted without sufficient evidence to establish their validity and therefore are merely prejudices. Conversely, some beliefs and ideas that are not obviously true at all ought to be accepted. It is not obviously true, to unenlightened common sense, that the surgeon's instruments must be thoroughly sterilized before the operation. It is not obviously true that the chair on which one is sitting is constituted of a swirling mixture of atoms; it is, in fact, mostly empty space. Although the contradiction of so-called obvious truths may injure or even offend one, the person intent upon improving his thinking will learn to cherish the truth more than his personal comfort. It is never easy to give up a cherished belief, but when an individual holds a cherished belief without sufficient evidence, he ought to be suspicious of it. To believe simply what we want to believe or what seems obvious to us is to contradict the testing and tentative attitude of the scientific mind.

It will also be well to be on guard against the human tendency to rationalize. To rationalize means "to find excuses for beliefs and behavior"; it is a means of justifying them. Some scholars maintain that most of conscious life is taken up with the activity of rationalizing. It is not necessary to go to this extreme to admit that we frequently do what we wish and invent ingenious reasons for our actions. One of the reasons the individual engages in rationalization is the desire to maintain a satisfactory self-image. Reason and thought are employed in the service of that end. In order to maintain a self-image that is not too painful to bear, an individual may erect defense mechanisms. These aid in presenting pictures of himself that he can respect. It is inevitable that an individual employs such devices.

One of the most familiar forms of rationalization is the defense mechanism called *avoidance*. The self feels threatened by a particular situation and escapes the threat simply by avoiding the situation. A student with a strong interest in the humanities, for example, may fear that science courses may prove too difficult for him and assiduously avoid them. Sometimes one avoids the threat inherent in a particular situation by deliberately forgetting. A routine laboratory task in the daily round of hospital duties may not appeal to the practitioner of nursing and thus is conveniently forgotten. It is not always the case that forgetting is the result of a deliberate resolve; rather, the subconscious self provides one with the mode of forgetting as a way of avoiding an unappealing task. The actual reason for failure to remember lies in the depths of the self.

Honesty with the self demands from each person a high degree of self-knowledge and, as philosophers from Socrates to the present have contended, self-knowledge is one of the most difficult kinds of knowledge to acquire. The ancient proverb, "Self-deception is the worst form of deception," still rings true.

Finally, one can improve the quality of his thinking by cultivating an awareness of the methods of propaganda and the means to combat it. The phenomenal development of the mass media of communication during this century has only too often bewitched and enslaved the human mind. Basically, there are three ways of influencing human belief. One is *to coerce* others into adopting desired beliefs, a method used mainly by authoritarians and totalitarians. Another, and much better way of influencing others, is *to convince* them by presenting evidence and reasons for the beliefs in question, an approach which is tendered lip service, at least, by most educated people. A third is *to persuade,* a method used by the propagandist. The propagandist attempts to influence belief without employing rational methods. His methods are essentially irrational. A clever propagandist uses a number of devices to persuade us to adopt certain ideas, beliefs, or modes of behavior. He provides his audience with convenient scapegoats by foisting the blame for ills that beset them upon particular persons, institutions, classes, races, or nations. In so doing he oversimplifies the vastly complex political, social, economic, and religious issues of the day. Providing scapegoats and oversimplifying the complex are ways of securing relief from frustration for many people; thus these methods of persuasion are unusually effective. It is much easier to think in terms of black and white than in infinite gradations of gray. The propagandist also capitalizes on the tendency of human beings to worry, and he is a specialist in helping them to rationalize, particularly when he is trying to influence them to believe or behave in ways that conflict with each person's conscience.

How does one detect the presence of propaganda and how can he check its influence? When one begins to suspect that he is the target of propaganda, it is sound procedure for him to attempt to determine the source of the material and to ascertain its purpose. Who controls the channel of communication and for what purpose? Also, he must be on the lookout for the misuse of analogy in the statements of the suspected propagandist. The use of analogies in the process of thinking can be exceedingly fruitful.

Indeed, it is difficult to conceive that thought can be fruitful without the aid of analogies. Analogies are useful in illustrating general principles and in demonstrating how complex processes actually work. One of the most useful analogies in the history of the natural sciences has been the comparison of the interior structure of the atom with a miniature solar system. Problems arise, however, when the use of analogy exceeds its lawful bounds. This usually happens when an analogy is carried too far or is used in an effort to prove something. In many respects electrons spinning in their orbits around the nucleus of the atom do not behave like planets revolving around the sun. This directs attention to the fact that because things are alike in certain respects does not mean that they are alike in all respects. In their most crucial aspects they may be entirely dissimilar. The propagandist is adept in the abuse of analogical thinking.

The more subtle the propagandist, the more subtle will be his use of words; particularly words with emotive power. The use of words with emotional content is not in itself a logical fallacy. Language would be impoverished if all emotive terms were removed from it. The fallacy arises when one allows emotion-filled words to stand in the way of clear thinking. Some words are honorific in their connotations, others are derogatory; the propagandist knows the power of each. Bertrand Russell's witticism is appropriate here: "I am firm; you are obstinate; he is a pig-headed fool." Recall that through methods of persuasion the propagandist attempts to control beliefs, attitudes, and behavior. He specializes in the use of words that will bring about the desired response, and he is not averse to playing on emotions.

Among recent trends in philosophy, one of the most stimulating concepts has been existentialism. The term itself is not easy to define, and there is no simple formula as to what existentialism represents. The purposes of this chapter will be satisfied by our stating that existential thinking forms a means of protest against vacuous metaphysics and against the numerous depersonalizing tendencies of our age. Man is viewed by the existentialists as a unique being who, as such, ought to take himself very seriously. This involves the recognition that man is more than consciousness, that he is threatened at every moment by the possibility of his own non-existence, and that he is the creator and sustainer of his own values. Some existentialist thinkers are atheists, whereas others profess belief in a Supreme Being. The denial of any supra-rational ground of being does not necessarily qualify a philosopher as existentialist. Reminding us of the precarious character of our existence as human beings, existentialism serves as a valuable corrective to excessive emphasis on science or to a superficial optimism about the nature of man. This thinking seems to be an outgrowth of the crisis of contemporary civilization.

The subject matter of this chapter can be summed up with the proposition that the person who has been influenced by philosophy has begun to learn what it means to be an individual. He realizes the worth of personal self-realization and therefore wishes to be himself, not a pale carbon copy of someone else. He holds the faith that each individual can make his finest contribution to society when he is most truly himself, at his very best, and as much of the time as possible. To be an individual implies resistance to the tyranny of obtuse conformity and, at times, to the despotism of public opinion or the heavy hand of the majority. It implies commitment to the rights of others, for they too are individuals, and to liberty of opinion, speech, and action, so long as the exercise of these liberties does not jeopardize the rights of others to the same liberties. To be committed to such democratic freedoms is right because only under these circumstances can the development of individuality flourish. To be an individual implies keeping one's mind open on questions until all the evidence is in and holding one's beliefs with tolerance and charity for the beliefs of others. One who is truly an individual is always asking himself these questions: "Do I really want to know the truth, or do I merely want to prove that my preconceived notions are right? Am I willing to lay aside the customs and traditions of my heritage, my community, and my church long enough to discover whether I ought to change my point of view? Have I ever set aside my prejudices, notions, and dogmas and examined the reasons for my most cherished opinions?"

To be an individual implies the humility to listen to the man who knows and the good sense never to laugh at new ideas, for the heresy of today may become the orthodoxy of tomorrow. The individual knows that thought is always the order of the day, that decisions must be made, and that machines for grinding out the right answers are not available. Infallibility is beyond the grasp of everyone, and there is no way of eliminating the risk inherent in the making of some decisions. The thinking individual is willing to take the risk and to act in the light of the best evidence available. If the foregoing criteria for living and thinking seem necessary components of the administrative personality, but difficult to achieve, remember the words of Spinoza: "All things excellent are as difficult as they are rare."

SUPPLEMENTARY READING LIST

Barrett, William, and Aiken, Henry (eds.): *Philosophy in the Twentieth Century,* 2 vols., Random House, Inc., New York, 1962.

Copi, Irving M.: *Introduction to Logic,* 2d ed., The Macmillan Company, New York, 1961.

Davidson, Robert: *Philosophies Men Live By,* Holt, Rinehart & Winston, Inc., New York, 1952.

Durant, Will: *The Story of Philosophy,* Simon and Schuster, Inc., New York, 1933.

Heineman, F. H.: *Existentialism and the Modern Predicament,* Harper & Row, Publishers, Incorporated, New York, 1958.

Kant, Immanuel: *The Critique of Practical Reason,* trans. by Lewis W. Beck, The Bobbs-Merrill Company, Inc., Indianapolis, 1956.

Plato, *The Republic,* trans. by Jowett, selected by Irwin Edman, Tudor Publishing Company, New York, 1954.

Spinoza, Benedict de: *Ethics,* trans. by Wm. E. White, edited by James Gutmann, Hafner Publishing Company, Inc., New York, 1953.

Titus, Harold: *Living Issues in Philosophy,* 4th ed., American Book Company, New York, 1964.

5

The Influence of Religion

by William Richard Stegner

Religion shapes the administrative personality because religion deals primarily with the quest for meaning and purpose in life. In contrast to religion, medical science does not involve a philosophy of life, but attempts to deal with natural phenomena and matters that can be studied objectively. In a certain sense it can be said that medical science deals with the *how* questions concerning man's health and physical nature. Russell Dicks makes this very clear:[1]

> Medical science, psychiatry included, is a technique, a method, an instrument, for achieving a given end; nothing more. It is not philosophic, nor concerned with the nature of living, nor the world in which it lives. It does not ask questions nor give answers concerning the why of life or living. It is not a method of living but an instrument or technique to aid living. When the physician, psychiatrist, general practitioner, or surgeon asks, "What is the purpose of life?" he has become a philosopher. Medical science strives to gain and maintain health for its subjects; religion strives to put meaning into health. Health without purpose is senseless.

RELIGION DEFINED

When the nurse, or any other person, asks questions about purpose or meaning in life, she leaves behind the realm of science and enters the realm of religion, for religion deals with questions of ultimate concern. By ultimate concern one means that which is of supreme importance in life: the core around which activities, standards of values, and one's life are oriented. Viewed in this broad perspective, every person who either consciously or unconsciously seeks the answer to questions of final importance in life deals with religion. Thus the great musician and missionary physician Albert Schweitzer defines religion in the following manner:[2]

[1] Russell L. Dicks, *Who Is My Patient? A Religious Manual for Nurses,* The Macmillan Company, New York, 1945, pp. 11–12.

[2] Albert Schweitzer, *Christianity and the Religions of the World,* 5th imp., George Allen and Unwin, Ltd., London, 1923, p. 37.

> In religion we try to find an answer to the elementary question with which each one of us is newly confronted every morning, namely, what meaning and what value is to be ascribed to our life. What am I in the world? I do not want to consider my existence merely as one which rises and perishes among the billions of billions of beings which constitute the universe, but as a life which has a value, if I comprehend it and live it according to true knowledge.

Thus by the very nature of being a human being the nurse asks religious questions since, in this broad sense, religion deals with one's total orientation to life. Although each of us attempts to ask and to answer fundamental questions about life, it is the function of religion to bring these questions to the level of conscious thought and to deal with them critically.

The definition of religion implied in the preceding paragraphs is broad enough to cover all particular forms and expressions of religion. In actuality, however, religion-in-general does not exist; only particular forms of religion, such as Christianity, Judaism, Islam, etc., exist. Consequently, in examining the relationship of religion to the nursing profession the discussion will be limited to one particular expression of religious faith, namely the Biblical, or as it is sometimes called, the Judaeo-Christian tradition. This seems proper, since the modern hospital and the nursing profession have arisen out of this tradition. Also, most of the idealism and motivation in present-day nursing derive from this tradition. One other qualification needs to be added. No attempt will be made to give a systematic treatment of the contents of the Biblical tradition; instead, religion will be emphasized as it immediately impinges upon the personality.

RELIGION AND INTERPERSONAL RELATIONSHIPS

Religion is important in the life of the nurse because religion, broadly conceived, is the "conviction by which one actually lives." There is probably no area where the practical importance of this statement is more evident than in the quality of the relationships the nurse forms, both with the patients she serves and the people with whom she works.

Chapter 3 singled out *respect* as the most desirable attribute of the administrative personality. For all administrators this involves respect for oneself. For the nurse in particular, it involves respect for the patient and for other hospital personnel. Also, respect is a fundamental concern of the Judaeo-Christian tradition, which has always addressed itself to the proper forms of human conduct.

For example, the new emphasis in nursing declares that the nurse is no longer to think of herself as one who treats "the cancer case in room 3," but as one who relates personally to "people who are ill." It is important to respect the woman in room 3 as a mother who is concerned about her children, her husband, and her home. Far from being a case history, a medical problem, or an object, this woman is a human being with hopes and desires and feelings, and in this particular case, a person with needs which the skill of the nurse can meet.

Nonetheless, it is much easier for the nurse to accept this insight intellectually than to live it in the daily routine of hospital activities, because this new view of a patient is contrary to the nurse's past education in the scientific disciplines. For the most part scientific education is based on abstract knowledge and statistical approaches, which tend to deemphasize personal elements. Scientific observation tends to be objective, detached, and general; objective measurements of quantity are used in place of personal qualitative judgments. In this world of the statistical average and abstractions, the unique concrete individual does not fit. In caring for her patients, therefore, the nurse must bring these two basic but contradictory attitudes together into a workable combination. The conflict between these opposing and contradictory ways of thinking can be solved only by "two-way" thinking. In speaking to psychotherapists in a context somewhat different from that pertinent to the nurse, the great psychiatrist, C. G. Jung, illustrated how two-way thinking must take place:[3]

> The doctor, above all, should be aware of this contradiction. On the one hand, he is equipped with the statistical truths of his scientific training, and on the other, he is faced with the task of treating a sick person who, especially in the case of psychic suffering, requires *individual understanding*. The more schematic the treatment is, the more resistances it—quite rightly—calls up in the patient, and the more the cure is jeopardized. The psychotherapist sees himself compelled, willy-nilly, to regard the individuality of a patient as an essential fact in the picture and to arrange his methods of treatment accordingly. Today, over the whole field of medicine, it is recognized that the task of the doctor consists in treating the sick person, not the abstract illness.

A homely illustration of this is the pleasure a hospital patient may exhibit when a member of the staff comes to chat with him for a few minutes and not to take his temperature or distribute a medication. Here the patient is not being treated as an object or an It, but as a person or a Thou.

[3] Carl G. Jung, *The Undiscovered Self*, trans. by R. F. C. Hull, New American Library of World Literature•Inc., New York, 1961, p. 20.

In addition to nursing education, the trend of present-day culture creates difficulties. The dehumanizing aspects of growing industrialization force human beings to regard each other as numbers, as units of work, or as objects to be manipulated and problems to be solved. Human beings are taught to manipulate other human beings as "things," or, in the case of much advertising, as units of purchasing power. One no longer looks upon the milkman, the elevator girl, or the bus driver as a person with hopes and fears and individuality, but as a kind of mechanism whose function is to satisfy human needs. Finally, a nurse who spends most of her working hours in a large hospital is made aware of "institutionalization," because much of her idealistic concept of health care has been replaced by discipline and routine. The same problems are dealt with over and over again. This trend in present-day culture points up the difficulty in treating patients and personnel as persons and not as objects. In view of the great difficulties that occur in attempts to show "respect for the individual," the basic problem is more and more becoming that of "why." Why should I bother to treat patients as persons? Indeed, if the nurse has had a liberal education she may raise the question on a philosophical level: Just what is the nature of man, or who is man that I should "put myself out" to be interested in him as a person?

The Biblical answer to these questions seems to be the greatest contribution the Judaeo-Christian tradition can make to the ethics of modern nursing. The Biblical ethic is concerned primarily with relationships between persons. The core of Biblical teaching stresses the quality of the relationships one forms with one's fellow man and with God. Perhaps the best modern interpreter of the meaning of the personal ethics of Biblical religion is the great Jewish theologian Martin Buber. According to Buber the two basic kinds of relationships open to human beings are (1) a relationship with another person, an *I–Thou* relationship, and (2) a relationship with a thing, an *I–It* relationship. These two kinds of relationships involve radically different attitudes. We use, experience, or study things. Perhaps a scientist, bent over a microscope to examine a culture, is the best example of an I–It relationship. On the other hand, an I–Thou relationship involves concern, not only with "myself and my feelings," or with another and his feelings, but also for both of us, for our ability to reach beyond ourselves and give of ourselves and enter into a relationship with another. Therefore, Buber implies that all real living is meeting.[4]

[4] Martin Buber, *I and Thou,* Charles Scribner's Sons, New York, 1958, p. 11.

This means more than a brief greeting or a handshake at a social gathering; it means two persons relating to each other in appreciation of each other's worth as unique individuals who have inherent worth and God-given dignity. This is what the Biblical ethic means by "loving thy neighbor as thyself." Ministers, nurses, or relatives who try to reduce this personal ethic to a series of formulas for conduct completely misunderstand the Judaeo-Christian ethic. At his deepest level of need a person does not crave words; he craves genuine creative relationships.

The Judaeo-Christian ethic is concerned primarily with personal relationships because God himself is personal. God is the Supreme Person, the Thou who relates to his children. This is very easy to illustrate from the Bible. In contrast to other religions of the ancient Near East, which tend to picture their gods as crocodiles or fish or other animals, the Bible always speaks of God in human terms. He chooses a people and loves them; he delivers his people from slavery and redeems them from the hand of the Pharaoh. At other times he judges his people in wrath and then turns to them in forgiveness. All these acts—loving, judging, forgiving, etc., are descriptive of personality. Moreover, God enters into relationship with man: He chooses Abraham to be the father of the children of Israel; He speaks to Moses from the burning bush and commissions him to lead Israel out of bondage; He enters into a covenant relationship with the whole people, and through the events of their history He judges them for breaking His commandments. While some prefer to think of God as an impersonal force, the Bible knows only a personal God who confronts man as a Thou. In placing His demands upon us in the Ten Commandments, God addresses us with the personal pronoun "Thou" and reserves the pronoun "I" for Himself.

In addition, the Judaeo-Christian ethic points to the importance of personal relationships in the process of healing because of the Biblical emphasis upon the unity of the personality. The Bible *and* medical science both view man as a psychosomatic whole. In contrast, many people have been taught that man is basically composed of two parts: an immortal soul and a perishable body. Sometimes, the mind-soul is contrasted with the material body. In contrast, the Genesis account of creation says that "God formed man of dust from the ground, and breathed into his nostrils the breath of life; and man became a living being." "Breath" is not another word for soul; it means the "principle" of life, that which makes a dead body come alive. In Biblical thought, then, there is no separation between the body and the soul. Rather, man is a unity, a whole person. The practical implications of this concept for healing lie in the interaction among the physical, emotional, and spiritual dimensions of a human being. The mind and body interact: one's state of mind affects one's body, and the condition of the body affects the mind. Thus good nursing no longer confines itself to the physical manifestations of disease only, for the mind, the body, and the spirit interact and create health. By the same token, Biblical religion is concerned with the whole person and his total environment, not just with a segment of the inner life that is designated "spiritual."

In the preceding paragraphs the importance of regarding a patient as a Thou rather than an It has been stressed. However this does not mean that the nurse must always "look for the best" in the patients and ignore negative and hostile feelings that may arise in the relationship. This is a sentimental attitude which is unrelated to real life situations. Frequently, hostile patients try to influence doctors, nurses, and relatives with almost any means at their disposal. To allow oneself to be so manipulated certainly is a denial of an I–Thou perspective of human relationships. A nurse who allows herself to be used as a tool in such a situation cannot regard herself as a Thou and will certainly lose the self-respect which is so desirable a trait of the effective nurse.

Just as important as the relationship between the nurse and her patients, but seldom stressed, is the relationship between the nurse and her coworkers. Here, respect for the individual and giving oneself to the situation at hand are just as important as treating patients as persons. When an individual considers persons in authority or those beneath him in rank as something less than human, his conduct becomes reserved and unnatural. He must frequently remind himself that behind the office, or behind the rather obvious questions of an untrained aide, is a person to whom a basic respect is due. This is especially true in decision-making situations, because one may not know all the factors that are involved. Many times the administrator or coworker brings to the decision a wealth of experience and background that others cannot see. Frequently, too, pressures of which one is not aware are being exerted.

RELIGION AND VOCATION

Just as important as the ethical system by which the nurse governs her conduct is the view she has of her vocation, or life work. While it is true that some nurses look upon their work as simply a means of making a living, the majority of nurses do not. Most young persons who enter professional nursing are motivated more by idealism and the desire to serve than by the lure of high salaries and ideal working conditions. But how is the idealism of the nurse to be maintained? How is respect for the job to be acquired? Again, the religious view of vocation seems to be the answer to this question.

Historically, nursing has been regarded as a specifically "religious" vocation. This was especially true during the Middle Ages when nursing was the responsibility of the religious orders. Also during the Middle Ages the meaning of the term *vocation* was largely restricted to the members of a religious order or community. Properly speaking, only the monk, the nun, or the priest had a vocation. Traces of this attitude toward vocation are found today in the tacit system many persons employ in evaluating different kinds of work. Jobs are labeled and evaluated in terms of their involvement with the "world." For example, Alexander Miller describes a four-class scheme of job classification and evaluation as *"impossible, dubious, satisfactory* or *uplift* jobs."[5]

This labeling of jobs has often worked to the detriment of the nursing profession itself. When people say that the nurse, like the minister or the priest, is "called" to her vocation, they sometimes think that she should make a special effort, in addition to her regular work, to influence people to live Christian lives. According to this kind of thinking there is the danger that the nurse who assists in an operation or directly serves the sick may falsely regard her work as "more" Christian than the work of the unskilled aide. Thus the profession becomes surrounded with a false aura of religious sentimentality, which tends to limit God to a so-called religious realm. It is questionable whether this view is true to the Biblical perspective.

How, then, is the modern nurse to look upon her vocation in the light of her own religious commitment? According to the New Testament, at any rate, mankind is called to total commitment; there is no part-time or full-time servant of God. Nor is there an occupation that is specifically religious when compared with other occupations or callings. Instead, all men are called to serve God in their own occupations. The meaning of the

[5] Alexander Miller, *Christian Faith and My Job,* Association Press, New York, 1959, p. 34. This little "reflection" book contains a balanced examination of the problems involved in the "religious" view of vocation in today's world.

word "vocation," then, is much broader than most persons suppose. "It does not refer to what a person might do of a religious nature while he is employed at some other task. It means that the work itself is a response to God's call: the dusting, or machine tending, or plowing or study." [6] According to this view there is no system of values by which one vocation is regarded as more Christian or more religious than another. All work which fulfills human need is included within the concept of vocation, and may be looked upon as a response to the call of God.

As it is used in the above context, the phrase "call of God" does not mean that a person should do only one single thing with his life, or that a person should wait for a voice "from above" before deciding on his life's work. Two factors constitute the call of God: need and ability. Many persons are aware of the needs of the world when it comes to choosing a vocation. On the other hand, each individual has some understanding of his own ability. This understanding may be enlarged through aptitude and guidance tests, and even through the counsel of wise friends. When the opportunity arises for the particular abilities of an individual to satisfy a need of the world for legitimate labor, the "call of God" has been fulfilled.

The view of vocation outlined above is based on the Biblical doctrine that God is the creator of this world. Through the agency of work—be it the work of factory hand, farmer, or nurse aide—God cares for His world and the needs of His creatures. Legitimate work is more than a way of making a living and more than one's own private business. Work is part of the order of creation, and through work each person is fulfilling the will of God in caring for His creation. According to this Biblical view of vocation, all necessary and useful labor is a glorification of God because it fits into His will and purpose.

This view of vocation has important implications for the nursing profession. With this ethical view of the importance of daily labor, the nurse cannot help but respect her job. This view of vocation also brings religious commitment and vocational responsibilities into the proper perspective. Religion is not something "added" to a nurse's regular duties, nor is "witnessing" something she must do to demonstrate her faith. As a member of the health care team, a nurse's primary vocational responsibility is to do her job well. Southard states,[7]

[6] Paul Hessert, *Introduction to Christianity,* Prentice-Hall, Inc., Englewood Cliffs, N.J., 1958, p. 337.

[7] Samuel Southard, *Religion and Nursing,* Broadmen Press, Nashville, Tenn., 1959, p. 145.

> Nursing is her profession, her God-given opportunity to prepare for service. Whether she ever speaks a specific word about religion or not, she has ministered as God's servant when she performs her nursing duties faithfully.

Thus the religious dimension which inevitably influences our interpersonal relationships and our view of vocation is one more facet of the administrative personality.

SUPPLEMENTARY READING LIST

Buber, Martin: *I and Thou,* Charles Scribner's Sons, New York, 1958.

Cabot, Richard C., and Russell L. Dicks, *The Art of Ministering to the Sick,* The Macmillan Company, New York, 1951.

Dicks, Russell L.: *Who Is My Patient? A Religious Manual for Nurses,* The Macmillan Company, New York, 1945.

Hessert, Paul: *Introduction to Christianity,* Prentice-Hall, Inc., Englewood Cliffs, N.J., 1958.

Hiltner, Seward: *Religion and Health,* The Macmillan Company, New York, 1943.

Jung, Carl G.: *The Undiscovered Self,* trans. by R. F. C. Hull, New American Library of World Literature, Inc., New York, 1961.

Miller, Alexander: *Christian Faith and My Job,* Association Press, New York, 1959.

Robertson, Josephine: *How to Help through Understanding,* Abingdon Press, Nashville, Tenn., 1961.

Schweitzer, Albert: *Christianity and the Religions of the World,* 5th imp., George Allen & Unwin, Ltd., London, 1923.

Southard, Samuel: *Religion and Nursing,* Broadman Press, Nashville, Tenn., 1959.

Weatherhead, Leslie: *The Will of God,* Abingdon Press, Nashville, Tenn., 1944.

6

The Influence of Art

by Rupert Kilgore

The study of philosophy is divided into three branches: logic, ethics, and esthetics. In the two previous chapters, logic and ethics (religion) were examined in terms of the contribution they make to the administrative personality as we know it. This chapter is concerned with the contribution that esthetics can make to that personality.

THE ESTHETIC EXPERIENCE

The term *esthetics* comes almost directly from a Greek word, *aestheitkos*, which means "perceptual." The Greeks used the word to distinguish between perceptual, or sensuous, knowledge and conceptual, or mental, knowledge. Mental knowledge usually consists of experiences that have been stored in our memories and which may be recalled when they are needed. At the mention of the word "rose," for example, one reaches into his mental storehouse and selects a mental picture of a rose. This seldom adds anything to the breadth of one's experience since it merely repeats an earlier experience. To gain perceptual or sensuous knowledge, one must examine an actual rose. Most people prefer to examine roses than to hear them discussed because the actual experience offers a higher level of excitement growing out of immediate visual sensation.

A truly esthetic response can develop only from the immediate experience with the object. An esthetic response to Beethoven's *Fifth Symphony* occurs only while one is listening to it. In the search for esthetic experiences one turns first to the fine arts. This is because the poet, the painter, and the composer create poems, paintings, and music in order to fulfill the human need for esthetic experience.

Works of fine art offer the opportunity for the most valuable and enriching esthetic experience. But it is possible to respond esthetically to any object or event. Under the pressures of a daily schedule, an individual usually responds to such things only in a practical way. When he leaves home in the morning to go to work, for example, he usually glances at the sky. If it is filled with dark rolling clouds, he may decide to carry an umbrella or a raincoat. This is a practical consideration. If he is particularly interested in meteorology, he responds to the sky in an intellectual way. He checks the wind direction and perhaps recalls from last night's paper the weather map with its high and low pressure areas in an attempt to understand the present cloudy condition. After he finds an explanation, he files it in his memory and forgets it. There is a third approach to the situation. He assumes the esthetic attitude and looks long and carefully at the moving clouds as a pure, visual experience. He enjoys the slow rhythmic movement, the variations in lights and darks, the harmonies and contrasts of subtle colors, and the effect all this has upon the landscape below. He becomes so absorbed in the various sensations arising from this experience that he forgets the practical consideration of threatening rain and the need to arrive at work on time. Low pressure centers do not enter his mind. Time stands still. He completely loses himself in the enjoyment of the immediate perceptual experience. Such experiences can be infinitely rewarding. They involve a feeling of an expansion of the self. For a few moments one seems to be in tune with the universe—a part of something much bigger and more important than himself. He gains a fresh and expansive approach to life, and a better understanding of its deeper meanings. He gains self-confidence and the desire to find and cope with bigger and more important challenges. For a brief time he has concentrated into a single transcending experience the characteristics that make him most human. Perhaps it is an expression of man's natural aspiration toward God.

CULTURAL AWARENESS

By the very nature of the education for the profession, students of nursing are required to concentrate on the natural sciences, particularly chemistry and biology. From such courses, they gain important and useful conceptual knowledge. In order to maintain a proper balance and ensure development of the whole person, schools of nursing also require certain cultural courses. These courses guide the development of the student's perceptual awareness and help her to integrate all areas of knowledge with her own developing philosophy of life. To the extent that the individual student is able to perform this integration, she gains knowledge of herself as a specific person. Graduation requirements are organized with two aims in mind: (1) to give a student the courses in theory and technique necessary to the successful performance of the many duties associated with nursing, and (2) to give a student an opportunity to develop cultural awareness through contact with all other areas of knowledge. The nurse who has cultural awareness has knowledge of herself as an individual, an understanding of her place in history, and a knowledge of her position in today's world.

The inherent characteristics that set human beings apart from the rest of the animal kingdom are curiosity, creative imagination, memory, the ability to reason logically, a desire for order, and the need for self-transcendence. Since they are inherited and are influenced by the environment, the quality and extent of these attributes are different in everyone. Some individuals have better memories, others are more creative, and still others have a greater need for self-transcendence. But all are equipped with these attributes and use them to some extent. Through profound self-analysis, an individual is able to determine his strengths and weaknesses among these inherent characteristics. The educative process enables him to overcome weaknesses and to develop strengths to their highest potential. Courses in the humanities, particularly in religion, philosophy, and the fine arts, enable a person to develop creative imagination and to satisfy his human need for order and self-transcendence.

Just as today's culture is a result of thousands of years of cultural development in the history of man, each individual is a product of his own specific cultural past. Such knowledge helps him to understand why he is what he is, and his self-awareness is increased. As one views the past from his place in time, he can take advantage of the cultural changes, progress, and errors he finds in planning his own future. He is also helped to understand his individual potential and its best possible future application.

All life experience offers the nurse the opportunity to become aware of her place in today's world. When she has acquired cultural awareness, she is not afraid of the future; nor is she afraid to face reality. Awareness of the human condition, and plans for the future in relation to it, will make life better for mankind.

THE ESTHETIC ATTITUDE

The ability to see specific events in relation to the whole is most easily developed through practice of the esthetic attitude. When an individual looks at a cloudy sky with no practical or intellectual considerations but for the pure joy of perceptual response, he is assuming the esthetic attitude. This is an attitude of detached, selfless, and disinterested contemplation. He is detached from his surroundings to the extent that he loses his sense of time. He becomes so absorbed in listening to a symphony orchestra or in watching a dramatic production that the evening slips by without his realizing it. He may lose himself so thoroughly in a book of poems or a good novel that he does not hear the doorbell or the telephone. He may also forget himself and his personal needs. He may become so intent in experiencing an art exhibition that he does not realize the room is too warm, or too chilly, for comfort. On the way to a restaurant, he may be attracted by an exciting sunset and temporarily forget his hunger. He is disinterested in the object or event from the practical and intellectual aspects. He does not care whether it is useful, where it came from, who created it, why it is happening, or how it is made. He contemplates it for the pure joy of listening or seeing. Children easily maintain this attitude when they discover something new to their experience. This means that the esthetic attitude is a natural and essential part of life itself.

Most human beings have been reared in a culture that emphasizes practical action and gives little attention to the art of contemplation. At first, a person must consciously assume the esthetic attitude while "experiencing" certain objects (preferably art objects) in order to enjoy an esthetic response. He must consciously detach himself from the pressures of day-to-day living, ignore himself, and forget all practical or intellectual meanings. He must direct his attention toward the particular object; the esthetic response will follow. The response is richest and most rewarding when it comes from experience with the complete work of art. One should stand far enough from a painting or sculpture to be able to see all of it at once. He must read the poem, watch the play, or listen to a musical composition all the way through. Works of art are made up of many parts and elements, all of which are integrated through harmony, contrast, and rhythm. When a person perceives that these parts are integrated into a total form or whole, he satisfies his desire for the experience of order.

As one learns to assume the esthetic attitude and discovers the pleasure and feeling of self-transcendence to be gained from the esthetic response to works of art, he finds it easy to use the same approach in front of events, situations, and objects in his day-to-day living. He discovers that there is integration and interrelationship between seemingly incidental happenings. If he examines the various ways in which these relationships are formed, he learns more about himself as an individual and he gains in self-awareness. Certain responsibilities that previously seemed to have no connection with the future he had planned suddenly become more interesting and meaningful. He finds that he has certain things in common with individuals who had previously been strangers because their interests were different from his. Through the interchange of ideas with new friends, he gains still more in self-awareness. He finds relationships between seemingly unconnected events in history and in today's world that will give him more respect for the continuity of life itself and inspire him to a positive dedication to the increasing purpose of his own life.

EMPATHY

Nurses and artists have more in common than would appear on the surface. Most human beings are afflicted with certain deeply based guilt feelings resulting from their knowledge of the evils that are part of the human condition. Some individuals are affected deeply enough to choose a profession or occupation that offers them the opportunity to cope positively with these existing evils. People who choose such professions include nurses, artists, doctors, missionaries, ministers, teachers, and social workers. Most of these professionals are underpaid, which means that they have chosen their professions because of the opportunity for service rather than for material remuneration. These professions are ones in which the individual can dedicate himself completely. There is no better way of giving meaning to existence than through a life of service to mankind. With the exception of the artist, individuals who choose these professions provide direct services to persons who need them.

Although the artist works alone, he does not, however, shut himself off from life but uses the time when he is not creating for experiencing life, responding to it, and increasing his understanding of its total meaning.

The nurse is a specialist who is prepared to take care of the immediate needs of her patients. The artist, however, is a specialist who is prepared to create permanent works that will offer others the opportunity to escape in a positive way from the chaos of daily living into an ordered world that calms the spirit.

The first responsibility of the nurse is to take care of the physical and mental needs of the sick and infirm. A good nurse knows that in most cases there is also a need for spiritual care. Through her experience with and sincere appreciation of the fine arts, she is in an excellent position to understand such needs and will not hesitate to search for solutions to problems that arise in this area. Without an unusual amount of sympathy for human beings in general, few individuals would enter the nursing profession. But sympathy is not enough. If she is to attend to the spiritual and social needs of her patients, a nurse also needs to be capable of empathy and understanding.

She learns sympathy through experience. At some time, she may have suffered physical pain; or she may have experienced mental suffering at the sickbed of a loved one. She is thus able to sympathize with her patients. Because she has many patients but limited time, she may be forced to take what seems to be an unfeeling attitude toward them in order to maintain her clinical perspective. Sympathy is not enough.

She can best learn empathy through her experience with the fine arts. Through the practice of "feeling herself into" the emulated postures of paintings and sculptures and the movements of dancers and actors, she learns to emulate them figuratively. When the nurse approaches her patient with the empathic attitude, she puts herself in his place and is then able to anticipate his needs, be they mental, spiritual, or physical. We cannot understand the application of the Golden Rule until we learn to approach human beings with the empathic attitude.

As one moves from one painting to another in an exhibition, assuming the esthetic attitude each time, he responds empathically without tiring because each painting gives him a new and different experience. As the nurse moves from patient to patient in the hospital, she can approach each one empathically without having to conserve her energy, because no two patients are alike. As patients they may be suffering from the same physical affliction, but as human personalities they are different and have different attitudes toward their illnesses and toward their nurses. Instead of tiring, the nurse will experience a feeling of self-transcendence because she is administering to the spiritual and physical needs unique to each patient.

LITERATURE AND EMPATHY

The nurse can broaden and deepen her understanding of human character vicariously through the reading of good novels. Anyone who remembers Tolstoi's description of the grandmother in *War and Peace* understands his own grandmother better than he did before. A true novel deals with reality—real people in real situations. It is not a romance in which the hero and heroine live happily ever after, nor is it a fairy tale where anything can happen and often does. It concerns human beings not unlike friends and relatives, and it reveals them in circumstances and situations similar to ones we have known. In vicarious experience with these differences in human experience, we increase our understanding of what it means to be human and to be involved in human situations. The task of a good novelist is to probe deeply into human personality and to reveal to his reader why the response of a given character is unique. Each character is a singular person with his own individual personality. As the reader recognizes this fact, she becomes more aware of her own uniqueness and grows in self-confidence. At the same time, the good writer will reveal what the characters he creates have in common with all people. This will make the reader more conscious of her own place in society and strengthen her feeling of responsibility toward society. She may find herself searching for the unique and individual characteristics among the people she meets and be able to gradually lose her tendency to prejudge. Because a writer is a trained expert in analyzing and reporting the motivations and reactions of people around him, we usually gain a better knowledge of human nature and its subtleties from good novels and plays than from personal experience.

The characters created by a good novelist are so realistic that the reader feels he actually knows them. For a few days after he finishes a book, the reader will miss the persons in it just as he misses friends who have moved away. This is because he has responded empathically to the characters in the novel to the extent that what happens to them happens to him. This is why we are able to gain a better understanding of the human condition from good novels than from the objective and factual reports of trained observers.

One of the best means to an understanding of human problems in our nation is through the novels of such writers as William Faulkner and William Styron. Each of these writers brings to his writing a lifetime of experience with human problems. We can respond emotionally to factual ideas and situations as they are reported by newspapers, but our response is much deeper and more vital when we experience it empathically while reading good novels. We are most deeply affected by experiences that involve our emotions. Each of Faulkner's and Styron's works is a complete entity—nothing happens that is not necessary to the plot, and everything that is necessary happens. If something seems out of place, it is because the reader has not yet found the connection.

Any good work of art requires imagination, effort, and involvement on the part of the person experiencing it. A good novel has depth meanings as well as surface meanings. An objective intellectual approach by the reader reveals only surface meanings, whereas emotional and empathic involvement discloses depth meanings. If we are able to discuss a novel with a friend who has also read it, we will undoubtedly gain new insights into characterization and will probably find more meanings. Since the nurse is in daily contact with all kinds of people, she should take advantage of every opportunity in works of art and in real life to learn all she can concerning human personality.

THE POSITIVE ESCAPE

The statement that the esthetic experience is a means to a positive escape needs further explanation. Occasionally, the complexities of our work and the frustrations from dealing with others accumulate until we need a temporary escape. Many of us turn to sensational novels, romantic movies, and television dramas because these require no effort and, consequently, no real emotional involvement. These works are usually so badly written, and the characters are so inept, that no subtle human tendencies nor any new insights into human personality are revealed. They often depict events that transpire without proper motivation. When one returns from these worlds of unrealities, he finds himself even more disappointed with the day-to-day conditions he faces.

Both religion and the fine arts offer a means to escape that can have positive results. As one enters the door of a house of worship on Sunday morning, he leaves a world of chaos and frustration and enters a world of prayer and meditation that offers a means to escape through self-transcendence into a strengthened faith. He is in a group with many others who are there for the same purpose. Through such an experience, he learns that the constant tendency of the human soul is to aspire toward something better. Through contact with God, as a group and individually, he experiences a kind of self-transcendence that renews his faith in the purpose to which he has dedicated his life and leaves him better equipped to solve the problems that are always a part of living in today's world.

As a person walks into an art gallery or a music hall, or selects a book of poems, he enters a world of art—a world where all things are ordered. All parts of a work of art are integrated into a whole; nothing takes place out of relationship with anything else. The motivations or explanations for what takes place are always found within the work. Such experience helps a person to realize the importance of integrity in his own personality. As one learns to enjoy listening to a symphony with its complexities, interrelated parts, and subsequent unification into a whole, he begins to realize that a similar order may exist in the real world. His job ceases to be just a job and becomes part of a larger organization that seeks order in departmental relationships and social interdependence. As he discovers the spiritual enrichment that becomes available to him when he spends a few minutes contemplating a painting esthetically, he also discovers that taking the same contemplative attitude toward objects and events in nature and in his daily life can elevate him to a high plane of existence and help him to cope with the disorders that are natural in today's society. Both religious and esthetic experiences offer a means to positive escape because they inspire one to transcend himself in a way that makes him a better human being for having had the experience. After such experiences, one never quite returns to the previous level of existence.

PRACTICAL ESTHETICS

As the nurse learns the advantages to be gained from her esthetic responses to works of art, she gains more respect for the artist as a creative individual. Here we are concerned with the serious artist who says what he must say in the style he has found best for his purposes. He is not influenced by considerations such as whether his work will sell or whether other people will like it. Someone once asked Picasso why he painted. He answered: "I paint in order to learn to paint better." To the artist, the challenge of art is the technical improvement of his ability. Incidentally, his ability to express more effectively his response to the world around him will improve at the same time. The artist seldom knows when he starts a work what it will express. As a work progresses, it begins to have meanings which he gradually emphasizes until the finished work expresses what he needed to say. One poet has said: "How can I know what I think until I see what I say?"

As the artist gains experience with the human condition, he develops toward that condition attitudes that determine the true meaning in his work. This meaning usually appears intuitively during the creative process. The painter, Baziotes, has said of his own work: "As I work, or when the painting is finished, the subject reveals itself." Certainly the artist, because of his great sensitivity, must have intuitive contact with something much larger than himself since, through specific individual works, he is able to express something universal.

As we experience the many different styles of painting, poetry, and music being created today, we realize that the artist has the courage to take advantage of the freedom of expression guaranteed by a democratic society. In each painting, we find that the artist is sincere and has imposed his own personal order upon his materials because he accepts the responsibilities that accompany his freedom. When we perceive several works by the same artist, we find that they are different yet similar enough to reveal a consistent philosophy and commitment on the part of the creator. When the artist's works are arranged in chronologic order, we learn that because of his need for self-transcendence the artist has tried to make each work more sincerely expressive and perceptively ordered than the previous one. Serious artists have a respect for their materials, for the society of which they are a part, for their own ability as creators, and for their potentials for future growth.

From her experience with the arts, the nurse can learn respect for the individuality of others as well as for her own. She will realize that she has a right to free creative expression in her own life and work provided she is willing to accept the responsibilities that accompany such freedom. She will gain respect for her job and for the people and materials she works with, and she will be aware of the need for a broad knowledge of all phases of the organization of which she is a part. The artist can teach her the value of self-confidence and humility, and the importance of keeping them in balance. She will learn the importance of complete dedication to the increasing purpose of her life, and reveal the sincerity of this dedication by her actions. She will find that her need for self-transcendence can be partially satisfied by a constant effort to improve her ability and that this attitude seems to be characteristic of successful practitioners of professional nursing. Constant efforts to improve performance have taken many paths, not the least of them being the development of an appreciation of the fine arts. It is suspected that the motivations for this choice were not always clearly recognized, but that the outcomes were as effective—the acquisition of respect for self, for others, and for the universe.

SUPPLEMENTARY READING LIST

Edman, Irwin: *Arts and the Man,* W. W. Norton & Company, Inc., New York, 1939.

Gotshalk, Dilman W.: *Art and the Social Order,* The University of Chicago Press, Chicago, 1947.

Guggenheimer, Richard: *Creative Vision in Artist and Audience,* Harper & Row, New York, 1950.

Jarrett, James L.: *The Quest For Beauty,* Prentice-Hall, Inc., Englewood Cliffs, N.J., 1957.

Langer, Susanne K.: *Problems of Art,* Charles Scribner's Sons, New York, 1957.

Mead, Hunter: *An Introduction to Esthetics,* The Ronald Press Company, New York, 1952.

Myers, Bernard S.: *Understanding the Arts,* Holt, Rinehart and Winston, Inc., New York, 1958.

7

The Influence of the Arts

by Marie J. Robinson

This book is in response to a specialized need—the need for qualified, competent nurses with administrative skill. Specialization is, of course, necessary in the light of the amount of knowledge that is now available.

In addition to the stress on specialization, there is heavy emphasis today on the scientific approach to knowledge. The government is spending hundreds of thousands of dollars to support foundations for improving the teaching of science, mathematics, and languages in high schools. High school teachers are being encouraged and subsidized to work toward higher degrees in these fields to improve the quality of teaching provided our future citizens, so that they may meet the demands of a space age and a world community. Undoubtedly this emphasis is essential if we are to survive in a world of increasing tensions. Equally important is the need for specialization. Our knowledge today is too vast to be absorbed meaningfully by any one person.

In the stress on the scientist and the specialist today, however, let us not forget that there is another aspect of man which deserves equal stress. Our technical skill, our nuclear and space know-how, our familarity with other languages, and our specialists will be of little value if we overlook the humanizing aspects of our culture. The liberal arts, the humanities, are what make our technologic aptitude valuable. Eric A. Walker, president of the Pennsylvania State University, emphasized this need in a report, *The Nation's Engineering Research Needs, 1965–1985.* The report recommends, among other things, that engineers acquire greater social, economic, and political understanding than they have.

As we gain in knowledge we must gain the wisdom to disseminate and utilize the knowledge we have acquired. We must learn to enrich our understanding, our appreciation, and our awareness of the world about us. We must learn to improve our relations with other peoples of the world not by dependence on our nuclear strength but by demonstrating to them that our culture has developed qualities and provided values that make our culture a desirable one to emulate. At the same time we must learn how human beings in our country and in other countries think and feel and act. We must be eclectic in our attitude.

Obviously, then, we must pay attention to our means of communication, so that what we say and how we say it conveys the best of what we know. We must also take advantage of the cultural climate in other universal fields of endeavor, such as music, drama, art, and philosophy, so that we may become the best human beings possible. Thornton Wilder, the noted American playwright, has suggested: "The editorial writers, social scientists, and ministers think they are infusing people with courage and meaning. But looking back to other ages and other crises, we know it was the artist who sustained the public ethos."

Consider the importance of the arts to the morale of the British people during the bombings in World War II and reevaluate the contribution of the USO companies who did so much, and still do, for the morale of our own troops. Is there anyone today who is not aware of the fine public relations work being done by performing artists from the United States in foreign countries? Is there anyone who does not realize that the triumphs they achieve overseas add to the prestige of our nation in these countries?

In common with all other professions, the nursing profession depends extensively upon the quality and the character of the persons in it. Any way in which the character of the individual is enhanced—any way in which a person is made more sensitive, sympathetic, and understanding to others—any way in which an individual is helped to communicate more effectively with his fellow human beings—cannot be considered unrelated to the field of nursing.

The contribution and importance of art and philosophy to the person in nursing are discussed in Chapters 4, 5, and 6. In this chapter speech, drama, and music as they affect us personally and professionally in the specialized field of nursing administration are considered.

SPEECH

If it has never occurred to you before, take a moment now to become aware that your speech reflects your personality more quickly, more vividly, and more truly than anything you may do. Unfortunately, your character does not show as instantly as your speech. In time, of course, it is your character that counts, and anyone whose character is not of the finest becomes ineffective as a speaker, but the effect of your speech is almost instantaneous with your appearance.

What impression does your voice give? Have you ever listened to it on a tape recording or a disc? If you have, did you react as the majority of people react upon hearing themselves: "That isn't *my* voice! Do I *really* sound like *that?*" Part of this unfavorable reaction is due to the physical impossibility of hearing yourself as others hear you. About this nothing can be done. The other aspect of the desire to reject the way you sound is due to your awareness that many voices are unpleasant. All too often voices may be harsh, shrill, breathy, weak, muffled, hoarse, or possess too much or too little nasality, so that they have an unpleasant whine or twang, or a breathy, fuzzy, raspy, or strained quality.

If the vocal quality is pleasant, other factors may make the voice less effective than it should be. Incorrect pronunciation or careless articulation suggests a lack of, or a disdain for, education and/or the existence of fuzzy thinking. A too smooth, too facile, too artificial tone may easily focus attention on the manner of speaking rather than on the matter of it, a situation which defeats the purpose of communication. It is important, then, that the quality of a voice be such that it gains favorable attention and puts the hearers in an agreeable mood for the thoughts and feelings the speaker is expressing.

A pleasant listenable voice is essential not only for persons who give speeches in courts, in legislatures, or at public meetings; persons who officiate at business meetings and social clubs; and persons who participate in committee meetings, but also for individuals who must speak frequently in the course of a normal day. Consider the nursing administrator in her contacts with her superiors and her coworkers. A controlled, pleasant voice can do much to facilitate the consultations, and the ability to speak clearly and effectively can be of inestimable value in explaining things and in giving instructions. The vocal quality employed by the administrator can do much to win cooperation and support. Instead of aggravating the listener it can soothe or build confidence, relieve tensions, and help maintain a pleasant and productive relationship. Naturally, the effect of a pleasing, well-modulated voice on a patient can be most helpful. Illness makes most individuals irritable. A raspy voice can add to that irritability. A pleasant voice may not eliminate the difficulty, but it certainly will not add to the tension.

Looking at speech from the other side, one should realize that speech can reveal a patient's mental outlook. A tense, restrained voice can indicate extreme nervousness; a monotonous voice may well reflect a depressed mental feeling. These observations cannot be considered accurate medical diagnoses, of course. Nevertheless, it may be of some assistance to the nurse who is attempting to make her patient more comfortable. There is an aspect of speech that is medical, however. Patients with speech defects such as baby talk and lisping, disorders such as uranoschisis and aphasia, and difficulties such as dyslalia, dysphonia, and cerebral palsy need skilled rehabilitative assistance from the speech clinician and the speech pathologist, in cooperation with the physician and the surgeon.

Although a nursing administrator cannot be expected to also be a trained speech clinician, it is not unreasonable to expect her to know of the assistance available to patients who need such help, and to endeavor to provide such trained personnel. She should know of the American Speech and Hearing Association, an organization that has constantly been working toward providing medically approved, competent specialists to work with speech and hearing difficulties. Hospitals are adding such trained personnel to their staffs. Public school systems are employing them at an ever-increasing rate in an effort to eliminate speech difficulties in the primary grades before the difficulties affect the child's personality and his ability and progress in his regular class work. Almost every large university has a speech clinic and therapy program where help is available to the surrounding community and training is provided for the additional workers needed in the field. The nurse who remains unaware of the work in this field is not adequately fulfilling her responsibilities.

There is no intention in this chapter to present speech as magic power. There is a definite intention to point out that Rudyard Kipling's statement that "words are the most powerful drug used by mankind" is true. They express you and your desires and hopes. They are one of the most effective and influential means of communication in the world today. They are one of the most powerful means by which civilized man has attained progress.

Anyone who has watched the almost painful struggle of a speech-handicapped individual to express himself to others is aware of this fact. Anyone who has seen the joy upon this handicapped person's face when communication is achieved is aware of this fact. Anyone who has been privileged to watch the happiness of a child when he discovers a new word and learns its power does not need to be reminded that the voice is still our most rewarding instrument in a humane world.

DRAMA

In the consideration of a humane world, we must take advantage of all that will increase our understanding of people. The arts contribute immeasurably in this respect, as an examination of one of them, drama, will indicate. The three great periods of drama are the Greek, the Elizabethan, and the Modern. Each period has shown man in conflict with something. In the Greek period it was man in conflict with divinity, as exemplified in Sophocles' *Œdipus Rex.* The Elizabethan era was concerned with man in conflict with himself, apparent in Shakespeare's *Hamlet.* The Modern period represents man in conflict with his environment, as in Ibsen's *Ghosts,* Chekhov's *The Cherry Orchard,* and Shaw's *Pygmalion.*

Although this classification is simplified, it has some validity. Oedipus tries to avoid a god's prophecy and thereby negates the influence of gods on the lives of human beings. Hamlet finds it hard to decide that his mother is partly guilty of the murder of his idolized father and is reluctant to avenge the wrong, because such a proceeding would condemn his mother. Mrs. Alving eventually discovers that the environment in which she is compelled to live by the mores of her society has destroyed her life and that of her son. Despite the truth of these dilemmas, a simplified classification overlooks the other qualities that make these dramas live.

There is in plays that have passed the test of time a dealing with human experience—with clashes of will, with tragic events, with humorous foibles—which we can recognize and for which we can feel some sympathy regardless of the time in which they were written. These experiences contain a quality of universality which is as evident today as it was when the plays were first written. We still have young lovers like Romeo and Juliet, ambitious men like Macbeth, proud men like Oedipus, rebellious women like Hedda Gabler, dutiful women like Mrs. Alving, and so on.

The extent to which we can find this empathic feeling with a character in a play, the extent to which a play says something meaningful about humanity, the extent to which it delights, entertains and, at times, inspires us to intellectual effort is the extent of its value, quality, and continued effectiveness.

Modern drama has, perhaps, stressed this dealing with reality in meaningful terms more obviously than dramas of the previous eras, not only in character and plot but also in stage setting and décor. Modern drama began in the 1860s with the self-styled "state satirist" Henrik Ibsen, whose mature dramas of ideas are clearly a departure from the well-made, artificially contrived plots of other playwrights of his day. Ibsen's plays are not the sentimental melodramas of sharp contrast between good and evil and oversimplification of character and situation of plays like *Love Rides the Rails,* and *East Lynne,* complete with their snowstorms, mortgages, mustache-twirling villains, fainting heroines, and manly heroes. He presented, instead, the gray blend of character and the realities of living—the compromises, temptations, and ambitions similar to the problems that beset everyone sooner or later.

Ibsen exemplifies the intent of artists and their concern with humanity. In letters to friends he pointed out that his goal in writing was his own "spiritual enunciation." In a preface to one of his early plays he wrote, "Much, around which my later writings center, the contradiction between ability and desire, between will and possibility, the intermingled tragedy and comedy in humanity and in the individual—appeared here in vague foreshadowings. . . ."

This insistence upon reality in drama is one of the universal facets of drama from Ibsen's time to our own. Anton Chekhov in Russia, George Bernard Shaw in England, Eugene O'Neill, Lillian Hellman, and S. N. Behrman in the United States are but a few of the modern dramatists who have brought reality to their plays.

There is another strong trend in modern drama which deals with reality in a different way, and which is also helpful in broadening our realization and grasp of human nature. This new trend, called *naturalism,* is the rebellion against the confining limitations of reality—the breaking away from rigid patterns in order to formulate something more meaningful in terms of human understanding.

Paralleling naturalism in drama have been the other arts. In painting the reality of Gainsborough, Whistler, and Vermeer was supplanted by the naturalism of Degas, Picasso, and Matisse. In literature, the reality of Charles Dickens and Sinclair Lewis was replaced by the naturalistic approaches of James Joyce, e. e. cummings, and T. S. Eliot.

In drama the attempt to avoid too confining a reality is most evident in the works of Luigi Pirandello in Italy, August Strindberg in Sweden, Bertolt Brecht and Frank Wedekind in Germany, Jean Cocteau in France, Irwin Shaw in England, and William Saroyan and Thornton Wilder in the United States.

Nineteenth century science and scientific methods strongly influenced naturalistic drama, for the scientific influence caused inquiring minds to question certain moral absolutes, original sin, the tie to human nature, the nature of evil in an abstract and absolute fashion. Once this questioning began it affected the treatment of character and motivation of conduct, for naturalism attempted to explain human conduct in terms of environment and heredity, and to explain man's place in the world scientifically. Older playwrights, e.g., Shakespeare and Molière, wrote from a Christian and absolute frame of reference and were not concerned with motivation of the original character. Iago, in *Othello,* is "evil," but there is no explanation of why he is so, beyond a casual reference to the fact that Othello preferred Cassio over Iago for advancement in rank.

With the break of modern drama from the traditional lines of the theatre in the questioning of basic moral, economic, and social concepts of the world, dramatists had to seek new theatres, for the commercial theatre, afraid to risk boxoffice losses in the face of criticism of concepts that are new, possibly shocking, and disturbing, denied the authors a hearing. Actually the nineteenth century commercial theatre was a direct ancestor of today's Broadway stage—nothing dangerous, immoral, or subversive, then or now, is approved, and it is concerned chiefly with entertainment and pleasure. While pleasure is an essential aspect of the theatre, it is not by any means the whole of it. We need to question and to decide, and to consider and to realize the mores under which we function, the beliefs that mold our lives, and the factors that influence and determine the society in which we move. Unless we do this, we are no more than children who will never be able to think for ourselves, much less govern ourselves or find the sense of satisfaction or completeness essential to our happiness.

Just how drama can help us in our quest for understanding and realization in the search for fulfillment may be easier to comprehend if we consider one dramatist and learn what he has done in his work to aid us in becoming finer and more sympathetic persons. For this purpose let us take the most important name of nineteenth century drama, Henrik Ibsen. He, more than any other playwright of the time, challenged the complacencies of the conservative thought of that period.

Ibsen saw most clearly the evolving of a drama of social fact and pressure in the life of the common people, although he did not go to the extremes his disciples managed. Past fifty when he wrote most of his plays, always having as his enemy the conditions and circumstances of life, possessed by the feeling that every man is responsible for his own self-realization and self-attainment, convinced that it was his job to attack the social shams and lies, the empty conventions, the complacency, the spirit of compromise and of cowardice, and the petrified moral beliefs he found in the life about him, Ibsen had the toughness of mind, the truculence of spirit, and the necessary imagination to see his job through to the end. Since he wrote only of what he knew, his own Norway became a symbol of social and moral cowardice, narrowness, and crippling smallness of spirit.

Brand and *Peer Gynt* were his first dramas of length, and in them he attacks the spirit of compromise, complacency, and acceptance of the second best. Brand is a hero; although he dies, he does not change nor compromise. Peer Gynt is the perfect symbol of compromise. At the end of the play he realizes that the practice of running away, the troll motif of going roundabout to avoid a clash, has brought his life to an exact cipher. Peer goes through life dodging purpose and responsibilities, and although he can think, wish, will and believe, he is incapable of action. He is aware that if he severed his trigger finger he could avoid military service, but to do it—no! He cannot. This prudential character of Peer's is what Ibsen attacks. Peer's life as a middling, timid, prudential man has made him an onion, which, when peeled to the "core," leaves nothing—a symbol Ibsen uses to call attention to Peer's progressive shriveling of mind and spirit as he avoids all responsibility. More than just a topical comment on Norwegian people, it is also a comment on big business machinations, language reformers, and ancestor worshippers. It is, then, not confined to the society of Ibsen's time; society like this is with us always, in all countries, in all cultures.

Peer Gynt is important in that it had in seed everything about which Ibsen was concerned in his plays—the individual's responsibility to himself; the right and wrong way of being one's self; the consequences of avoidance and compromise; the possible redeeming force of selfless love; the right to adhere to the ideal. It is important, too, in that these problems concern everyone today as well, especially individuals who are interested in more than merely existing.

In *Ghosts,* Ibsen portrayed topics that had been forbidden—the effect of heredity and environment, which makes Oswald, the son, a victim of paresis. Here we have the destructive influence of the past upon the present. There is no easy way to avoid the stark ending. Mrs. Alving's fulfillment of duty to husband, because society frowned on divorce and separation, prevented her from a joy in life that might have saved both husband and son. The ghosts triumph at the end.

In *A Doll's House* Ibsen presents the conventional wife of the times, treated as a pet and a doll who plays at taking care of home and children. Her revolt against the denial of her individuality, of her being a person, woman or man, results in her leaving husband and children, a shocking resolution indeed to the people of that day. Nora's demand for rights as a human being was a blow to conventional marriage. But human beings have a right to destroy that which would destroy them as human beings, to insist upon a recognition of individual rights, a part of common humanity.

The Wild Duck heralds the shift from the flaws in society and tradition to the flaws in the individual, to the personal source of defeat within the individual, a shift apparent in all of Ibsen's later plays. In *The Wild Duck* Ibsen gives us the reformer, obsessed almost pathologically with the claim of the ideal, with the need for reforming everyone he meets, without any sense of the nature of human beings or any understanding that each person is an individual—this is the main character, Gregers. Ibsen in this way exposes the false Messiah, the pitiable and contemptible travesty of the true Redeemer, as the man Gregers tries to save is not worth saving.

Today we have human beings like those Ibsen portrayed, and we still need his penetration and insight to help us understand them and ourselves. We have men with a mission but without sense or courage. We have individuals who shrink from duty and responsibility. We have women who have not yet realized their own potentials. We have the speaker who is not the doer. We have men struggling for achievement. We have the person who compromises. We have doubters who are concerned with what you have gained if you have lost love and happiness in achieving what you thought you wanted. All these elements of common human experience are as topical today as they were when Ibsen wrote of them.

In addition to its meaningful comments on human nature, which should be of value in understanding patients, coworkers, superiors, and the self, there is another and perhaps more specifically applicable area of drama for the administrative personality. Psychologists and psychiatrists have found that creative drama, when enacted by a patient, is often invaluable as an aid in locating the source of the patient's disturbance or the type of problem confronting the patient. Just as painting and doodling are often helpful in exposing the viewpoint of an emotionally disturbed person, adult or child, so is drama helpful in revealing the difficulty or distortion causing the disturbance. The possibility of such aid for patients should also be part of the knowledge of the administrator, and some understanding of the area would facilitate conferences with staff psychiatrists and psychologists.

One further comment seems essential. Drama is not just serious in purpose. The theatre, motion pictures, and television are important means for relaxation and enjoyable respite from the tensions of everyday living. To be entertained by an evening at the theatre, to spend a few hours of pleasure at a motion picture, to relax in front of a television set, and to be amused by the skilled artists on the screen can be a most welcome means of maintaining a stable outlook on life. There is validity in the Greek idea of catharsis, the purging of the emotions of pity and fear through the medium of plays.

MUSIC

What has been said about the ability of drama to relieve tensions can be more strongly applied to the field of music. If there is anything more relaxing than an evening of music, it is difficult to name it. One can find music to suit every mood—a gay gavotte, a soothing sonata, a sentimental waltz, an inspiring opera. Music can reinforce a mood, or it can change it. Often, when one is discouraged, an hour of music can alleviate the sadness. When one is elated, music serves to release the happiness. Music is readily available through recordings, radio, television, concerts, and recitals, and through individual efforts, which often enhance the effects. Learning to play a musical instrument takes time, but the reward is well worth the effort involved. When one plays an instrument he experiences a catharsis of the emotions and the enjoyment of playing with a group of other musicians in a companionship that is pleasing and stimulating and adds to one's sense of fulfillment.

Music also has a gratifying effect on the mentally ill. The sound of music calms patients; the playing of it helps to bring them a measure of return to reality.

Music has been a part of all cultures from the beginning of time. Primitive races used drums and reed pipes, clapped their hands, and stamped their feet for the rhythmic accompaniment to their ritualistic dances. Music has reflected national traits and hopes, longings, and history from time immemorial. Music of some sort has been irretrievably woven with religion, dance, celebration, mourning, and leisure throughout every age of man, and it has richly added to the tapestry of life in each era.

SUMMARY

One cannot overlook the vital function of the arts. For centuries, speech, drama, music, painting, sculpting, and literature have been means of communication for persons, countries, and cultures. Artists have been sensitive enough to perceive and gifted enough to record life as we live it; our moral beliefs, hopes and aspirations, failures and regrets, triumphs, and history are found in their works. Their means of expression have varied, but the intention of each artist has been the same—to communicate that which he has perceived in a clear and meaningful form.

If the painter did not wish to communicate his perceptions to others, why does he not destroy his work once he has completed it? If the writer did not want his words to endure, why does he not use disappearing ink? If the sculptor has no interest in a lasting impression, why does he expend time scoring marble and stone? Obviously, artists use enduring means to preserve their works so that they may communicate to fellow human beings regardless of time and space.

We are fortunate indeed that the desire to make their contributions lasting has been the concern of artists. Think how much pleasure the world would have missed had it never had Rembrandt, Matisse, or Vermeer. Consider the enjoyment that Brahms, Bach, and Beethoven have brought with their music. Reflect on the loss the world would have to sustain were it denied Shakespeare, Goethe, or Benét.

More than pleasure is at stake here, though. We have learned much from artists, and we will continue to learn more as our own lives and experiences grow and change. Artists have opened our eyes to hitherto unnoticed beauty. They have opened our minds to unrealized wisdom. They have strengthened our morale with unknown richness. They have instilled in our hearts an unlimited humanity.

Through the artist and the medium he employs we are made truly aware of the world in which we live and of the people who inhabit it. Without art we can exist. We can earn our bread, build our shelters, clothe our bodies, and raise our families; but this is being without meaning. To live with meaning we need more than material necessities. We need a humanity to feed our souls. Harold Weston, chairman of the National Council on the Arts and Government, Inc., concretely expressed this, when he said, ". . . the arts provide fall-out shelters for the human spirit vastly more essential—more urgently needed—and at infinitely less cost than those for the human body."

The arts enrich our lives and instill in us all that is best in our culture. They represent the best of which we are capable, the highest to which we can aspire. They are at once our strength and our joy. They reflect us more completely, more penetratingly, than all our technical ability and specialized skills. Although we cannot all become artists, we can all benefit from an appreciation of the value and the contribution of art to life, to personal development, and to the ability to understand and to cope with the complexities of this modern world.

Whatever our profession, we all need to rededicate ourselves to the ideals that Louis Pasteur had in mind when, on his seventieth birthday, at a celebration in his honor at the Sorbonne, in Paris, he recommended to those present:

> Say to yourselves first, "What have I done for my instruction?" Then, as you gradually advance, "What have I done for my country?" Until the time comes when you may have the immense happiness of thinking that you have contributed in some way toward the progress and good of humanity.

SUPPLEMENTARY READING LIST

Anderson, Virgil A.: *Training the Speaking Voice,* Oxford University Press, New York, 2d ed., 1961.

Bentley, Eric: *The Playwright as Thinker,* Meridian Books, New York, 1946.

Bentley, Eric: *In Search of Theater,* Alfred A. Knopf, Inc., New York, 1953.

Gassner, John: *Masters of the Drama,* Dover Publications, New York, 1945.

Getzels, Jacob W., and P. W. Jackson: *Creativity cnd Intelligence,* John Wiley, New York, 1962.

Gorelik, Mordecai: *New Theatres for Old,* Samuel French, New York, 1949.

Gray, Giles Wilkeson, and Claude Merton Wise: *The Bases of Speech,* Harper & Row, Publishers, Incorporated, New York, 3d ed., 1959.

Macgowan, Kenneth and William Melnitz: *The Living Stage,* Prentice-Hall, Inc., Englewood Cliffs, N.J., 1955.

Wallace, Karl R. (ed.): *The History of Speech Education in America,* Appleton-Century-Crofts, Inc., New York, 1954.

West, Robert, Merle Ansberry and Anna Carr: *The Rehabilitation of Speech,* Harper & Row, Publishers, Incorporated, New York, 3d ed., 1957.

part 3

The Place: The Hospital Yesterday and Today

8

Administrative Theory in Relation to Social Structure and Forces

by D. Paul Miller

The importance of the influence the environment has on one's ability to perform the administrative process is stated in Litchfield's third major proposition and the two minor propositions derived from them (Chapter 2). It is interesting to note that *environment* refers to both the place of employment as well as the community in which the place is located. But theories growing out of these propositions have not yet been formulated and tested. Descriptions of environment represent judgmentally derived knowledge instead of scientifically identified facts, leaving in their wake many incomplete explanations and few predictions.

Knowing that environment exercises a tremendous effect on the performance of the administrative process is a beginning, however, and compels one to attempt to describe environment in terms of the best available knowledge and within the historical framework of the following reference points: (1) individual behavior; (2) organizational behavior; (3) environmental events (events outside the organization, such as events that occur in the community); and (4) interactions of all three.

When we view modern society we are invariably impressed with its dynamic nature. It is constantly changing, interacting, and "on the go." Since social institutions are a product of society, and since society is dynamic, it is only to be expected that the emerging institutions will also be dynamic. The social institutions of health are no exception to this rule. In this chapter attention is focused on the hospital, because the hospital is the environment in which the greatest number of nurses today spend most of their time. Since the hospital is essentially dynamic in nature, the nurse must recognize the importance of maintaining a dynamic attitude in her learning experience if she is to keep pace with her work environment.

There is no place for set methods in the nursing field. At any given time the facilities and techniques in use and the general conditions in force are likely to be different from those in use and in force at another time. Also, there may be wide variations from place to place at a given time. The skills and knowledge the nurse acquires today may be replaced tomorrow with new skills, new knowledge, and new techniques. An understanding of the past, therefore, is important in understanding today, and an understanding of today is important if one is to be able to anticipate and understand the future.

THE EARLY HOSPITAL

From the earliest days down to the present day man has tended to show compassion for and interest in the well-being of his fellow man. He has offered his ill and suffering neighbor his favorite remedies, and he has administered his healing skills in one form or another. He has selected adaptations that have contributed to his chances for survival from the perilous Stone Age to the present day equally perilous but vastly different space age. The anthropologist Marshall D. Sahlins has pointed out that the origin of human society must be attributed to man's subordination of qualities such as selfishness, brute competition, and individual interest, which were dominant in the prehuman organism, to cooperative kinship relationships and acceptance of "morality over might." [1]

The early civilizations—Egypt and India—had treatment methods that utilized what may be considered an unwrought prototype of the hospital. As early as in the dynastic period, which began in 3100 B.C., Egypt had specific methods of treating her ill and of administering drugs. Although the common place for treatment was the home, the temples in some instances served as hospitals. In some of the early Egyptian temples both medical and faith healing were administered. In India, in the sixth century B.C., "Buddha appointed a physician for every ten villages and built hospitals for the crippled and poor." [2]

The early Greeks and Romans carried on with further advances in medical treatment. Following the ways of their Egyptian predecessors, the Greeks also used temples as places of refuge for the sick. Inscriptions found on the columns of some of the early Greek temples are sometimes referred to as the first clinical records. These inscriptions indicate the names of patients, the nature of their conditions, and the type of disposition made

[1] Marshall D. Sahlins, "The Origin of Society," *Scientific American*, vol. 203, pp. 76-86, September, 1960.

[2] Malcolm T. MacEachern, *Hospital Organization and Management*, rev. 3d ed., Physician's Record Company, Chicago, 1957, p. 1.

of the various patients. As civilization spread westward into the Roman Empire, so also did the various techniques and treatments for the ill.

Hippocrates was born in Greece in 460 B.C. His diagnoses of various human pathologic conditions, and his remedies and treatment methods, together with his emphasis on fact instead of on faith, are the reasons he is considered the father of medicine. He treated fractures, performed surgery, and was aware of and attempted to explain conditions such as epilepsy, ulcers, and tuberculosis. Advances in medical treatment continued in the Empire and in time were felt in Europe proper and eventually in the New World. The modern Western hospital has grown more directly out of the medieval institutions that had the same name but different functions.

During the medieval period, an institution which was more definitely separated from the temple was developed. Even though apart from the temple, it was still a definite function of the religious spirit of the day. This new institution was called *hospitia,* from the Latin adjective *hospitalis,* or the noun *hospes,* which means "host." The English *hospital* comes from the French *hospitale.* The words "hospital," "hostel," and "hotel," although each has a different meaning, are derived from the same Latin source and at one time had the same general meaning.[3]

In medieval times, approximately A.D. 1000 to 1500, as it had been since the beginning of the Christian Era, the total life of the people was still oriented within the framework of religion. Political loyalties, economic considerations, educational responsibilities, and health matters were subject to the official Church. Great emphasis was placed on pilgrimages during this period. Commercial inns and travel accommodations had not been established as yet. Since the church emphasized the pilgrimages, it seemed to be the responsibility of the church to provide temporary shelter for weary pilgrims. Ordinarily these shelters were adjacent to the monasteries. As a consequence, the hospital became a sojourn for many travelers. Commonly the travelers who resorted to the hospital were often in such a serious state of illness that they never recovered. The hospital served to make their lives as comfortable as possible until their days were spent.

This traditional view of health care suggests a dichotomy which can be detected in the patterns man has devised for the care of the sick. Namely, insofar as it is humanly possible, the church will attempt to perpetuate eternal physical life, i.e., prevent death by every possible means, as long as possible and for as many persons as possible, and at the same time prepare each person for a pleasant life to follow.

[3] *Ibid.,* p. 6.

After the hospital had assumed the role of caring for the ill, it operated in what may be considered a negative role for several centuries. The role was negative in the sense that hospital confinement was considered undesirable and was to be avoided if home care could be obtained. The ill person always preferred home care to hospital care; relatives also preferred that their dependent ill receive home rather than hospital care. This preference for home care was not for financial reasons but because the needed facilities were more readily available at home. Also, because of the inadequacy of the facilities and personnel in the hospital, it was generally believed that the chances for recovery were greater in the home than in the hospital. Individuals who could not obtain home care surrendered themselves to the hospital as a last resort. General acceptance of the hospital was not realized until science and medicine had made notable strides.

The first incorporated hospital in the United States was the Pennsylvania Hospital, established in Philadelphia, chartered in 1751, and opened to the public in 1755. In some respects it was a genuine forerunner of the modern hospital. It had features that are still a functional part of the modern hospital. The primary reason for the establishment of this hospital was to provide a place where local physicians could treat their private patients. Even at this early date it was recognized that to bring a number of patients into a single place would facilitate the medical care for these patients. This, probably more than any other factor, is the core function of the modern hospital. Also, some of the early leaders in the field of medicine realized that such a center could become a highly desirable place in which the finest facilities would be available to large numbers of patients. Services could be increased to an extent that could never be matched by the home-care practice that had been commonplace heretofore. It was realized, however, that before this system could become practical much antihospital prejudice on the part of the public had to be overcome.

The number of hospitals increased steadily, hospital services became more and more specialized, and surgery became more commonplace. Nevertheless there was a "dark age" in hospital history in the first half of the nineteenth century. Mortality from surgery was exceedingly high. Treatment, in some instances, regressed to a point lower than that of the ancient and medieval periods.

The twentieth century, however, has witnessed an upturn in hospital developments. The number of hospitals has mushroomed, and a new aura of sophistication has become associated with the hospital. The modern hospital is a sharp contrast to its nineteenth century counterpart, and it continues to change. The changes reflect adaptations of a spontaneous but evolutionary nature, not deliberate and rational planning.

The modern hospital is still in formative and, in some respects, experimental stages. Its changes have been many, and the corresponding adjustments are many. In no sense can the transition be considered complete. Such a view would be both unwise and dangerous. It is perhaps truer today than at any time in the history of hospitals that changes and adjustments are being both sought and wrought. Although some changes are inevitable and must necessarily be faced, there are definite indications in hospital organizations today that persons with policy-making power are advocating deliberate change. These changes are not always of the type which is necessary for immediate survival; they are, instead, of a type which prevents the difficult situation from occurring in the first place. The changes tend to be preventive in nature, indicating the modern approach to health.

SOCIAL CHANGE AND HOSPITAL ORGANIZATION

Based on the assumption that the nature of any organization is systematically related to (1) its goals and purposes and (2) its environmental situation, this discussion is an examination of the environmental factors that affect the hospital organization most and the relationship that exists between the environment and the hospital.[4]

Hospitals have changed tremendously through the centuries and today they are vastly different from what they were yesterday. Modern changes in hospital organization and operation have transpired as a result of changes in the social and cultural aspects of the environment. Another point that needs clarification is the inclusion of both *society* and *culture* as facets of the environmental setting.

Society is people and their interaction and interrelationships. For the purpose of this discussion, the concerns are with groups of nurses, doctors, administrators, members of the custodial staff, patients, and so forth. The common denominators are the interaction and the organizational relationships among the persons involved. Whenever the behavior of one person affects the behavior of another person there is interaction and a social situation.

Culture is not people but something used, possessed, and carried on by

[4] Richard L. Simpson and William H. Gulley, "Goals, Environmental Pressures, and Organizational Characteristics," *American Sociological Review*, vol. 27, pp. 344-351, June, 1962.

society's members, yet distinct from the people themselves. Culture is the design for living and acting; the plan, or blueprint, for human action. Culture within the hospital includes the rules, regulations, policies, and patterns that are a vital part of a hospital. Specifically, hospital culture encompasses the admissions policy, the requirements for financial arrangements, ward assignments, routine requirements for patients of various types, the knowledge, skills, and practices of the medical and nursing staff, and even the patterned activities of the maintenance employee.

In addition to the abstract or nonmaterial culture described above, included in some definitions of culture is the man-made physical, or material, environment. This includes, for example, the buildings, communication devices, and equipment of all sorts. These are vital components of a hospital. Culture then is defined as the man-made environment, both material and nonmaterial. In relating culture and society, the distinction to be kept in mind is that *people constitute the society;* and the *design for behavior,* together with the artifacts produced, *constitutes the culture.*

In actual operation a society and its culture are inseparable. For this reason it is appropriate to use terms such as *environment, situation, setting,* or *circumstances* to include both culture and society. Certain circumstances in the sociocultural setting play a significant part in determining what the hospital is and what it may become.

Today many types of human ailments are not ordinarily treated outside the hospital. With the exception of some rural areas and the occasional personal preference, today we seldom hear of the expectant mother who would consider giving birth to her child outside the hospital. Major surgery is dealt with almost exclusively in hospitals. Most illnesses of a serious nature are observed and treated in the hospital. For adequate treatment of many conditions the hospital has become a necessity, and it has become possible to carry on with this "hospital-a-necessity" policy in society only because certain environmental adaptations have been made. Hospital treatment is effective and consequently is attractive. Also, various plans for financing health care make hospitalization possible for most persons. The underlying principle of these plans, whether public or private, is that the public at large contributes premiums or taxes, and the person in need realizes the direct benefit. Within such a system of medical and hospital plans and provisions, hospitalization becomes a reality for an ever-increasing proportion of the population. The consequence is the general attitude that the hospital must be available for all who need it.

SPECIALIZATION AND DIVISION OF LABOR

It is difficult for a person today to participate in a service vocation without having to consider the demands of the increasing pressures to specialize. The general practitioner in medicine is being replaced by the obstetrician, the pediatrician, the throat and ear specialist, the brain surgeon, and the like. The nurse is being encouraged to specialize in fields such as maternity nursing, nursing of children, public health nursing, teaching, administration of nursing service departments, and the like. In other areas of hospital work there is the dietitian, the physical therapist, the psychologist, the social worker, the chaplain, and even the plumber and the electrician, all of whom are specialists. To an increasing extent responsibilities are delineated and assigned in accordance with the special training or background of an individual. Without special training, an employee is at a decided disadvantage. In many instances it is impossible to practice or find employment without legal license or certification in a field of specialty. Concomitant with the increased emphasis on specialization, it is expected that the hospital organization will be managed with increasing efficiency.

A major drawback in this specialization-division-of-labor program is the accompanying monotony, which tends to wear heavily on the personality. It appears that the psychological makeup of the human personality may be better adapted to a variety of activities than to the specialized monotonous routine. The nurse who was trained two decades ago, for example, is experiencing the transition of the hospital from its role as a small operation with informal primary-group relationships and general duty responsibilities to the larger operation with formal relationships—encompassing specialized duties and persons known by the functions they perform instead of as individuals—and frequently is unable to make the proper adjustment. This, of course, creates additional problems for the administration and for other policy-making personnel of the hospital. It sometimes becomes necessary to weigh the disadvantages against the advantages and perhaps slow the rate of change in order to achieve the greatest degree of efficiency in the total operation.

POPULATION MOBILITY AND URBANIZATION

Another circumstance which has an impact on the development of hospitals is the ever-expanding population. The world population is increasing at a rate that promises to double the total population within forty years. The natural population increase (i.e., births over deaths) is approximately 34 million per year; 93,000 per day; 64 per minute. In other words, there is an increase of more than one person per second in world population.

The natural increase in population in the United States in the decade 1950 to 1960 was 30 million; 3 million per year, 8,200 per day, or an increase of approximately 5½ persons per minute. This rate is not diminishing in the present decade. From these figures it becomes obvious that if the hospital maintains its "necessity" quality, and if the population continues to increase as expected, the need for a greater number of hospitals or, at any rate, facilities to accommodate a greater number of patients, is inevitable.

There is a remarkable similarity between the social patterns in the Middle Ages and the social patterns in society today. During the Crusades it was the travelers who had no access to home facilities or home treatment who, when illness struck, needed attention. This led to treatment in inns and in private homes, which later developed into various forms of public accommodations designed to meet the illness-away-from-home needs of the day. Treatment for the ill, of necessity, became increasingly institutionalized during this period. In modern America it is also the mobile society which creates the need for hospitals. The surge in hospital development in the Middle Ages and the surge in hospital building today are not merely coincidence. Several other considerations support this thesis.

A considerable proportion of society's illness seems to be psychological in nature, a kind of need for illness. It is not uncommon to find "patients" in the hospital today because they want to rest, "to get away from it all." Such rest is possible because they have hospitalization provisions. Also, persons are sometimes ill because they have sick leave or because they crave attention. These attitudes reflect sociocultural conditions that cause a type of somatic illness the primitive or frontier society could not afford to bear. The modern and complex society not only can afford it but would not function normally without it. Further, there is a greater degree of personal and social insecurity among travelers in strange places as compared with home community persons with well-established primary-group relationships. It appears that stay-at-home persons may actually not have as high a frequency of illness as the mobile society. Another factor involved is that in the home community, where persons know one another and interact more freely, there may conceivably be more reciprocal aid from person to person.

Although land frontiers have virtually disappeared, mobility still remains a major process. The population still moves. In the United States, for example, in 1930, 5 million persons born east of the Mississippi River were living west of the Mississippi River. At this same time 25 million persons were living outside the state in which they were born. In the period 1941 to 1945, 12 per cent of the population changed counties and between 1940 and 1947, 70 million persons moved to a different house.

The Bureau of the Census makes an annual survey of about 25,000 dwelling units and reports the results in *Current Population Reports*. According to these reports, one person of every five moves to a different house each year. Annual migration across county lines in recent years has been more than 9 million per year. By comparison this figure is more than three times as great as the total annual growth of the counties. The number of persons who change residences across state lines annually is 1½ times as great as the country's annual population increase. This high rate of mobility means, in essence, a high frequency of impersonalization. The human interaction in these mobile circumstances is not in general intimate and informal; it lacks the personal and friendly relationships that are established when contacts and interaction are of a more permanent nature.

The modern conditions of mobility and impersonalization are closely intertwined with the process of urbanization. Urbanization is the movement city-ward. Human behavior today is predominantly an urban way of life. Even rural residents have, to a large extent, adopted urban ways. Large numbers of people live in small areas with a great deal of cultural complexity and a somewhat formal state of interdependence. In the total societal operation there is a large number of specialists, each performing his particular role. In addition to the agricultural producer there is an array of "general" specialists such as manufacturers, wholesale distributors, and business retailers; and service specialists, such as physicians and nurses, schoolteachers, insurance salesmen, airplane pilots, politicians, policemen, garbage collectors, electricians, hairdressers, and TV repairmen. This total array of specialists distinguishes modern society from the earlier and more traditional society. Emil Durkheim refers to it as *organic solidarity*. He thinks of each of the parts or specialists as organs performing a necessary function in the operation of the total organism (society). There is a high degree of interdependence among specialists. The relationships tend to depend upon the functions performed rather than upon the personalities involved.

TRANSPORTATION AND COMMUNICATION

It is important in hospital operations today that ready and rapid transportation be available to virtually all persons. Furthermore, it is important that communications be developed and available to the extent that one is as nearly in contact with the hospital as his nearest telephone. All-weather roads are being developed at increasing rates. Only a relatively small and ever-diminishing proportion of the American population is isolated because of impassable roads.

The paved streets, improved highways, throughways, and one-way arteries make it possible to travel efficiently and with great dispatch. Highly efficient ambulance service is available at a moment's notice and on twenty-four-hour call. Notice is usually given by telephone which, with its improved dialing systems, makes efficient communication available to most persons. Intrahospital communication lines increase the efficiency in hospital operation as hospital units become larger and personal contacts less possible.

Developments that may be considered scientific in the sense of modern science were occurring with the discoveries and inventions of Galileo, Newton, and other scientists in the sixteenth and seventeenth centuries. The newly acquired knowledge, discoveries, and inventions were a result of scientific inquiry, theory, and research. This sociocultural environment proved to be technically vital to hospital operations.

Scientific activity itself does not bring about social changes. It is only when this activity is applied toward specific goals that the developments and changes occur. It is the engineering and the application of the scientific knowledge acquired which bring about improvements in medical practice and in hospital operations. The application of this knowledge as such is not science but activity which involves the use of science. In effect the physician is a medical engineer, and other hospital personnel may correctly be considered engineers of various types as they use and apply their knowledge.

INSTITUTIONALIZED HEALTH PLANS

Various developments, particularly in the areas of political and economic culture, have had a real impact in making hospital services available to the public. Through tax-supported programs, public aid is provided at various levels of government: township, municipal, county, state, and federal. This aid is ordinarily channeled through social welfare departments that have been established by political provisions. In recent decades there has been increasing pressure to expand tax-supported public aid for medical and hospital care. This type of aid has increased significantly, and from appearances today it will continue to increase. This increase in public aid is a response to social needs. Resistance to increased aid comes in the main from persons who feel that further Federal provisions tend to destroy individual responsibility. The opposition contends that aid should come through programs in which the individual assumes the responsibility of participating in and of paying premiums.

Numerous private insurance companies provide hospital plan features in their policies in response to this pressing need. The Blue Cross plan initiated at one university hospital included only schoolteachers in its original form. It has since developed into a plan open to the public and is operated on a nonprofit basis. One fact that should be recognized in regard to these programs is that usually the person who needs the hospital service and medical treatment is less able to pay for it at the time of the need than at the time he is healthy and employed. These programs permit him to realize the benefits at the time of need. Without a health insurance program he may be unable to pay and thus be at a decided disadvantage in obtaining the services.

The modern hospital is no longer a place the patient approaches with reluctance, apprehension, and the fear of death. Instead, he enters the hospital willingly and anticipates improved health and longer life. The public today accepts the hospital and considers it a necessity.

SOCIAL STRUCTURE AND SOCIAL PROCESS IN HOSPITAL OPERATION

To clarify the terms *social structure* and *social process*, and in order to understand how *process* may conceivably become *structure*, it may be helpful to make some theoretical applications. Social structure is considered a composite or complex whole made up of various elements, such as the status and roles of individuals as they interact in groups. Since social structure has specific and identifiable components, it has specific form. This form also can be identified as the whole of the structure, whatever it may be. Social process is patterned change. The observer can see a specific quality in the pattern; for example, the process of conflict or cooperation. One may also contend that the process too has specific *form*, thus giving it the quality of structure, i.e., patterned change with specific and identifiable parts. In the sense that it is a composite whole made up of parts, process may correctly be considered structure. In other words, it is *structured process.* Structure is the snapshot; process the motion picture.

The nurse is one of the many parts of the social structure in the hospital as well as a person who participates in the various behavior patterns of the hospital. Thus she is a vital part of both structure and process. It would be realistic insofar as hospital operation is concerned to consider the staff nurse as a sort of home base. In any hospital today she is a central figure. She is the one person who contacts and must communicate with virtually all hospital personnel, from the physician to the janitor. She is also required to contact, communicate with, and submit to at least four different lines of authority. This places her in an extraordinarily difficult position. She must be a diplomat, a counselor, a servant, a housekeeper, an errand boy, and a medical authority. At times, she must be all of these at the same time. She is, for example, subject to the authority of the nurse supervisor and the nurse director. She is indeed subject to the physician's orders and must work with him directly on many occasions. Furthermore, since she is an integral part of the hospital personnel she is subject to the hospital administration and must on occasion answer directly to the administrator himself. In addition to these persons in authority, she has direct contact with and must meet the needs, the whims, and fancies of the patient. In fact, service to the patient is seen as her primary responsibility. She is often the hospital's liaison with the public and with the patient's friends and relatives. In each of these relationships there is the administrative function. In some instances she is administered to, in others she is the administrator.

So long as all goes well, so long as she is able to carry out the orders of the physician and the supervisor without violating hospital policy and the patient is "doing well," all is well with the staff nurse. It soon becomes obvious, however, that these various circumstances do not and, in fact, probably cannot all exist at the same time for any notable length of time.

In some instances it may be necessary for the nurse to bear the brunt of a careless order given by one of her superiors. She may be forced into a difficult and, at times, impossible situation. She must consider her various lines of responsibility: the physician, the supervisor, the hospital administrator, the patient, and relatives and friends of the patient as well as her own moral responsibility. Although the nurse's role is unique, satisfactory disposition of the problems the nurse encounters is not impossible. As a matter of fact, the prevailing attitude of the nurse appears to be one of an eagerness to grapple with the difficult situation. She generally accepts the encounter in fine order. She sees the crying need for her services and accepts the challenge.

Problem situations in administration at whatever level they occur usually suggest the need for improvement. These problems usually occur because of inadequate adjustment to changing circumstances. Today's biggest problems often imply the need to improve on the last generation's solutions. If efficient hospital operation is to be maintained and improved, the persons involved in this operation must be aware of and sensitive to the dynamic nature of modern society. The hospital does not and, in fact, cannot operate in a vacuum. It is a part of the total societal operation and must always be viewed in context. The human aspects of the hospital, with its various qualities and in its various relationships, is the subject matter of this section, and will be discussed under two headings. The first considers the hospital classifications and personnel groupings that are essential to the formal organization of the hospital. The second considers the personnel and social status. Although the activities related to the various statuses will be discussed in greater detail in the section on social process, status relationships as such are a part of the structure.

Hospital Classifications. Every hospital has several major groupings. Each group has distinctive characteristic functions. The administration formulates and enforces hospital policy. The professionals and their assistants are the only group which has essential and direct contact with the patient. Members of this group perform specialized functions according to their training and qualifications. The nonadministrative nonprofessionals perform important service tasks for efficient operation of the hospital, but do not formulate policy nor have essential patient contact. The patient is the total object of service of the entire working staff, although in much of the work the relationship with the patient is indirect.

The classification of hospitals is usually done either according to their clinical function or on the basis of ownership and control. The American Hospital Association uses these two criteria plus a third criterion, the type of care—long- or short-term.

Malcolm T. MacEachern suggests that the combination of clinical classification and ownership and control classification gives the most nearly correct description.[5] Insofar as clinical types are concerned, hospitals are either general or special. The general hospital admits and treats many different kinds of patients with a wide variety of needs: medical, surgical, obstetrical, chronic, etc. The special hospital accepts patients of only one type. There are, for example, hospitals that admit and treat only

[5] *Op. cit.*, pp. 34 and 35.

patients with mental and nervous disorders, or tuberculosis, orthopedic conditions, cancer, and the like.

Hospitals classified by ownership and control fall into one of the two major categories, government-controlled and privately controlled. The government-controlled hospitals include Federal, state, county, and municipal hospitals. The privately controlled hospitals include church, community, fraternal order, and independent institutions. The most common type of hospital today is the general hospital, controlled by either church or community. The church-controlled type is perhaps found more frequently than the community-controlled type. In fact, the community-controlled hospital often has at least indirect, if not direct, ties with the churches in the community.

The organizational structure, the general operation, and the care rendered in any of the differently controlled types of hospitals are not necessarily or significantly different. The difference lies more in *how* they are run than by *whom* they are run. The hospital analyzed in this chapter may well be one of a number or a combination of types. It should perhaps be nearly correct to consider this hospital a nongovernmental or independent general hospital. This would perhaps be the most representative of the environment in which the nurse today is most frequently found.

Hospital Personnel. The medical staff includes all physicians who treat or administer to patients in the hospital. It includes general practitioners, internists, surgeons, obstetricians, pediatricians, radiologists, and other specialists who are licensed to practice. This group has no official connection with the hospital's administrative organization. Any influence or connection it has in administering hospital policy is without formal provision. Technically the responsibility of the physician is limited to the care of his patients within the provisions of the hospital. It is needless to say, however, that in reality the medical staff exerts a very real influence on the total hospital operation including, in many instances, matters that affect formulation and re-formulation of hospital policy.

The nursing staff includes registered professional nurses, licensed practical nurses, and nurse aides. Among the registered nurses there are some with diplomas, some with degrees from junior or senior colleges, some with graduate degrees, and some with advanced training and practice as specialists in various fields. It is the staff nurse who has the most direct contact with the patient; ironically, she is usually the registered nurse with the least amount of training and experience. That is, nurses with the greatest amount of training and experience are more likely to be moved into the higher administrative positions. As a result the administrative positions carry increasingly less patient-contact responsibilities as one moves upward.

The nonprofessional and nonadministrative personnel category is self-explanatory. Included in this group are the housekeepers, maintenance men, cooks, laundry personnel, and so forth. In general their responsibilities are not making decisions or policies so much as simply following orders that have been authorized.

There are undoubtedly certain other personnel workers who have not been indicated here. The purpose of this discussion, however, in no sense is to be all inclusive. At best it should be a representative picture of the general hospital. The personnel groups indicated above, and patients, constitute the major portion of the human resources of any hospital.

Patients are a unique part of the hospital social structure. This is an element of the human resources which, in some situations, is an interacting part of the hospital personnel; in other instances, it is completely oblivious of even the presence of other persons.

In analyzing the patient relationship to the hospital social structure, it should be noted first that the patient is the main focus of attention. In a very literal sense all attention, all performance by other workers, whether professional, administrative, or service, is directly or indirectly focused on the patient. Thus the patient is the central figure around which the entire hospital operation tends to orbit. The production goal in the hospital is unique in that failure in its goal means that the person disappears from the scene. This is not the case in any other social institution today.

Another unique situation in relation to the patient is that in some normal hospital situations he is totally incapable of any social interaction. For example, when the patient is anesthetized for surgical intervention or for other types of treatment he loses total function of the sensory apparatus and social interaction is carried on among doctors and nurses entirely without the patient's participation. In this situation the interaction takes on a theoretically limited aspect. When the patient regains consciousness, however, the interaction again becomes total.

In other normal situations the patient is a very real part of the social interaction. He converses, he requests, he complains, he demands and, oftentimes, he simply visits with the attending doctor or nurse or other patients. The uniqueness of the patient's part in the social structure is that although he is the major concern, he sometimes participates and interacts socially and sometimes is a totally nonparticipating member and even is completely unconscious of the situation of which he is the focus.

Personnel and Social Status. Significant in the structure of any organization is the status arrangement of its personnel. There is the tendency among all societies to classify their members into categories and to place the categories above or below one another and consider the members superior or inferior on the basis of the position occupied. The status of any particular person is a reflection of the respect others hold for him. It also reflects a self-image. That is, for a person to occupy a particular social position, two circumstances must exist: (1) others must recognize him as occupying that position, and (2) he must be aware of, and assume with proper role playing, the position he occupies.

Another principle of social stratification relates to the limitations, or restrictions, a society imposes upon members of the various status categories. In some instances the limitations are inflexible. In these situations it is difficult to move out of a particular class, either up or down. In other instances movement up or down is relatively easy; few, if any, limitations are imposed and change in status is easy and frequent. The former tends to be caste-like; the latter is commonly referred to as an open-class system.

It is sometimes helpful and, in fact, quite realistic to note these two forms of stratification as points on a continuum. Caste represents one extreme and open class the other. The implication then, is that stratifications—all grouping and subgrouping related to social class—would fall at some point on the continuum. Some societies tend to be caste-like in general, with definite limitations on vertical mobility; others tend to be open–class-like with a great deal of freedom for moving up or down, depending on the qualities that are important as class determinants.

It should be noted also that although the larger society may fall at some particular point on the continuum, often there are subgroups that are different. Some groups, professionals and others, for example, may tighten their requirements and make it more difficult and even impossible for a person to enter another group whereas the greater society may be quite flexible in its requirements for upward mobility. Because the principles of social class and stratification are also a part of the hospital society, some well-known and rigidly defined lines are properly observed, although there may be no formal provisions for any of them.

Definite status lines can be found between and among physicians and nurses. Also one finds distinct lines among various service and maintenance employees. In some instances formal symbols are used to indicate status lines even in rank. When formal symbols are not used, the persons concerned are usually and easily made aware of the distinctions. For example, in the case of nurses, the nurse with the graduate degree has the highest status. This is usually symbolized by her administrative or other functions. She may be a director, a supervisor, an instructor, or clinical specialist. The nurse with the baccalaureate degree is next in rank. Assignment, rate of advancement, and salary rate may distinguish her. The diploma nurse is next in line. She is a registered nurse, has the uniform, and wears the "pin" of the institution in which she received her training. Although the uniform or other outward symbols may not indicate rank, it is commonly known among her "workers," associates, and even patients that the diploma does not rank as high as the baccalaureate degree.

The licensed practical nurse generally wears a white uniform, a pin and, in the majority of agencies, a cap with a mark or symbol that identifies it as the cap of a licensed practical nurse. The nurse aide usually wears a pastel uniform. The duties of each of these members of a nursing staff are clearly defined, and it appears very important to all members that the permitted and prohibited functions be adhered to rigidly. Among doctors the distinctions are perhaps less commonly known, yet in many instances specific distinctions are made among chief resident, assistant resident, and intern. Sometimes status among physicians is symbolized by a knee-length coat for the chief resident, a waist-length coat for the assistant resident, and no coat for the intern. Status among physicans is also reflected in the classes of patients they serve. If a physician's patients are, in the main, members of a high socioeconomic level, this factor tends to reflect his high status.

Distinctions among other employees, although they do exist, are perhaps of less importance to this discussion. It is difficult to make generalizations among these personnel since there are no formal symbols to reflect differences in status. Differences in status are important only to individuals who are directly concerned. It may be correctly stated that when there are no formalities to reflect status, status tends to be imposed by persons of high status and is recognized, though perhaps resented, by persons of low status. The criteria for status may vary widely from one hospital to the next. It may be important, for example, for a person to have a record of long tenure. In another instance one particular job may be respected and recognized as being higher in rank than another job.

Albert F. Wessen gives a clear picture of occupational status in the hospital.[6] He outlines five general classes, each containing several subgroups. First in rank are the physicians, in order of rank: the visiting staff physician, the resident physician, and the intern. Second are the nurses, in order of rank: the clinical supervisor or instructor, the head nurse, the staff nurse and the student nurse. The third group he terms *paramedical professionals* and *technicians*. In this group are dietitians, laboratory technicians, x-ray technicians, social workers, occupational therapists, and physical therapists. The fourth group is composed of semiskilled (trained) workers: licensed practical nurses, medical technicians, dietitians' aides, ward receptionists, and clerks. In the fifth and final group, unskilled workers, he lists nurse aides, male aides, ward helpers, floor service maids, cleaning maids, and janitors.

The total number of subgroups of hospital workers within the five general groups is twenty-three. The chief criticism of this classification is that it represents only ward workers. Other workers, who are a vital part of the hospital operation, are not included. Among these are the administrator and his staff, hospital receptionists, switchboard operators, maintenance and "engineer" personnel, auxiliary workers, and others. Within its limitations, however, Wessen's classification appears to be an accurate presentation of occupational status.

In summarizing the class situation, it should be stated that every organization, by virtue of its being organized, has its criteria for determining rank. These criteria may vary from organization to organization; however, usually there are criteria that are recognized as being fairly universal in hospital settings. Insofar as there is social class, each person is aware of his position; others in the ranking, whether above or below, are also aware of each person's position.

The hospital is essentially an organization of interacting human beings. Although the physical structure and the specialized techniques are essential components, the core of the hospital operation, human relationships and human interaction, suggests social processes.

The Conflict Process. In this discussion several processes are considered in an attempt to give a comprehensive picture of the "goings on" in the hospital. Perhaps most significant is what is called the inherent conflict process. At least this stands out as a major process which involves practi-

[6] "Hospital Ideology and Communication Between Ward Personnel," from E. Gartly Jaco (ed.), *Patients, Physicians, and Illness: Behavioral Science and Medicine*, The Free Press of Glencoe, New York, 1958, p. 460.

cally every person connected with the hospital and virtually every department of the hospital. Many lesser processes take place within this greater process. The tendency is for one group in the hospital to pit against another group until the entire hospital operation seemingly becomes involved. There are other processes of a perhaps more minor nature but which are still particularly significant to the nurse in the hospital setting. These are the processes of association, professionalization, communication, mobility, and extra-hospital organization. The nurse is a participant in and/or related to these processes in a specific way.

If competition and conflict are basic to survival, then the hospital will undoubtedly survive. There is a situation in the hospital organization which almost inevitably engenders a major conflict. It is discussed widely among hospital personnel. It is described in the literature on hospital operations, trends, or problems. This conflict is ordinarily referred to as the conflict between hospital policy and physicians' orders. It focuses around procedures in fiscal matters and goals in the service aspects. Money and service each have symbolic meanings. Each is desirable and necessary in hospital operation, but in the practical sense it appears that the procedures necessary for attaining each are in inevitable conflict.

The conflict oftentimes is an essential opposition between the medical staff on the one hand and the hospital administration on the other. It is not an opposition between these two groups in any exclusive sense; that is, the conflict is not limited to them. Other personnel in the hospital enter the picture at some level and to some degree, but it would perhaps be clearer to confine it, in the main, to a conflict between the physicians and the administration.

Chester I. Barnard has analyzed the roles of persons in authority.[7] He has devised the concepts "scalar status" and "functional status," which are helpful in the analysis of the inherent conflict situation found in the hospital. Scalar status is always associated with a position in a hierarchial system, in which the position itself implies authority. In applying this concept to the hospital the administrator, by virtue of his position and regardless of any inherent service rendered, is an authority and must be considered as such. He is by virtue of his office a part of the policy-making process, or is oftentimes the policy-maker. His authority is felt by all; physicians, nurses, technicians, and others in the hospital setting. The term *administrator* implies that he has authority. In essence his function is to

[7] Chester I. Barnard, *The Functions of the Executive,* Harvard University Press, Cambridge, Mass., 1938.

make decisions, grant permissions, and delineate prohibitions. His job is to coordinate the entire hospital operation so that it will function efficiently and within the budget and regulations that have been established. He is then, by Barnard's concepts, scalar status.

In contrast, functional status is the position held by an individual by virtue of the kind of work he performs. His work and performance are respected and, in a sense, revered to the extent that he is regarded as high in status and thereby a person of authority. He performs in an unusual capacity and consequently demands respect. There is also the scarcity factor associated with his skills. This is the status realized by the physician.

There is a unique aspect in the power structure at this point. Here is the medical doctor, a person who in American society is accorded a great deal of respect. He enjoys high prestige and has highly specialized training. He enjoys a great deal of independence and has a general dislike for authority. He is without question a man many persons voluntarily look to with respect. In the minds of many he is even God-like. Despite these circumstances the medical doctor does not have a formal relationship with the hospital administration. He is, as it were, a guest who, insofar as hospital policy is concerned, does what he is told; he must work within hospital policy, which he does not have the authority to make. It is actually not so much a matter of his doing what he is told, since few persons may tell the doctor how to carry out his work. It is more a matter of his being on the outside or, at best, serving in an advisory capacity instead of performing in a formal capacity in the administration of the hospital.

Because of his position in the social structure and because of his functional status the physician has the authority that is enjoyed by a person who has followers. A great many persons believe that the physician *is* the healing power. They attribute to him superhuman power. Consequently this means inherent conflict within the hospital so long as hospitals have lay administrators and so long as physicians are attributed superhuman power. A possible solution to the inherent problem may, hypothetically, at least, be an M.D. administrator. As a matter of fact, this has been tried and may even be considered a trend. Although it may reduce conflict, this arrangement is not without problems. The administrator is still the administrator with administrative problems, even though he may be a medical doctor. It is still a fact that both the administrator and the medical doctor, each in his traditional role, are authoritative figures, although their roles are different and basically conflicting. One person, even though he may be a medical doctor-administrator, cannot play contradictory roles simultaneously. This may be compared with the laborer now foreman. He goes to the "other" side. In such instances the person is usually known by his function rather than by his personality or his credentials.

The conflict described need not necessarily be a major problem. It is necessary for each of the forces involved to recognize the existence of the other. Not only this, but each of these forces represents a vital part of the structure, neither of which could survive without the other. The doctor is a service to the hospital, and he has a real need for the hospital service. If relationship between the hospital and the physician for any reason should be severed, undoubtedly health treatment in any modern community would be reduced. Even though each has its particular interest and each uses a different method, the hospital and the physician are nonetheless bound together by the common goal of adequate patient care.

The Associative Process. In the previous section the process of conflict was discussed. The process of *association* is an opposite of conflict. The conflict and competition processes have their merits. It is often contended, and correctly so, that these processes provide man with the incentive to strive for higher and greater goals. Undoubtedly a great deal of social and cultural advancements results from the various processes of opposition. On the other hand, it is conceivable that the results may be much the same even though each situation is different. The results may be social and cultural advancements in the case of either process. The association process tends to provide its participants with a type of personal satisfaction not found in the oppositional processes, whereas the oppositional processes seem to demand a situation with unfilled goals, an inevitable quality of dissatisfaction. The oppositional processes of conflict and competition cannot operate if all persons involved are satisfied. The difference is mainly in method of procedure.

The hospital has numerous associative processes operating constantly. In essence these processes are relationships in which the members have common interests. Their relationships become informal as the association process operates and tend to take on a quality of permanence. As a result of the association process, the persons involved oftentimes become "friends." The relationship is one in which, instead of a mere functionary segment, the total personality becomes involved. A degree of familiarity and even intimacy may occur. The sociologist uses the term *primary group* to describe this relationship. The primary group relationship is the friendly, intimate, informal relationship. In the *secondary group* the contacts are limited to the formal, strictly business or functional, type of relationship.

As the association processes operate, the group relations tend to shift from secondary to primary-group relationships. In the hospital the associative process is found in wards, on entire floors, in the operating room, and among occupational therapy groups, office workers, nurses, and other hospital workers.

In comparing social interaction on the medical floor with that on the surgical floor, Temple Burling et al. suggest that there are "little world" formations.[8] Each floor has particular characteristics that distinguish it from another floor. The patients differ generally, even in their outlook on life. The workers, nurses, doctors, and aides approach each floor differently, and in general the give and take within each group is of a different but readily observable nature. In any case, there is the tendency for the associative process to work when persons are required to be in close contact over sustained periods of time. As stated earlier, it is possible for both the associative and the conflict processes to operate at the same time and involve the same persons, although the situations for each process are different.

Professionalization. The term *profession* is usually used to signify the activity of individuals who, because of training and acquired skill or knowledge, can perform a particular type of service. Earlier, *specialization* in modern society was related to hospital development. Specialization is closely related to the professionalization process. Harvey L. Smith points out that the hospital is a seedbed of professionalization.[9] Technicians, librarians, nurses, and aides all work toward recognition as professionals. Their problem is unlike that of the labor union that strives for increased wages. Their concern is the development of a set of skills that will enable them to serve in a specialized capacity and gain higher recognition. Furthermore these groups desire membership in an organization which will be recognized universally and will give its members a greater sense of security. Their goal is perhaps more that of prestige than increased wages.

Eli Ginsberg contends that the greatest challenge of the nursing profession today is its need to deepen its understanding through research.[10]

[8] Temple Burling, Edith Lentz, and Robert Wilson, *The Give and Take in Hospitals,* G. P. Putnam's Sons, New York, 1956, pp. 244-259.

[9] Harvery L. Smith, "Two Lines of Authority: The Hospital's Dilemma," *The Modern Hospital,* March, 1955, reprinted in E. Gartly Jaco (ed.), *Patients, Physicians, and Illness: Behavioral Science and Medicine,* The Free Press of Glencoe, New York, 1958, p. 475.

[10] Eli Ginsberg, "What Nurses Need Is A Chance To Grow," *The Modern Hospital,* vol. 98, pp. 103-106, 186, 188, April, 1962.

The implication here is that any mature profession does its own research and contributes to its own field of knowledge. When this is not possible, and to the degree that a "would-be profession" must rely largely upon sources outside its own group for its body of knowledge, to that degree it is not a mature profession. Many would-be professions are still infants in their development toward recognition. Groups that are more recently moving toward professional status include the various technicians, dietitians, and librarians. Although not as mature in professional status as medical doctors, for some time nurses have been recognized as professionals. The primary need for further development in the nursing profession is perhaps for them to sever their dependence upon the medical profession and to develop their own profession with independence and confidence.

Communication Problems in Delegating Authority. In any bureaucratic organization there seems to be an everlasting need to improve the lines of communication. Personal dissatisfactions, unfair treatment, and the like are usually attributed to misunderstandings; and misunderstandings occur among persons who do not communicate satisfactorily. Whether in the college or university organization, the industrial plant or the hospital, frequently a person or a committee is assigned to serve as liaison between the administration and the people being administered. There has perhaps been less attention given this problem in the hospital than in either industrial organizations or educational institutions. The reason is not because of a lesser need but because of the nature of the channels of communication in the hospitals.

Harvey L. Smith, in his article "Two Lines of Authority," referred to earlier in this chapter, describes the basic communication problem in hospitals in masterful fashion. The problem is basically that of orders from two sources which, oftentimes, have conflicting goals. This problem, the inherent conflict, was discussed earlier and need not be pursued further here. It amounts to a situation in which orders come from "above," and in the hospital there are two or more "aboves." It is perhaps the nurse more than any other hospital employee who is caught in this cross fire and has difficulty in defining her situation.

Whether administrator, doctor, patient, nurse, technician, or other worker, every hospital employee is inevitably involved in the communication process. Each must be in touch with someone else. There are those who give and those who receive orders. The significance of communication lies not in what is communicated but rather in the existence of open lines of communication. Anyone, regardless of his job, should have at his disposal the proper lines that will enable him to make requests, give orders, or voice complaints. Because the nurse is involved in so many different avenues of the hospital operation, open communication lines would perhaps be as pertinent to her as to other persons in the direct-service category of hospital staff members.

The Nurse and Upward Mobility. In our institutionalized and highly organized society today upward mobility is an important incentive for nearly all persons, regardless of the occupation or the status level in the structure. The prevailing feeling in society is that one must constantly advance in order to be successful. Advancement usually comes by way of changing to a position with greater responsibility or higher prestige, or perhaps by advancing on the salary or wage scale within the same position.

In the case of mobility within the hospital the situation is again different from that of mobility in the factory. One sometimes hears of the "log-cabin to White-House" type of mobility in the factory, in politics, and in other areas of endeavor. The individual starts as a floor sweeper, for example, and through a series of advancements in the prescribed period of time moves to the "top." Advancements of this type are virtually impossible in the hospital since the work here is largely in various fields of specialization. Only persons with special training and experience are qualified for the top jobs. Examples include physicians, nurses, technicians, bookkeepers, and dietitians. A person in the housekeeping department, for example, who has served long and well, may be a person of exceptionally high esteem, may have performed her task well, and may be regarded as deserving of promotion. Regardless of how deserving she may be and how much the administration would like to favor her, it is still impossible to advance her to the rank of laboratory technician or chief bookkeeper, because of the special training required for these positions. Harvey L. Smith refers to such a situation as "blocked mobility."

It is probably true that the nurse more than any other hospital worker enjoys possibilities of upward mobility. She starts as a student nurse or a nursing major, advances through the various levels of the student (first, second, and third year), and in the case of the graduate of a baccalaureate program, fourth year, and R.N. After this she may be a staff nurse, assistant head nurse, head nurse, supervisor and, finally, nursing director. The positions are clearly delineated, and generally the nurse is clearly identified either formally or informally. Although the "symbols" are not always obvious or formal, it is generally clear to the hospital personnel, and even to the public, who holds which position. The mobility pattern is less

part 4

The Process

9

Administrative Theory in Relation to Process

In Chapter 8 the third major proposition stated by Litchfield was explored in terms of the person who performs the administrative process and the setting in which the administrative process is performed. In the present chapter the administrative process, the actual doing of the job, will be considered. In his first major proposition Litchfield proposed that the administrative process is a cycle of action which includes decision-making, programming, communicating, controlling, and reappraising (Chapter 2). In summarizing the minor propositions related to the above activities, he suggested that the degree of success enjoyed by the person who utilizes the administrative process is directly dependent upon the degree to which a decision is interpreted in the form of a specific program and communicated to those of whom action is required, the establishment and enforcement of standards of performance, and the review and revision of decisions as rapidly as change occurs. Essentially he identified the action cycle as the *administrative process,* and *administration* as the performance of the administrative process by an individual in the context of an enterprise functioning in its environment.

The second person referred to earlier, Dr. Daniel Griffiths (Chapter 2), has not only formulated a theory of administration but has also researched one of the hyoptheses therein derived. In 1959 he formulated a theory of administration—administration as decision-making—which has generated considerable thinking, discussion, speculation, and research. He lists and explains the following assumptions [italics supplied]: [1]

> 1. *Administration is a generalized type of behavior to be found in all human organizations.* Administration is a term used to describe an aspect of life in a social organization. Since there is no aspect of living unrelated to a social organization, administration is an integral part of all human

[1] Daniel E. Griffiths, *Administrative Theory,* Appleton-Century-Crofts, Inc., New York, 1959, pp. 71-74, 89-94. Reprinted by permission of the publisher.

life. A logical deduction from this assumption is that the adjectival varieties of administration are more alike than different . . .

2. *Administration is the process of directing and controlling life in a social organization.* This assumption means that administration is the implementation of the purposes for which an organization is designed through such procedures as establishing criteria for the performance of individuals as they live in the organization and establishing controls to make certain that performance agrees with plans. Administration is not an artificial function superimposed on the normal activities of human beings; it is rather a process (cycle of events) engaged in by members of a social organization in order to control and direct the activities of the members within the organization. Administration occurs whenever the life processes of an organization are being controlled. In contrast to this, it can be said that administration is not the production of the organization. Barnard indicated this quite clearly when he said, "Executive work is not that of the organization, but the specialized work of *maintaining* the organization in operation." [Chester I. Barnard, *The Functions of the Executive,* Harvard University Press, Cambridge, Mass., 1938, p. 215.]

3. *The specific function of administration is to develop and regulate the decision-making process in the most efficient manner possible.* It is sometimes assumed that the function of the chief executive officer is to *make* decisions, generally by himself because others are incompetent. This is not the basic assumption of this theory; rather it is the assumption that it is the function of the executive to see to it that the decision process proceeds in an effective manner. . . .

4. *The administrator works with groups or with individuals with a group referrent, not with individuals as such.* An administrator interacts with others in the organization primarily in terms of the *group* to which others belong. The school administrator's perception of X is of a member of a teaching group, rather than Miss X as an unique individual. . . . In other words, administrators are oriented to groups, not individuals.

From these assumptions Dr. Griffiths develops the concept that "Decision-making is becoming generally recognized as the heart of the organization and the process of administration."

From the theory of administration as decision-making the following testable propositions resulted:

Major Proposition. The structure of an organization is determined by the nature of its decision-making process. . . .

Minor Proposition. An individual's rank in an organization structure is directly related to the degree of control he exerts over the decision process.

Minor Proposition. The effectiveness of a chief executive is inversely proportional to the number of decisions which he must personally make concerning the affairs of the organization.

Minor Proposition. Differences in the organizational structure of military, industrial, educational, business and public administration institutions are related to differences in decision-making processes rather than such conventional concepts as private enterprise.

Major Proposition. If the formal and informal organization approach congruency, then the total organization will approach maximum achievement.

Major Proposition. If the administrator confines his behavior to making decisions or the decision-making process rather than making terminal decisions for the organization, his behavior will be more acceptable to his subordinates.

Major Proposition. If the administrator perceives himself as the controller of the decision-making process, rather than the maker of the organization's decisions, the decisions will be more effective.

Griffiths did not include in his statement of the second assumption a description of the process (cycle of events) when he stated that administration is a cycle of events engaged in by the members of a social organization in order to control and direct the activities of the members within the organization. Since description of this cycle or decision-making process is basic to understanding the second assumption, he later presented it in detail:

1. Recognize, define, and limit the problem.
2. Analyze and evaluate the problem.
3. Establish criteria or standards by which solution will be evaluated or judged as acceptable and adequate to the need.
4. Collect data.
5. Formulate and select the preferred solution or solutions. Test them in advance.
6. Put into effect the preferred solution.
   a. Program the solution.
   b. Control the activities in the program.
   c. Evaluate the results and the process.

In analyzing the points of commonality made by Litchfield and Griffiths we may say they agree that:

1. All administration takes place within the context of an organization.
2. Administration is the performance of the administrative process (cycle of events or activities).
3. The administrative process is performed by an individual or a group.
4. The adjectival varieties of administration are more alike than differ-

ent. Or stated differently, administration and the administrative process occur in substantially the same generalized form in industrial, commercial, civil, educational, military, and hospital organizations.

The approach to administration taken by Litchfield is extremely broad; consequently he gives somewhat more attention to facets of administration other than the process, which is Griffiths' primary focus. In so doing Litchfield emphasizes the attention that must be given to the person who performs the process, the place in which he performs the process, and the larger community in which the enterprise is located.

With the above summarizations, the origin of the direction of this text becomes apparent. The assumptions, still to be tested, coincide with the beliefs of the authors and are based upon empirical observations and experience.

The most interesting fact, however, that becomes identifiable through a study of the work of these two authorities is that the administrative process described by Litchfield and the decision-making process described by Griffiths are essentially the same process. In essence, each outlined the facets of the scientific method that can be applied to all administrative operations. The authors of this book propose that *the administrative process is the scientific process.*

The theory is not in final form and is only a beginning in nursing. It is offered to nurses for consideration, experimentation, elaboration, and criticism. The assumption upon which the theory that the administrative process is a scientific process is based, and from which hypotheses may be derived, is that prescribed techniques alone are no longer sufficient for the complicated administrative tasks at hand. All of us have learned that in order to prepare an annual departmental budget, for example, an accurate inventory of supplies must be maintained. This is a technique and in no way reflects the philosophy underlying the budgetary functions.

Undoubtedly theory formulation plays a valuable role in the quest for new administrative knowledge; knowledge that has its basis in fact and scientific inquiry. Some hypotheses have been stated, others must be stated; all of them must be tested. Nursing is urged to use the findings of other investigators in this field, but there is much else to be done and nurses are expected and obligated to participate in research efforts. Only in this way can administration become something more than the application of common sense to administrative operations. Research, however, takes time. If there is any support for the claim of many persons that theory is impractical, it is in relation to the element of time. The need is now. Consequently, in the absence of complete or exhaustive administrative theory, the *administrative blueprint,* described in Chapter 11, is offered as a source of guidance to nurses who, in the meantime, must continue to perform administrative functions without the benefit of theories that have been validated. But first it must be determined what the administrative functions of nurses are, and by whom they are performed.

10

The Administrative Functions of Nurses

Many authors have identified a so-called dilemma in nursing—in fact, the word, as a result of overuse, now precipitates some of the same kinds of emotional responses that the phrase "shortage of nurses" elicits. The dilemma seems to be, primarily, the conflict nurses are experiencing due to the gap which exists between the objectives of educational programs in nursing and the expectations of the employers of graduates of these programs. It has been said that educators instill in their students that "the sacred value in the profession is the welfare of the individual patient." Consequently, students feel that their "highest function is to give compassionate, tender, personal and technically competent care to sick people." [1] We would hope that the educators are successful in this effort. But this is just one objective of an educational program. The student must also be taught how she can best perform this function and retain this value in its position of supremacy.

A review of the university bulletins of accredited baccalaureate programs in nursing will make it apparent that educators are aware of the professional role of the nurse as well as of the needs of employing agencies. Every program has in its bulletin a statement of its philosophy in relation to the preparation of the student for employment in first level positions, and the curriculum offerings give credence to the statement. Without exception the courses offered are designed to prepare the graduate of the program to achieve her "highest function," either directly or indirectly, through other persons. Courses such as Human Relations, Communications, Principles of Health Teaching, and Introduction to Administration all have as one of their objectives promotion of the student's ability to function with and through people.

Educators are no longer unrealistic in their preparation of nurses

[1] Lyle Saunders, "The Changing Role of Nurses," *American Journal of Nursing*, vol. 54, p. 1097, September, 1954.

now that they have some direction from the nursing profession. The Divisions on Practice units of the ANA anticipate having described what and how the nurse practices in the five broad areas of community health, geriatrics, maternal and child health, medicine and surgery, and psychiatric and mental health by the end of 1969. In the meantime, the profession has identified the functions for which nursing students need preparation. And the significant factor is that these 1956 statements of functions were not prepared *for* nurses. They were prepared *by* practicing nurses, and they reflect the consensus of the thinking on the nature of the nursing functions in any given position.

Inasmuch as attention is focused in this text on hospitals as the predominant setting in which the nurse performs her functions, an item analysis was made of what all nurses in hospitals describe as their functions. The results seem to indicate that the prediction of sociologists and psychologists that the role of a nurse increasingly will become that of an administrator is now recognized by the membership of the nursing profession. The statement prepared by the directors and the associate and assistant directors of nursing service enumerates the following administrative functions:[2]

A. To provide for nursing care of patients.
B. To provide personnel for nursing care of patients.
C. To provide for personnel policies which will allow for job satisfaction and growth of personnel.
D. To provide adequate physical environment for patients and personnel in the nursing service.
E. To provide a budget which will allow for adequate personnel, supplies, equipment and physical facilities.
F. To provide means and methods by which the nursing personnel can work with other groups in interpreting the goals of the hospital and nursing service to the patient and the community.

A *function*, as this group defines it, "is a broad area of responsibility composed of many activities pertaining to a position."[3] In analyzing the statements of functions of the general duty nurse, the head nurse, and the supervisor, it was found that essentially the same functions were included. The differences seemed to be in degree only: (1) the degree of responsibility one assumes for the final performance of the function, and (2) the degree to which one participates in the performance of the function.

[2] "Functions, Standards and Qualifications for Practice of Nursing Service Administration," American Nurses' Association, New York, 1956, p. 1.

[3] *Ibid.*, p. 1.

The second function, for example, to provide personnel for nursing care of patients, is perhaps the function which is least commonly considered a function of the general duty nurse. But general duty nurses have stated that the following functions are theirs:[4]

> Teaches and directs nonprofessional nursing personnel for whom she or he is assigned responsibility.
> Assumes responsibility for contributing to the educational program of any student who is having clinical experience under the nurses' guidance.

Are these functions not "providing personnel" for nursing care? They do not compare in degree to planning a master staffing pattern, for example, but they contribute to the professional development of two levels of personnel and they allow the general duty nurse to assist in the performance of the function of providing personnel for the nursing care of patients. From the analysis then we learn that the profession says that all nurses perform the same functions to a greater or lesser degree. Recalling that the interest at the moment is primarily in the administrative functions performed by nurses, however, are all these functions administrative functions?

Are the functions stated by the directors of nursing service necessarily administrative functions? If to provide for nursing care means that the director can personally give the nursing care, would the performance be administrative in nature? It would, if she does the planning, organizing, coordinating, etc., that enable her to give the care. The directors of nursing service have stated what they consider to be the administrative process and what many others have labeled "functions" or "principles" of administration. These are the administrative functional elements of the job: planning, organizing, directing, controlling, and coordinating. It is the extent to which one can apply these elements to the performance of a function that determines the administrative nature of the function. The definitions of the elements of the function, as accepted by the profession, are: [5]

> To plan is to define an objective and develop an outline of a course for action. This outline should be formulated through cooperative effort with all those involved in achieving the objective.

[4] "Functions, Standards and Qualifications for Practice of the General Duty Nurse," American Nurses' Association, New York, 1956, p. 3.
[5] *Op. cit.*, p. 1.

To organize is to translate the course for action into a method of accomplishment.

To direct is to put the method developed into effect.

To control is to evaluate the effectiveness of the methods in terms of results produced, and to revise as necessary.

To coordinate is to relate the action with other departments.

In a restudy of the statements of functions in an effort to determine the presence or absence of factors that determine the administrative nature of the functions, it was found that directors and their associates apply all the functional elements of the job to the performance of each function. In order to perform the function of providing for the nursing care of patients, for example, the director plans, organizes, directs, controls, and coordinates. Thus the function, as it is performed by the director, may be assessed as being completely administrative in nature; this, one would anticipate. But interestingly enough, it was also found that the general duty nurse applied at least one of the functional elements to the performance of each general duty function, and the head nurse and supervisor, one or more. Consequently, it may be concluded that the functions of nurses in all positions are administrative to some degree. The distinction to be made here is in the area of the scope of the activity. To plan for the care of a single patient is delimited as compared with planning for the care of all patients. But the fundamental knowledges necessary to the planning activity are identical.

An appropriate analogy seems to be in the area of research. Prepared researchers are equipped to engage in the investigation of an extremely complex problem, but they acquire the knowledges necessary to the investigation by initially investigating a problem of very limited scope. The processes, nevertheless, are the same in both situations. Knowledge of the principles of the process of research as they apply to an uncomplicated problem generally enables one to adapt their application to a complicated problem. The same obtains in the performance of administrative functions. The knowledges used by the general duty nurse are the same as those used by the director in the performance of any administrative function, and these must be learned by all.

It thus may be said that nursing has defined and widely publicized the functions of nurses and has concluded that the functions of nurses in all categories are essentially the same. The differences are factors of degree: the degree of responsibility one assumes for the total performance of the function and the degree to which one participates in the performance of the function. Furthermore, all the functions of nurses in all positions are administrative to a degree; the degree in this case being determined by the scope of the activity. Despite the scope of the activity, however, the same knowledge, skills, and abilities are needed by all nurses in the performance of their administrative functions.

In the absence of adequate administrative theory and in the belief that assistance is available to all nurses who perform administrative functions, the *administrative blueprint* is introduced.

11

The Administrative Blueprint

The *administrative blueprint* can best be described by stating initially what it is not. It is not another taxonomy. It is in no way in competition with POSDCORB or APOSDCORB, which have served satisfactorily through the years as systems of classifying the administrative functions. It is not a theory of administration; it does not describe the administrative process. Nor is it a philosophy of administration. Values, as such, are not involved.

Simply stated, the blueprint is a design for doing the job; it is an organized arrangement of interdependent parts. It is theory oriented, and if it is followed, considerable success in the performance of the job may be assured. The blueprint's effectiveness has not been verified by experimentation, but it has been verified by observations. The important concept to acquire in relation to the blueprint is its totality as a guide to action. The activities involved are not sequential; they are concomitant and interdependent, and they must be applied to the performance of each administrative function.

The blueprint provides the framework within which each function is approached. How-to-do-it techniques have no place in the blueprint, but what to do to be prepared to do the job—how to prepare oneself and others for the successful performance of administrative functions is its inherent value. It allows complete freedom of action in terms of originality, imagination, judgment, resourcefulness, initiative, curiosity, sageness, and intellectual heritage.

The guide to the action that must be taken in the performance of any function of administration is the following blueprint, which recognizes that each activity is an intellectual one and that all of them are continuous and simultaneous:

Step 1. Thinking
Step 2. Planning
Step 3. Communicating the proposal
Step 4. Gaining group acceptance of the plan
Step 5. Organizing for the execution of the plan

Step 6. Delegating for the execution of the plan
Step 7. Guiding for the execution of the plan
Step 8. Evaluating

Basic to each activity in the *administrative blueprint* is the scientific process—the process which is inherent in the administrative theory we propose. In thinking about the function of staffing, for example, the scientific method is applied to the activity of thinking, and the same is true of planning, communicating, etc. The blueprint is not intended as a substitute for the theory, but rather for the novitiate in administration; the two in combination seem to provide the necessary assistance for the performance of the administrative functions. The scientific process is applied to each activity in the blueprint, and each activity in the blueprint is applied to each administrative function.

STEP 1. THINKING

The activities of the blueprint have not been listed in the order of their importance to the performance of the functions, frequency of usage, value to the user, or any other criterion, inasmuch as the interrelatedness and recurring nature of the activities preclude their being considered in this way. All content in this text, however, has placed an exceedingly high value on the activity of thinking. This has been deliberate, inasmuch as the art and act of thinking seems to have fallen into some kind of disrepute.

In a college freshman class of forty students, for example, when the act of thinking was discussed, not one of the students revealed an example of ever willfully or voluntarily engaging in thinking about anything more consequential than what to wear, how to groom the hair, and the like. If this example is a representative picture of a national trend, the situation exists only because most individuals have not learned what an exciting experience thinking can be.

The attention given by Dr. VanderWaal to what thinking is (Chapter 4), to methods of thinking, to obstacles to thinking, and to ways of improving the quality of thinking was purposeful to the end that an ability to think reflectively is basic to the implementation of the blueprint. He has said that the scientific method is reflective thinking. Hence the emphasis upon thinking. But the thinking intended as an activity in the blueprint encompasses more than reflective thinking.

Depending upon one's definition of a problem, all thinking need not be problem-centered, unless every situation is regarded as being a problem situation. A pleasant and satisfying situation can also supply the motivation for the most stimulating and rewarding kind of thinking. To deliberately indulge in an internalized kind of brainstorming in relation to an acceptable situation and to blend it with a degree of imagination can produce remarkable ideas; ideas that must then be subjected to the reflective thinking process. Creative thinking is incontestably the most gratifying type of thinking, the most highly prized, and the most attainable. It may be done at leisure, when there is no pressure to resolve an identified problem. It may be done in a preselected environment. All that is needed is the willingness of the individual to give time and effort to the process; the productivity of the mind can be virtually guaranteed.

An acquaintance who is public relations manager with a large public service company schedules a time daily for this kind of thinking. Before his family awakens he takes a cup of coffee into the living-room, sits and smokes four cigarettes, and thinks. This activity is unencumbered by the newspaper, the radio, people, or a pressing problem; those he saves for the hours at the office, and he attests to this early morning ritual as the most productive time of his entire day.

Thinking, then, in relation to the performance of an administrative function is the essence, the core from which action originates. It must readily exemplify that each activity must be applied to every other activity of the blueprint. Certainly thinking must be a part of planning, communicating, etc., if the administrative function is to be performed successfully.

STEP 2. PLANNING

Planning as an activity of the blueprint has to do with planning for the performance of an administrative function, not with planning it. Planning, as such, is a continuation and extension of the thinking process, which includes reflective thinking as well as creative thinking. The outcome of the thinking and planning activities of the blueprint yields the plan and provides the setting in which the plan for the performance of the function can be implemented.

Inherent in the planning activity is the obligation of all nursing personnel to become thoroughly familiar with the agency in which the administrative function is to be performed. It involves a restudy of the philosophy, objectives, and organization of the institution and of each department within the institution. The details of the organization of the institution are identified in terms of authority and responsibility, physical or plant organization, and departmental organization, including identification of the functions of each department.

A good example of the latter is the personnel department in a hospital. For years nursing service considered the personnel department a service department for all departments of the hospital except nursing. True, it is important that each prospective nursing employee be interviewed by a responsible person in the nursing department, but the activities of obtaining references, transcripts, payroll processing, etc., may well be in the province of the personnel department.

The initial phase of the planning activity is designed to ensure complete knowledge of the situation as it exists, but this is just the beginning of the planning activity. The important aspect of this phase is that elements within the institution that need further study and perhaps change become identifiable. The best performance of a given function is dependent upon the identification and subsequent amelioration of impending factors. In other words, thinking and planning are preparatory activities that facilitate the performance of the administrative functions.

STEP 3. COMMUNICATING THE PROPOSAL

The point to be kept in mind in this step in the blueprint is that the *proposal,* not the plan, is being communicated. All involved personnel in the institution must be made aware of this fact and that the reason for communicating the proposal is to involve them early in the thinking process and, possibly, to elicit from them ideas in relation to the thought being proposed. As Dr. Dan Davies frequently reminded his students in administration at Columbia University, "There is no limit to the amount of good that can be done, if you don't worry about who will get the credit." There is no limit to the assistance that can come to the administrator if all persons involved and all suggestions made are taken into consideration regardless of the source. The essence of the success of this step is the element of timing; from the first thought forward, all must become a part of the activity.

STEP 4. GAINING GROUP ACCEPTANCE OF THE PLAN

If the proposal has been skillfully communicated and the suggestions of all have been considered and incorporated, when feasible, in the plan, much is already accomplished toward gaining group acceptance of the plan. There is, however, additional theory of merit that can be brought to bear in this step. In the process of gaining group acceptance, forethought must be given to the sociologic content presented earlier by Dr. Paul Miller. A knowledge of the dynamics of all groups operating within the institution and their ability to influence the degree of acceptance that a plan will receive is invaluable information. Equally important to this step in the blueprint is knowledge of human relations. It has been said that the human element in administration cannot be negated, and most certainly this is true in relation to this step of the blueprint: The characteristics of the administrator in relation to his treatment of human beings dictate the employee response he will receive.

A deep-rooted respect for all human beings, which may be evidenced most obviously by an ability to listen and to hear, is necessary to gaining group acceptance. The crucial facet of this step is that group acceptance does not just happen; it takes concerted effort to achieve. A trial run is sometimes useful.

STEPS 5 AND 6. ORGANIZING AND DELEGATING FOR THE EXECUTION OF THE PLAN

Organizing and delegating for the execution of the plan are discussed jointly inasmuch as these two activities of the blueprint occur in combination. Again, these are not the administrative functions of organizing a nursing department nor delegating the authority and responsibility for achieving the objectives of the department, although the processes may be similar. The activities are identified in the blueprint primarily because they are so frequently treated inadequately in the process of preparing for the execution of an administrative function.

A classic example of this omission occurred during the introduction of team nursing as a method of assigning nursing personnel to patient care. Few nursing departments organized this plan of care for continuation around the clock; the organization provided for the execution of the plan during the day tour of duty only. Furthermore, the responsibility and authority necessary to the performance of the functions of the team leader were not relinquished by the head nurse. This plan was built upon a basically sound philosophy of care of the ill, but it failed all too often because all the steps of the blueprint were not applied to the execution of the plan in each situation.

STEP 7. GUIDING FOR THE EXECUTION OF THE PLAN

The definition of leadership used in the Hagen and Wolff study,[1] "Those behaviors perceived by superiors, peers, and subordinates which facilitate achievement of group goals," states precisely the philosophy of the blueprint step, guiding for the execution of the plan, or facilitating the execution of the plan. The need to make all nurses acutely aware of this activity as it applies to the performance of an administrative function derives from the same study. The data indicated that the leadership in nursing evidenced by the directors of general hospitals was primarily in relation to "things," i.e., equipment, supplies, etc., not in relation to promoting nursing as a profession. The directors showed a lack of concern for long-range planning. They did not evidence leadership in promoting a sense of unity either within the nursing service department as a whole or within the hospital as a whole. Unfortunately, the same role was identified for the supervisors in these hospitals. If this is the situation as it existed in hospitals in 1959, there is cause for some doubt that the situation has changed remarkably in the interim; consequently the inclusion of this activity in the blueprint.

To facilitate is to "make easier" or to make possible. Is this not the catalyst that activates the blueprint? Its presence may of necessity be felt prior to the thinking phase. There may be individuals who need help with learning how to think or about what to think. Or perhaps it would not be felt until the plan has been formulated and is ready for implementation, and then only by way of supplying the experiential background necessary to the inauguration of the venture. Conceivably, it may never be felt at all. But the consequential fact is that it is always there—someone is always readily available—with the level of assistance needed by the group.

STEP 8. EVALUATING

Evaluating is the process of measuring, of determining the extent to which the outcome compares with the stated goal. Evaluation as it is used in the blueprint embraces intrinsically the scientific method applied to each step of the blueprint as well as to the plan which evolves. The evaluation process can be remarkably simplified if there are valid and reliable instruments of measurement available. If there are none, then the process is either im-

[1] Elizabeth Hagen and LuVerne Wolff, *Nursing Leadership Behavior in General Hospitals*, Institute of Research and Service in Nursing Education, Bureau of Publications, Teachers College, Columbia University, New York, 1961, pp. 9, 80.

possible or a matter of judgment. The latter has been the situation in nursing until very recently, and remains so in many areas that need to be evaluated. For example, the old problem of evaluating personnel performances meaningfully remains. At this point an evaluation of one person by another is nothing more than a judgment. But the quality of the judgment can be improved, if the person making the evaluation collects all the information he can get from all the sources he can find and objectively considers the facts. If sufficient facts are not available, the judgment cannot be made. It is inexcusable to base an evaluation on the findings obtained through the use of an inappropriate instrument of measurement, and it is possible that some evaluators are unable to be objective or lack the sensitivity and understanding necessary to make an evaluation. The contribution that this last step makes to the blueprint is its promotion of the use of the scientific method in evolving and in evaluating the final plan for the performance of an administrative function.

SUMMARY

In observing nurses in the practice of administration we have found that some adhere meticulously to many of the steps in the blueprint, others seemingly ignore most of them. It is our hope that the blueprint will make each nurse consciously aware of the need to engage in all the suggested activities in preparation for improved performance of her job. There is considerable evidence to support the statement that "animals, human and subhuman, must learn to think." [2] Perhaps such progress may be achieved if all nurses learn to think reflectively during each step of the blueprint and then apply the blueprint to the performance of all administrative functions. A detailed description of the application of the blueprint to one facet of one administrative function, staffing, is presented in the following chapter.

[2] Harry Harlow and Margaret Kuenne, "Learning to Think," *Scientific American,* vol. 415, p. 6, August, 1949.

12

Application of the Administrative Blueprint to the Staffing Function

The staffing function is the most exciting and most gratifying of all the administrative functions. It is the process through which personnel are made available for the giving of care to people. It is the function for which all other administrative functions are performed. It is also the function through which the hopes, aspirations, ideals, and dreams of nursing personnel come to fruition. Scarcely a single patient contact fails to attest to the significance of this function; the patient's appearance, attitudes, actions, condition, and comments all reflect the effectiveness of the staffing pattern.

Recognition of the importance of the consequences of the performance of this function is basic to the acquisition of the skills necessary to the successful management of the function. No other function demands the adherence to the *administrative blueprint* to the degree that staffing does. No step can be safely omitted, and no amount of time is too much to have spent in *thinking*—Step 1 prescribed in the blueprint—in relation to the process appropriate to the function.

THINKING

Considerable attention has been given to the thinking step in relation to the staffing function. A review of the literature will disclose the present state of the staffing function and give direction as to what changes and/or improvements are needed.

Structured efforts to solve staffing problems were underway in nursing as early as 1937. These efforts have been of value to the profession, and evidence of progress in relation to the staffing knowledge available as well as to the development of research acumen can be traced through these previous attempts to solve staffing problems.

The findings of the first six staffing studies in nursing [1–6] were based on surveys of then-existing staffing practices. From the information obtained from the surveys, staffing guides were prepared for the various types of hospitals and types of patients. Publication of what the authors considered the best current practices gave all nursing service administrators new thoughts and new ideals.

The Bredenberg [7] report, in 1951, of four staffing studies conducted by Catholic University nursing students demonstrated the feasibility of using the experimental method of research in a hospital situation. Each student had used the one-group method of experimental research; the single variable had been variations of the team plan for nursing service. In each of the four studies an attempt was made to control all essential factors, save the single variable, which was manipulated with a view to determining and measuring the effect of its operation; effect being defined as improved quantity and quality of nursing service. In each instance effectiveness was measured by means of observations made by the researcher or of opinion expressed by the subjects. The conduct and report of these studies made two major contributions to the progress of nursing research: (1) the introduction of a heretofore unused methodology in nursing service research, and (2) the identification of the need for valid and reliable instruments for measuring the effectiveness of the factor being studied.

The Kellogg Foundation study reported by Herman Finer in 1952 listed the following "administrative consequences of a numerical shortage of personnel": [8]

[1] National League of Nursing Education, Committee on Studies, *A Study of the Nursing Service in Fifty Selected Hospitals,* New York, 1937.

[2] National League of Nursing Education, Department of Studies, *A Study of Nursing Service in One Children's and Twenty-one General Hospitals,* New York, 1948.

[3] Margaret K. Schafer, *Staffing the General Hospital 25 to 100 Beds,* American Hospital Association, Chicago, Ill., 1949.

[4] Alice Bell, "A pattern for a Nursing Staff in a General Hospital," unpublished report.

[5] Rochester Regional Hospital Council, *Average Nursing Hours per Patient in Member Hospitals,* Rochester, New York, 1953.

[6] Tuberculosis Advisory Nursing Service of the National League for Nursing, Tuberculosis Nursing Advisory Service, *Cue to Staffing Tuberculosis Units in Hospitals,* National Tuberculosis Association, New York, 1952.

[7] Viola Bredenberg, *Nursing Service Research: Experimental Studies with the Nursing Service Team,* J. B. Lippincott Company, Philadelphia, 1951.

[8] Herman Finer, *Administration and the Nursing Services,* The Macmillan Company, New York, 1952, p. 48.

> 1) Quality of service is a function, that is, an inherent factor, of quantity. 2) The number of people in the job bear a direct relationship to the time and energy that each unit must spend as her arithmetical share of the work to be done, assuming the standard of service is not lowered. 3) It may even be uneconomical to have too few nurses in relation to the quantity and standard of the work to be performed, though the fewer the numbers of nurses, the smaller the salary bill. 4) Better quality personnel may be able to investigate successfully the causes of scarce quantity. 5) The shortage of personnel enforces devices for the more efficient use of prevalent numbers. 6) Very many members of the profession have lifted up their eyes from the grinding daily routines to assert firmly that the caviling about shortage of personnel is exaggerated.

These statements have precipitated considerable thought and action, as is evidenced by the following reports found in the literature.

Two consecutive studies of a large general hospital, begun in 1952 by the Urban Life Research Institute of Tulane University and completed in 1954, helped to clarify the conditions and forces that created and sustained the shortage of nurses.[9] The editors of the report, Reissman and Rohrer, credit the profession with having tried to alleviate the "felt shortage" by increasing the efficiency in the recruitment programs of schools of nursing. They proposed that one of the best solutions to the problems raised by the shortage of nurses is better utilization of nonprofessional employees. They seem to agree with the suggestion of Lyle Saunders [10] that nurses would do well to "stop being envious of and encroaching upon the doctors' functions on the one hand and reluctant to release functions to less skilled people on the other." To "substitute a new conception of the role of the nurse based upon the nurse as a teacher, administrator and specialist," was offered as a realistic approach to the future functioning of the nurse.[11]

The Harper Hospital Study reported by Marion Wright, in 1954, served nursing service administrators well by pointing up the practicality of applying method improvement techniques used in industry to the operation of a hospital nursing service.[12] The contribution of the study that has a direct bearing on the present discussion is the forcefulness with which the multi-

[9] Leonard Reissman and John Rohrer, *Change and Dilemma in the Nursing Profession,* G. P. Putnam's Sons, New York, 1957.

[10] Lyle Saunders, "The Changing Role of Nurses," *American Journal of Nursing,* vol. 54, p. 1097, September, 1954.

[11] Reissman and Rohrer, *op. cit.,* p. 16.

[12] Marion Wright, *The Improvement of Patient Care,* G. P. Putnam's Sons, New York, 1954.

faceted problem of staffing was defined. It was made quite clear that all aspects of hospital organization and functioning must be considered vital components of any staffing considerations. To staff a unit without full awareness of the extra-nursing departmental servicing provided that unit can only evidence uninformed thinking and planning.

The literature thus far has demonstrated the magnitude of the problem of staffing and the approaches that were used in previous attempts to solve the problem.

Imagination and an interest and willingness to experiment are forerunners of basic research and contribute toward marked progress in professionalization. The George and Kuehn study is a noteworthy example of these characteristics.[13] This study was an attempt to determine the desirable size and composition of the nursing service group. The determination was not based upon what was being done in hospitals evidencing good practices but upon what was envisioned as sound practice. The researchers experimented with nine combinations of professional nurse and nonprofessional worker groups caring for from six to sixteen patients each. The decision as to which of the nine combinations was the pattern of choice was based upon the opinions of the patients, professional nurses, and observers and the outcome emphasized the value of instruments for determining needs, solutions, and direction for a course of action.

The Mullane study has several implications for the staffing process in the administration of nursing service.[14] Eight criteria of excellence were identified by the researcher, and the relationship between the existence of the criteria and job satisfaction of the nursing staff in twenty-three hospitals in Michigan was explored. "A relatively high and positive relationship was found to exist between the degree to which each of the criteria was found in the hospital and the level of job satisfaction expressed by the nursing staff, the relationship being highest for the criteria relating to the staff, budget and conservation of energy and materials." [15] This finding most certainly gives assistance to the administrator in determining the relative importance of his many functions and their expected outcomes.

At about this same time the relationship between turnover and staffing

[13] Francis George and Ruth Kuehn, *Patterns of Patient Care,* The Macmillan Company, New York, 1955.

[14] Mary K. Mullane, *The Identification and Validation of Some Criteria of Excellence in Administration of Hospital Nursing Service,* Ph.D. dissertation, University of Chicago, Chicago, 1957.

[15] *Ibid.,* p. 175.

became an area of interest to several researchers. In 1957 Levine reported turnover figures from a study of the Public Health Service and the American Hospital Association in sixty non-Federal general hospitals.[16] The study measured turnover in terms of the instability factor, i.e., voluntary termination of employment within a year of employment. Analysis of this measure indicated that "professional staff nurses had the highest instability rate of all groups of hospital personnel: 50 per cent employed at the beginning of the year quit before the end of the year." [17] Certainly the implications of this finding for staffing are obvious.

In the same year Wright reported on the relationship between turnover and job satisfaction.[18] He found that ". . . although 'leavers' were significantly more dissatisfied with job conditions in general than 'stayers,' the difference was not great." [19] Does this indicate that the stayers too are dissatisfied, and that there is a fine line separating the stayers from the leavers? Additional information that was helpful to the consideration of this question was soon made available.

In 1958 the Diamond and Fox study made a rather unique contribution to nursing research and to the problem of turnover and staffing.[20] Staffing studies which had been done during the years 1943 to 1954, and which had attempted to systematically answer pertinent questions (listed below) by studying staff nurses themselves, were now studied for the purpose of integrating the findings of all five studies.[21-25] The questions about which

[16] Eugene Levine, "Turnover Among Nursing Personnel in General Hospitals," *Hospitals,* vol. 3, pp. 50–53, September 1, 1957.

[17] *Ibid.,* p. 53.

[18] Stuart Wright, "Turnover and Job Satisfaction," *Hospitals,* vol. 31, p. 47, October 1, 1957.

[19] *Ibid.,* p. 47.

[20] Lorraine K. Diamond and David J. Fox, "Turnover among Hospital Staff Nurses," *Nursing Outlook,* vol. 6, p. 388, July, 1958.

[21] Mary Barbara Ann Annster, "Ninety-nine General Duty Nurses Say," *American Journal of Nursing,* vol. 53, pp. 59–61, January, 1953.

[22] Louis Hough, "What Are the Reasons for Nursing Service Turnover?," *Hospital Management,* vol. 79, pp. 43–46, 106, January, 1955.

[23] Ruth L. Lotspeich, "Why Do General Duty Nurses Resign?," *American Journal of Nursing,* vol. 51, pp. 468–469, July, 1951.

[24] Virginia M. Null, "Facts Tell a Story," *Nursing Outlook,* vol. 3, pp. 418–423, August, 1955.

[25] U.S. Public Health Service, Division of Nursing Resources, *Planning for Better Nursing in Michigan,* Washington, D.C., 1953.

information had been sought by the studies were: (1) What is the extent of turnover among hospital staff nurses? (2) Why do they resign? and (3) Is turnover among staff nurses avoidable or unavoidable? The findings of all five studies indicated that approximately two-thirds of the resignations by staff nurses were motivated by the following personal reasons: marriage, pregnancy, husband's plans, educational plans, etc. About one-third of the resignations were motivated by job dissatisfaction related to the following factors: salary, hours, work load, general personnel policies, security, opportunity for advancement, and interstaff relationships. Thus, if we accept the premise that resignations due to personal reasons are unavoidable since we cannot control them, the findings suggest that perhaps one-third of the resignations by staff nurses may be avoided and would improve the staffing picture considerably.

The acclaim given the tool [checklist] developed by Abdellah and Levine is a natural phenomenon.[26] A need, crucial to the future progress of research in nursing, had been identified. The United States Public Health Service instrument, a checklist designed to measure patient and personnel satisfaction with nursing care, appeared in response to that need. The development of this tool was a beginning in an area where much more needs to be done.

The literature up to this point had identified staffing as a consequential problem and had suggested the experimental method of research. Finally, the Abdellah and Levine report provided the instrument of measurement necessary to the method of research and to the next effort made to solve staffing problems. In 1958 the Shanks study experimentally determined the effects of staffing patterns on patient and personnel satisfaction with nursing care.[27]

This study served to reaffirm the suitability of the experimental design to research in nursing, and to support the previously nonresearch-supported judgments of directors of nursing service departments. The data supported the hypothesis that as the proportion of graduate-nursing hours is increased the level of patient satisfaction with nursing care increases. The second experimental hypothesis of the study, related to personnel

[26] Faye G. Abdellah and Eugene Levine, U.S. Public Health Service, Division of Nursing Resources, *Patients and Personnel Speak*, Public Health Service Publication no. 527, Washington, D.C., U.S. Government Printing Office, 1957.

[27] Mary D. Shanks, *The Effects of Experimental Staffing Patterns on Patient and Personnel Satisfaction with Nursing Care*, doctoral project, Teachers College, Columbia University, New York, 1958.

satisfaction with nursing care, was not statistically supported by the checklist scores (the Abdellah and Levine instrument). Analysis of the checklist items and the recorded patient and personnel comments revealed that the level of doctor and nurse satisfaction with nursing care increased as the proportion of graduate-nursing hours increased. The level of practical nurse satisfaction with nursing care increased as the proportion of practical-nursing hours increased.

During this period a staffing study was being conducted by the Public Health Service.[28] Based on a sample of 57 general hospitals with a daily average of between 100 and 500 patients and considered homogeneous with respect to standards of patient care, this study was designed to define how omissions in nursing services as perceived by patients and personnel are influenced by the number of nursing hours available. This study was interested primarily in nursing hours for the purpose of projecting a staffing pattern, whereas the previously mentioned study concentrated on the proportion of professional and nonprofessional personnel.

The Budzyna study contained an interesting statement, one which reflects the continuing existence of findings first reported by researchers ten years ago. [29] "This study shows that many of the folk in this nursing folk regional society are reluctant to change their traditional concepts of nursing care." This study also concluded:

> From the norms suggested by the folk in the nursing folk regional society it follows that the basis of a staff-constructed master staffing pattern is possible:
>
> *a.* Nursing care: Comprehensive
> *b.* Standard of practice: Optimum
> *c.* Method of personnel assignment: Team
> *d.* Method of patient assignment: Progressive care.

The second finding is somewhat more encouraging than the first. Some progress is being made in this difficult area of willingness or ability of nurses to accept changes.

In May of 1961 members of the operations research division of the Johns Hopkins Hospital developed a direct care index based upon the time

[28] Faye G. Abdellah and Eugene Levine, *Effect of Nurse Staffing on Satisfactions with Nursing Care,* American Hospital Association, Hospital Monograph Series, no. 4, Chicago, 1958, p. 35.

[29] Anna Helen Budzyna, "Cultural Lag in the Concepts of Nursing," *Nursing Research,* vol. 10, pp. 132–140, Summer, 1961.

needed to give care to the patients in the following three categories: (1) self-care (2) total care, and (3) partial care.[30] In its present form the Direct Care Index is a gross indicator of shifting needs for nursing time, based on current practice as an acceptable standard of care. "The most significant reaction that can be taken to changes in the index is movement of nursing personnel or patients so as to match nursing resources to the changing need for them." [31]

Much of the research that has been done in nursing is beginning to dovetail. For example, the work being done with Progressive Patient Care is based upon the principle that the patient who requires care and the person who is able to give that care must be brought together.[32]

One of the more recent staffing studies is the Levine investigation of staffing in one Federal and two non-Federal hospitals.[33] The main difference between the hospitals is that non-Federal hospitals employ more than twice as many nursing personnel per 100 patients than Federal hospitals employ. Five factors were delineated as the quantifiable factors that affect staffing: the patients receiving the services, the personnel providing services, the adequacy of services being provided, the organization in which the services are provided, and the efficiency of the organizations. A description of the methods and tools used in measuring the effect of each factor is included in the report.

It is interesting to note that the Abdellah and Levine checklist has been used in four of the studies discussed in this survey of staffing research, including the present study. This fact seems to indicate the scope of the dearth of instruments available to the researcher in nursing. The statement of the findings is noteworthy: "Thirty per cent of the difference [in staffing needs] was estimated to be attributable to practices and policies which, according to the definitions of this study, did seem to be indicative of greater administrative efficiency in the Federal hospital. This is a sizable proportion since it represents nearly 20 nursing personnel per 100 patients." [34] Also administrative efficiency was described as being ". . . those

[30] Robert J. Connor, et al., "Effective Use of Nursing Resources: A Research Report," *Hospitals,* vol. 35, pp. 30–39, May 1, 1961.

[31] *Ibid.,* p. 38.

[32] Jack C. Haldeman, M.D., *Elements of Progressive Patient Care,* U.S. Department of Health, Education, and Welfare, Public Health Service, Washington, D.C., 1959.

[33] Eugene Levine, "Nurse Staffing in Hospitals," *American Journal of Nursing,* vol. 61, pp. 65–68, September, 1961.

[34] *Ibid.,* p. 68.

practices, policies, or procedures that enable a hospital to provide as adequate nursing services as another with fewer nursing personnel per patient and which can feasibly be adopted by the other hospital." With this dramatic example of nurse power conservation, it seems appropriate to pause and reflect.

In reviewing what has been said and done, a justifiable conclusion is that progress has been made through research. As recently as 1950 staffing patterns were evaluated in terms of consensus. If the hospitals included in a survey agreed upon a pattern, the pattern was accepted as right. This method no longer suffices. The answers to questions are now being sought through thoughtful, well-designed investigations. It is the obligation of the administrator to think about these studies, analyze them, and make the appropriate applications of the findings to the staffing function. "The process of analysis reduces answers to a level of understanding. It is the only procedure that forces upon one the need to question every thought and act."[35] If the intellectual process has been neglected in nursing, this step in the *administrative blueprint,* the objective consideration of available evidence, will reinstate it.

The initial statement of the status of the staffing function among all functions of the administrator has been verified in terms of the job satisfaction of nursing personnel. Three of the reports found that there is a positive relationship between staffing and personnel satisfaction with nursing care.

Considerable hope and encouragement have been offered administrators who have experienced an excessive number of resignations or who find that perhaps their administrative efficiency can be improved and result in a reduction of staffing needs by as much as 30 per cent.

The national picture indicates that nursing has increased its numbers in order to meet the increasing demands of society, even though it frequently is difficult to know where the additional numbers are. However, identification of the factors that make it seem that there are fewer rather than more practicing professional nurses helps to emphasize the immediate need to define roles for all nursing personnel in all health agencies.

Perhaps the most significant fact that has been revealed by the literature is that there is no single answer to the problem of staffing, no standardized ratio of hours of professional nursing care per category of patient per

[35] Robert Eddy, *An Evaluation of the Role of Scientific Method in Doctoral Programs in Education Administration,* doctoral dissertation, Rutgers University, New Brunswick, N.J., 1959.

twenty-four-hour period. This determination of staffing needs must be made by the nursing personnel in the given situation. And the inevitable question, Is there a shortage of nurses, can be answered only in relation to the degree of skill the administrator possesses in performing the staffing function. As has been said, the most critical shortage today is not manpower, but "intelligent management." [36]

PLANNING

The *planning process,* the second phase of the blueprint, is a continuation and extension of the thinking process. Planning is the conscious thinking which precedes the actual performance of a piece of work. Admittedly, in the busy day of the administrator of a nursing service department, it requires considerable self-discipline to allow oneself the opportunity to indulge in the pleasurable act of planning. However, having accepted that staffing must be evolved from a given situation by the nursing service personnel involved, perhaps some of the guilt that accompanies the taking of time to indulge in the process of planning will be removed.

The significance of the need to plan for adequate staffing has been rather forcefully demonstrated by the following example of the influence of adequate personnel on the death rate of two hospitals. Both hospitals were well-equipped, with the same medical staff treating the same class of patients. In one, the ratio was one nurse to six patients, and the postoperative death rate was 5.5 per cent; in the other, the ratio was one nurse to one and one-half patients, and the postoperative death rate was 1.8 per cent. The only appreciable difference in the two hospitals was the ratio of nurses to patients.[37]

This is rather a nice tribute to nurses, but exception must be taken with the conclusion. The ratio of nurses to patients may not have been the important consideration in this situation. At least some consideration must be given to the possibility that not all nurses perform at the same level. Many factors affect staffing, and certainly one factor is that the quality of nursing care and the quantity of nursing care are directly influenced by the knowledge, judgment, skills, and values of those participating in the care.

The fact then emerges that staffing is not merely a consideration of

[36] Richard T. Viguers, "What It Takes to Be a Good Supervisor," *The Modern Hospital,* vol. 91, pp. 63–66, July 1958.

[37] Malcolm T. MacEachern, *Hospital Organization and Management,* rev. 3d ed., Physicians Record Company, Chicago, 1957, p. 526.

numbers of people but a way of life, a reflection of the philosophy and objectives of the agency, of the department of nursing functioning within the framework of the agency, and of all the nursing personnel employed by that agency. This will be true of staffing only to the extent that the nursing service administrator allows for broad personnel representation from hospital administration and nursing service for participation in the planning stage. If it is the philosophy of the agency that any person who presents himself for admission be admitted and be given care, then the preparation of the staff must be such as to accommodate a diversity of patient conditions and needs. Other staffing decisions will be contingent upon the statements of belief regarding the kind of care to be given (custodial, technical, rehabilitative, or all three), the administration of patient-centered care, the use of the team method of assignment, the placement of patients in terms of the acuity of the illness (the concept of progressive patient care), and the participation of the hospital nurse in interpreting home nursing to patients and initiating referrals (continuity of nursing services). In fact, the formulation of the philosophy and objectives of nursing and nursing service in a carefully detailed way is fundamental to any consideration of staffing patterns. An excellent example of such a statement was prepared by the Harper Hospital and can serve as a guide for other nursing service departments.[38] There is no better source of direction for planning in relation to staffing than an item analysis of the philosophy and objectives of the agency and the department of nursing service. For example, if it is a belief that there is a need for teaching patients and that the nurse is the one to assume this responsibility, then time must be provided for her to do this teaching. If the nurse is to participate in research, time must be provided for this participation. It is in this way that the philosophy and objectives give constant, consistent, operational assistance to the administrator in the performance of the staffing function. Complete acceptance of these philosophical considerations by all nursing personnel will dictate the effectiveness of the ultimate staffing pattern.

A second factor which influences staffing to a marked degree and which must be considered during the planning for the execution of the function is the organization of the agency and the nursing service department. Actually, this factor is influential in direct proportion to the extent to which

[38] Department of Hospital Nursing, National League for Nursing, "Here Is One Hospital's Philosophy of Nursing," *Department Hospital Nursing Doings, Highlights, News,* vol. 4, p. 2, October and December, 1959.

the nursing service administrator is prepared to function in her position. It reflects the ability to establish good working relationships with the administration, the department heads, the medical staff, and nursing service personnel and may result in the establishment of an autonomous nursing department with the accompanying administrative status that allows effective organization.

As a function of organization, a clear statement of the philosophy and objectives has been mentioned. Other functions include the availability of a departmental organizational chart which illustrates the lines of authority and channels of communication for inter- and intradepartmental functioning, agency and departmental policy manuals, job descriptions and specifications, nursing practice manuals, in-service education, periodic evaluations of facilities, appraisals of nursing care, and the opportunity to participate in committee activities and professional meetings. Only through these functions of organization can all nursing personnel know precisely what is expected of them and the administrator know how the personnel can achieve these expectations. For example, if the structure of the organization does not allow for supervisors, then certainly this has implications for staffing in relation to the functions and qualifications of head nurses and assistants or associates in nursing service administration. Or, if the job description of the team leader does not provide the authority necessary to the guidance function of the position, the functions of the head nurse and all team members will be affected. Probably the most classic example of organization as a factor influencing staffing is in the area of interdepartmental functioning, the extent to which each patient area is serviced by all other departments of the hospital not only in terms of delivery to the unit, but an automatic re-supply on the basis of established quotas. The foregoing seems to be related to administrative efficiency, and establishes the positive relationship between this factor and staffing through research findings.

Another organizational factor affecting staffing is the architectural design of the hospital or the physical organization of the plant. Much experimentation is being done in this area, the objective always being increased efficiency and convenience for nursing service personnel. Such items as placement of patient areas in view of the nurses station, increased numbers and more centrally located bathing and toilet facilities, supply storage spaces, and service areas are being considered. Laborsaving devices such as wall oxygen and suction apparatus, pneumatic tubes, two-way intercommunication systems, dumb-waiters, and data processing systems to guide staffing patterns are being built into the new hospitals.

The final organizational factor to be considered in the planning for effective staffing is, of course, the broad area of personnel administration. The personnel department of the agency must provide leadership for the personnel program, but every nurse in the organization is, to some extent, a representative of the personnel department. As such, much can be done by the individual to improve personnel policies and practices, job satisfaction, qualifications for employment, motivation, quality of performance, and productivity. These facets of personnel administration bear directly upon staffing needs and vary widely from agency to agency.

In summary it may be said that the greatest amount of work involved in the staffing function is in the preparatory phase. One must be thoroughly familiar with the agency that is to be staffed. Much guidance in this process will come from reviewing records and reports: records of meetings of the board of trustees, administrative committee minutes, departmental minutes, admissions records, medical and nursing audits, ward census reports, patient condition reports, personnel records, etc. In the last analysis, however, the only way to have all the needed information is to study in a structured way each unit that is to be staffed in terms of the factors that affect staffing and the effect they have on the unit as it is presently staffed. This then is to say that to staff a unit effectively, efficiently, and economically is to apply the scientific method of inquiry to the blueprint activity of planning in order to forecast the staffing needs of a unit. As the necessary information is gathered the pattern for a given unit begins to evolve. The pattern is an outgrowth of the analysis of the collected data together with the information that is brought to the process from previous staffing research.

Before proceeding further, it must be emphasized that staffing is a large, joint effort. Perhaps the first thought in relation to staffing originated with the director of nursing, but not necessarily. Certainly, however, all nursing service personnel are involved in the function, to a greater or lesser degree. The thinking of all is needed—the reading, studying, and participation in the collection and analysis of the data gathered for any given unit.

At this point, with a pattern evolving, there is still one more facet of the planning step of the blueprint. What is evolving are the staffing needs as the unit exists, but should not some thought be given to possible changes in the situation? Are there better ways of performing functions? Is a redefinition and reallocation of activities and functions indicated? Is a reclassification and relocation of patients a possibility? Perhaps the purchase of timesaving equipment such as physiologic monitors warrants consideration. At any rate, the important point here is that now is the time to really stir up some thinking, especially the employees' imaginations, by giving every one an opportunity to paint with a big brush; by not allowing any present practice to go unquestioned; by expecting few answers but many ideas. The natural and desirable outcome of this process is experimentation. A willingness to experiment is vital to progress.

With the completion of the experimentation and the adoption of the changes consistent with the findings, a given unit is ready for the application of the question: What are the staffing needs in terms of the factors that affect staffing and the effect they are having on the unit as it is presently staffed? The pattern that emerges in response to this process is to be the pattern of choice for the unit. The same methods, in all of their time-consuming completeness, must then be applied to each unit for which one has the staffing responsibility. The aggregate of the patterns for the units then provides the information for the composition of the master staffing pattern: the plan that portrays, in terms of numbers and categories of personnel, the philosophy of nursing care of the agency or institution. From planning a plan is formulated, or, the function of staffing a unit is under way.

COMMUNICATING THE PROPOSAL

Communicating the proposal is a step in the *administrative blueprint,* and as such it does not fall into a sequential arrangement. This step originates with the first thought about staffing and will be ever present throughout the performance of the staffing function. Before the use of the word "communicate" became popular, it was commonly used to mean "relaying of information," and this was fairly consistent with the process and with autocracy. In relation to staffing, the person involved was told what his assignment was to be. In recent years, however, the director of nursing service rarely has had the opportunity to "tell" anyone anything, but has had to spend an endless amount of time in communicating, not only to relay information but to discuss or exchange ideas and information.

Nothing beyond the thinking phase is done without the beginnings of communications. Communicating the proposal has to do not with the final plan, the master staffing pattern, but with the nucleus of the idea. The many techniques appropriate to this process are individual and group discussion sessions; brainstorming sessions early in the thinking and planning phase; in-service education programs geared to the problem of staffing, establishment of special interest groups such as groups interested in library research, action research, or planning in relation to the application of the findings of the first two groups to a given situation. Informed leadership is necessary to the successful utilization of any one of these techniques. Ultimately, of course, the final pattern which evolves from this process will also be discussed just as widely. That time becomes a factor to be considered becomes obvious, but it has been found through experience that if the amount of time given to this phase is generous, it is more than compensated during the ensuing phases of the performance of the staffing function, and most especially during the next step of the administrative blueprint, *gaining group acceptance of the plan.*

GAINING GROUP ACCEPTANCE OF THE PLAN

Two factors seem to be directly related to group acceptance: accurate and complete information, and a thorough grasp or understanding of the plan. The causes of both of these factors are furthered in direct proportion to the degree that individuals have been personally involved in the project. Simply offering an individual the opportunity to participate allows him to recognize that he is considered worthy and competent enough to contribute to plans that are vital to the agency. Furthermore, after having participated in planning it is extremely difficult to be negatively critical of the product of one's own efforts.

A pilot study is a technique that has been used quite successfully in promoting group acceptance of a staffing plan. The staffing plan is implemented on one unit only, and if the plan is as satisfactory as the planners had expected it would be, the enthusiasm with which it is received will be contagious. Another advantage of this technique, of course, is that it allows for evaluation and the making of any necessary adjustments while the implementation of the plan is still on a small scale.

ORGANIZING AND DELEGATING FOR THE EXECUTION OF THE PLAN

Step 5 in the administrative blueprint, *organizing for the execution of the plan,* has a built-in sixth step, *delegating*. Within a democratic administrative framework, the one step does not exist without the other, as each pertains to the execution of the plan for the performance of an administrative function; in this case the execution of a master staffing pattern.

A point of consequence in relation to these two steps is their dependence upon all previous steps of the blueprint. A thorough treatment of all previous steps is necessary to the management of these two. Upon reaching Step 5, in following the blueprint, one will find that the groundwork for the completion of Steps 5 and 6 has been established along with many of the activities inherent in organizing and delegating.

The *organization* is the structure through which the staffing pattern will be implemented, and the *delegation* is the identification of the people through whom the pattern will be implemented. The structure, being one of the factors influencing staffing, will have been evaluated during the planning step. Its present form will allow for immediate execution of the plan. Had the structure and the proposed staffing pattern been incompatible, the differences would have been recognized and resolved during the planning stage. For example, if the structure had not provided for the position of In-service Education Director nor ascribed the functions of that position to any other position, but the proposed staffing pattern included an increased number of nonprofessional personnel who would need extensive on-the-job training, the incompatibility would have become apparent at the time the proposed staffing pattern was evolving from the process of analyzing all factors that affect staffing.

The organization also provides for delegation of the authority and the responsibility necessary to the performance of all activities of the agency. The need for this provision has long been recognized, but the ability of the individuals involved to comply with the provisions varies greatly. The ability and willingness to delegate seems to be a function of the personality of the individual. One who can intellectualize the most freely on the merits of delegation may be the greatest offender. And the most unfortunate aspect of this facet of the staffing function is that of the number of persons who must be willing to carry out the process to its completion. It is a little like the game of hand ball—the authority and responsibility for implementing the staffing plan passes through many hands. The extent to which the total effort is successful depends upon the completeness with which each individual is able to relinquish to others the proper share of authority and responsibility. It has been demonstrated that the process can be interrupted at any point; in fact, it has been known to never have been started.

The scope of this particular problem is such that all nursing personnel must be constantly aware of it. The somewhat discouraging element of this particular problem is that it seems to be uncontrollable. The best approach at this point has been early recognition of the individual who is unable to delegate. The procedure following recognition is adapted to the individual: counseling, psychological testing, encouraging additional education, and, unhappily, removal of the individual, if no improvement is evidenced. Organization and delegation are vital to the effective performance of the staffing function, particularly in relation to personnel satisfaction, and, ultimately, to patient satisfaction with nursing care.

GUIDING FOR THE EXECUTION OF THE PLAN

In the performance of the foregoing steps of the blueprint—the thinking about staffing, the formulating of a staffing plan, the communication of the plan, the gaining of group acceptance of the plan, and the organizing and delegating for the execution of the plan—the entire process has assumed the presence of *guiding for the execution of the plan,* Step 7 in the blueprint. Any activity which relies on intelligent group planning instead of on external authority for determining courses of action implies the availability of guidance or leadership.

Leadership may come from many sources, and it is the responsibility of the status leader, be it the head nurse, supervisor, etc., to stimulate and recognize the development of leadership qualities in all nursing personnel; guidance and leadership being used interchangeably. It has been the experience of many persons that throughout the developmental stages of any project there is considerable guidance available, but when the plan has been in operation for a period of time, the enthusiasm for the plan subsides, and with it goes much of the guidance that has been so readily available.

A study by the National Research Council revealed that the most important single determinant of morale and performance is leadership.[39] This finding establishes the relationship between staffing and leadership, and supports the thesis that guidance must be constant, consistent, and continuous to the extent that it is a readily felt force within the organization, emanating from several directions and all levels.

Every nurse has an obligation to work toward the maximum development of her own leadership qualities. Every nurse has the opportunity to set the pace for some member of the health team. Technical competence is no substitute for the ability to accomplish through people.

EVALUATING

Evaluating, the eighth and final step of the blueprint, is a stimulating process, and a necessary one. An evaluation is made for three reasons: (1)

[39] Lynn R. Timmons, "Qualities of a Leader," *Hospital Management,* vol. 91, p. 81, February, 1961.

to learn where you have been, (2) to learn where you are, and (3) to learn where you are going. The two essential steps in evaluation are:

1. The measurement of quality.

2. The establishment of the relationship between quality and purpose. Herein lies the problem in evaluating the effectiveness of a given staffing pattern. Quality nursing care has yet to be defined, and until it is, there is no way of measuring the effectiveness of a staffing pattern in terms of quality.

The statement which most accurately describes this basic need in nursing is the following quote from Lord Kelvin ". . . when you can measure what you are speaking about, and express it in numbers, you know something about it; but when you cannot measure it, when you cannot express it in numbers, your knowledge is of a meager and unsatisfactory kind. . . ."

The adequacy of a given staffing pattern can and must be continuously appraised in terms of the purposes and objectives of the nursing department and the institution; the satisfaction of the patients, nurses, and physicians with the care the patients are receiving; and the morale of the personnel.

Some of the tools available for use in systematically evaluating the effectiveness of the staffing pattern are the nursing audit, the budget (which reflects and controls the plan) for staffing, self-evaluation processes, and integrated group evaluation of the staffing situation. In using these tools, however, uppermost in mind must always be these questions: For what purpose is measurement or evaluation being done? Do the units of measurement fit the ultimate objective? Do the facts allow for the making of judgments?

The evaluation process, or reflective thinking, is applied to the first thought in relation to evolving a master staffing pattern, continued with the proposal, and, finally, with the plan. This kind of approach to staffing makes the evaluation process take on a complete circuit effect, the purpose of evaluation—a continuous appraisal.

This delineation of the way the blueprint may be applied to a single administrative function is sufficiently detailed to serve as a model for the application of the blueprint to any administrative function. Attention is now directed to concrete cases that identify the other administrative functions of the nurse and offer an opportunity for controlled experience in applying the blueprint to the performance of these functions.

part 5

Cases in Administration in Nursing

13

An Introduction to Case Analysis

A profound respect for theory compelled the authors to devote the preceding portion of this text to academic and conceptual considerations of the philosophy, the person, the place, and the process involved in nursing service administration. However, they also agree with Robert Dubin, who says, "You can learn this [administrative] theory and yet feel a sense of emptiness about it because it is at a level of abstraction removed from the *acts* of administration about which it is generalizing." [1] Knowledge concerning the practice of administration in nursing, therefore, is presented through the description and discussion of actual incidents in nursing service. The cases have been drawn from actual experiences in administrative positions in various hospitals in several sections of the United States. The names of the personnel, the patients, and the places have been changed. A hypothetical hospital is the setting for two reasons: to prevent the identification of any particular institution and to encourage an appreciation of the complexity of a single setting rather than isolated aspects of several settings.

The particular situations were selected because they represent some of the everyday concerns of nurse administrators, concerns to which the *administrative blueprint* can be applied. They place the nurse in contact with the realities of facilitating nursing care for people, and give the neophyte in administration, the student, an opportunity to learn first "from the arm-chair," from reflection on the actions and the problems of others. This arm-chair administration can serve as preparation for the actual practice of administration. The cases offer the practicing administrator a respite from the pressing problems of her own situation, an opportunity to gain insight through the experiences of others, and an opportunity to use the

[1] Robert Dubin, *Human Relations in Administration: The Sociology of Organization*, Prentice-Hall, Inc., Englewood Cliffs, N.J., 1951, p. 384.

administrative blueprint in vitro prior to using the proposed design for action.

A case record of an actual happening, at first reading, may seem relatively simple, but after close scrutiny it will be found to contain all the rational and irrational aspects and complex interrelationships one finds in his own work situations. Obviously, no case record can contain all the minute details of the events described. But when one pauses to consider his own perceptions of daily activities and events, he realizes only too well the minute details that eluded his notice. It is within these limitations that one must function in reality; it is in spite of these limitations that one can learn from the analysis of a case.

The primary purpose in using the case method of presenting the practice of nursing service administration is not simply to convey facts and principles, but to encourage and stimulate the nurse administrator to think in the presence of new situations and to demonstrate the application of the proposed blueprint for administrative action. This method has proved to be extremely effective as a medium for teaching law, medicine, business, and social casework. It has also been used in education for nursing through studies of patients in clinical nursing courses and through case studies in courses in nursing service administration.

One element of the usual case method of presentation will be missing from the discussions of the case situations—the element of "class" discussion. The printed discussions may seem one-sided. There will not be an opportunity to disagree in person with the authors' perceptions of the situation or the suggestions for action or for solutions. It is hoped that each reader will first read the case, analyze it, seek the information necessary for the formulation of possible actions, discuss the case with peers and colleagues, and then read the case discussion.

The authors recommend that as each case is read the reader make notes in the column headed "Case Notes," adjacent to the text. In the first case, the authors have indicated in this column the aspects which seem to them to be pertinent. The reader may wish to exclude some and to emphasize others and is encouraged to do so, keeping in mind the setting and the person or persons involved in the situation.

After the above has been done and the case presentation reread, the situation should be examined in light of the philosophy of administration, the person, the purpose, the place, and the application of the blueprint. The following questions may be raised:

What is going on here?

What are the separate and distinct elements of the situation as reported?

What facts are explicit in the situation?

What information, what attitudes are implicit?

What is the responsibility of the nurse administrator in relation to his patient, to himself, to the nursing service, and to his employer, the hospital?

What elements of the administrative process are involved?

Then, and only then, is one adequately prepared to suggest actions that should be, or should have been, taken in the situation described.

As each reader asks these questions, she should first limit her attention to the case data, to an appraisal of the situation described. In attempting to do so, several reactions may develop. First, she may be inclined to regard the case as lacking in relevance to her own position; she may be a head nurse, not a staff nurse. Another reader may say that the cases concern a teaching hospital, not a community hospital similar to the one in which she works. Another may claim that there is no relationship between the incident described and her own functions in a public health agency. For these readers the authors would point to the concepts of the universal application of the administrative priniciples and of the blueprint for the approach to the process and to the concept that all professional nurses have administrative functions, the difference being only the degree of involvement.

When presented with a situation that occurred in another locale, with other persons involved, many individuals have a tendency to proclaim such a situation as unlikely in the nursing settings with which they are familiar. Perhaps, at the initial reading, this would seem to be true; yet the analysis of such incidents will inevitably provide insight into seemingly unrelated areas and will indicate attitudes and reactions that may be operating in circumstances familiar to the reader.

It is conceivable, and indeed highly probable, that no two individuals would present the same analysis of a case or propose relatively identical solutions. If this is true, some may immediately say that it is futile to study the situation, to propose the use of the blueprint, or to plan to apply the process. Such a reaction would fail to consider the causative factors in variability. Each person brings to the reading of the case and to any real-life situation an individual way of construing facts and perceiving ideas, because of past experiences and current preoccupations. This is inevitable. This is desirable. This is what creates the challenge for the administrator. This is what prohibits the establishment of ready-made solutions to administrative situations. And yet it should not forestall the proposal of appropriate alternative courses of action and the eventual selection of a course of action most fitting in the situation, the course of action indicated by the relevant administrative principles. In "real life," decisions must be made, action must be taken.

The process of case analysis is not immediately satisfying; initially, it may be extremely frustrating. It requires effort, perseverance, reflective thinking, creative thinking, and the pursuit of additional facts. It can be particularly distressing to the person accustomed to passive reception instead of active participation in the process of learning. It has been the experience of the authors in using this method with students that as each student is guided through the first case (and occasionally the second case) she begins to feel a sense of achievement in analyzing the case, in proposing solutions, in discovering that some of her conclusions agree with, and others differ from, those drawn by peers, perhaps because of the elements of independence and creativity inherent in case analysis. Many readers undoubtedly have had this experience in discussing clinical nursing problems with new practitioners or with students.

With these admonitions and recommendations in mind, the reader is asked to consider the place, a 750-bed hospital, as the setting of the reported incidents in nursing service administration. The authors believe that the result of these reflections on practice will lead individuals to formulate generalizations about the administrative process, to appreciate the proposed theories of administration, to broaden their perceptions of the behavior of persons in administrative situations and, above all, to develop new ways of thinking, with the ultimate goal of improving the quality of nursing care.

SUPPLEMENTARY READING LIST

Andrews, Kenneth A. (ed.): *The Case Method of Teaching Human Relations and Administration: An Interim Statement,* Harvard University Press, Cambridge, Mass., 1960, pp. 175–192.

Dubin, Robert: *Human Relations in Administration: The Sociology of Organization,* Prentice-Hall, Inc., Englewood Cliffs, N.J., 1951.

Kepner, Charles H., and Benjamin B. Tregoe: "Developing Decision Makers," *Harvard Business Review,* vol. 38, pp. 115–124, September-October, 1960.

Pesznecker, Betty, et al.: "Testing Students' Ability to Grasp Principles," *Nursing Outlook*, vol. 13, pp. 57–59, January, 1965.

Pigors, Paul, and Faith Pigors: "The Incident Process–A Method of Inquiry," *Nursing Outlook*, vol. 14, pp. 48–50, October, 1966.

Tribou, Marita: "The Incident Process in Teaching," *Nursing Outlook*, vol. 13, pp. 36–39, January, 1965.

14

The Charles Evans Memorial Hospital

The setting for each of the case incidents in nursing service administration is the Charles Evans Memorial Hospital. This hospital is a 750-bed voluntary, nonprofit, general hospital in a city with a population of 500,000. Every year 19,750 patients enter the hospital. The clinics conducted by the hospital serve many medically indigent persons. The total operating costs average $18,685,000 annually. A total of 1,860 full-time personnel serve an average daily census of 722 patients. The hospital is situated on well-landscaped grounds in a suburban area and is readily accessible by public and private transportation.

The hospital was established in 1908 with a threefold purpose: to care for the sick while engaging in teaching and conducting research. The hospital conducts a diploma program in nursing. Its facilities are used by the medical, dental, and nursing schools of a large university and by the practical nurse program of the local vocational high school.

The ultimate direction of the activities of the hospital rests with its Board of Trustees and the board's Executive Committee. Three members of this twelve-member self-perpetuating board are relatives of the original benefactor, Charles Evans. The one top-level administrative position is held by John Alexander, whose title is Director of the Hospital. There are five assistant directors. Three of these administrators direct the activities in the areas of professional services, business management, and special services, respectively. The other two assistant directors are responsible for directing the activities of all departments during the evening and night tours of duty.

The Nursing Service Department, the largest department in the hospital in numbers of personnel, has 975 full-time employees. The Director of Nursing Service and Nursing Education, Ann Elliott, is directly responsible to the Assistant Director of Professional Services. She is assisted by an associate director in charge of nursing education and by four assistant

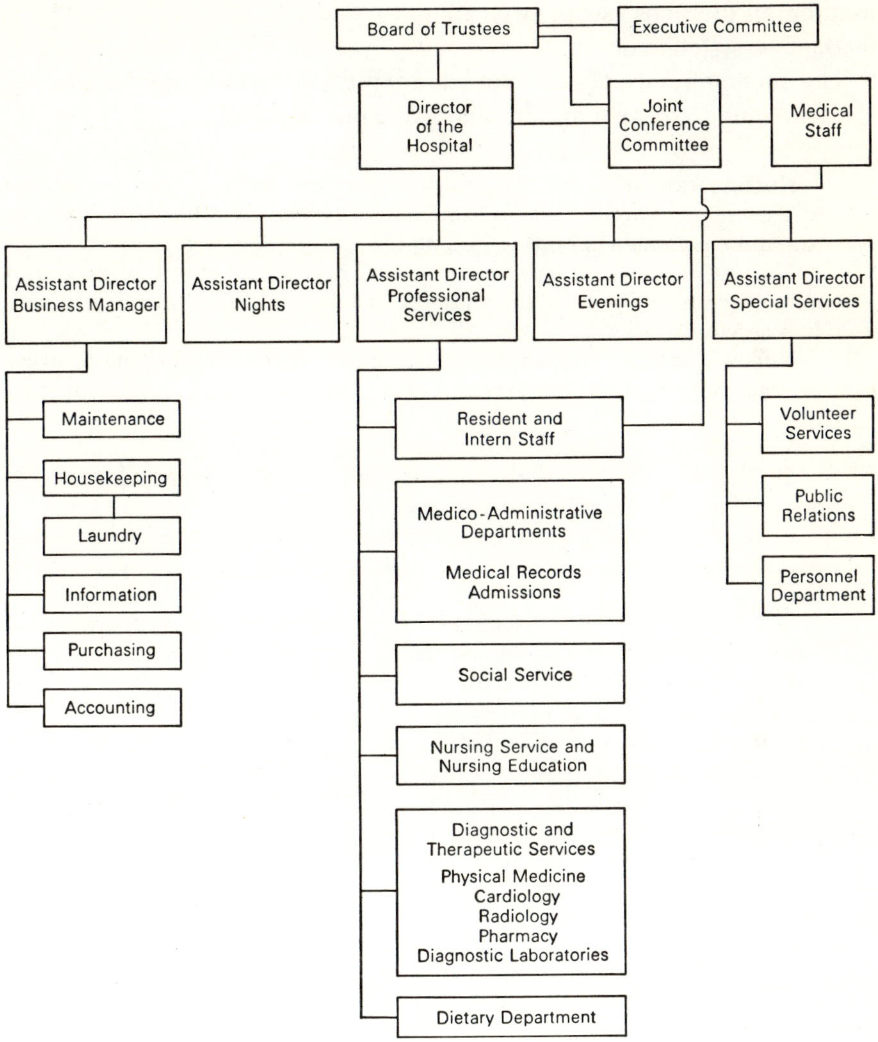

FIGURE 1. Organization chart, Charles Evans Memorial Hospital.

directors of nursing service. There also are administrative supervisors, who are responsible for the direct supervision of activities in the separate nursing units for maternity, pediatric, psychiatric, clinic, medical, surgical, orthopedic, and rehabilitation patients. The case method of assignment is used on all divisions except two. These two nursing units utilize the team method of assignment.

The nursing service department has adopted as its philosophy of nursing the following basic assumptions and principles of care.[1]

> Nursing care encompasses health promotion, the care and prevention of disease or disability, and rehabilitation, and involves teaching, counseling and emotional support as well as the care of illness.
>
> Nursing care is an integral part of total health care and is planned and administered in combination with related medical, educational and welfare services.
>
> Nursing personnel respect the individuality, dignity, and rights of every person, regardless of race, color, creed, national origin, social or economic status.
>
> The patient has a right to expect:
>
> 1. That he will receive the nursing care necessary to help him regain or maintain his maximum degree of health.
> 2. That the nursing personnel who care for him are qualified, through education, experience and personality, to carry out the services for which they are responsible.
> 3. That the nursing personnel caring for him will be sensitive to his feelings and responsive to his needs.
> 4. That, within the limits determined by his doctor, the patient and his family will be taught about his illness so that the patient can help himself, and his family can understand and help him.
> 5. That plans will be made with him and his family, or if necessary, for him, so that, if possible, continuing nursing and other necessary services will be available to him throughout the period of his need. These plans will involve the use of all appropriate personal and community resources.
> 6. That nursing personnel will assist in keeping adequate records and reports and will treat with confidence all personal matters that relate to the patient.
> 7. That efforts will be made by nursing personnel to adjust the surroundings of the patient so as to help him maintain or recover his health.

The Charles Evans Memorial Hospital is an agency organized to serve the community and the physicians by providing facilities for a compre-

[1] National League for Nursing, "What People Can Expect of Modern Nursing Service," National League for Nursing, New York, 1959.

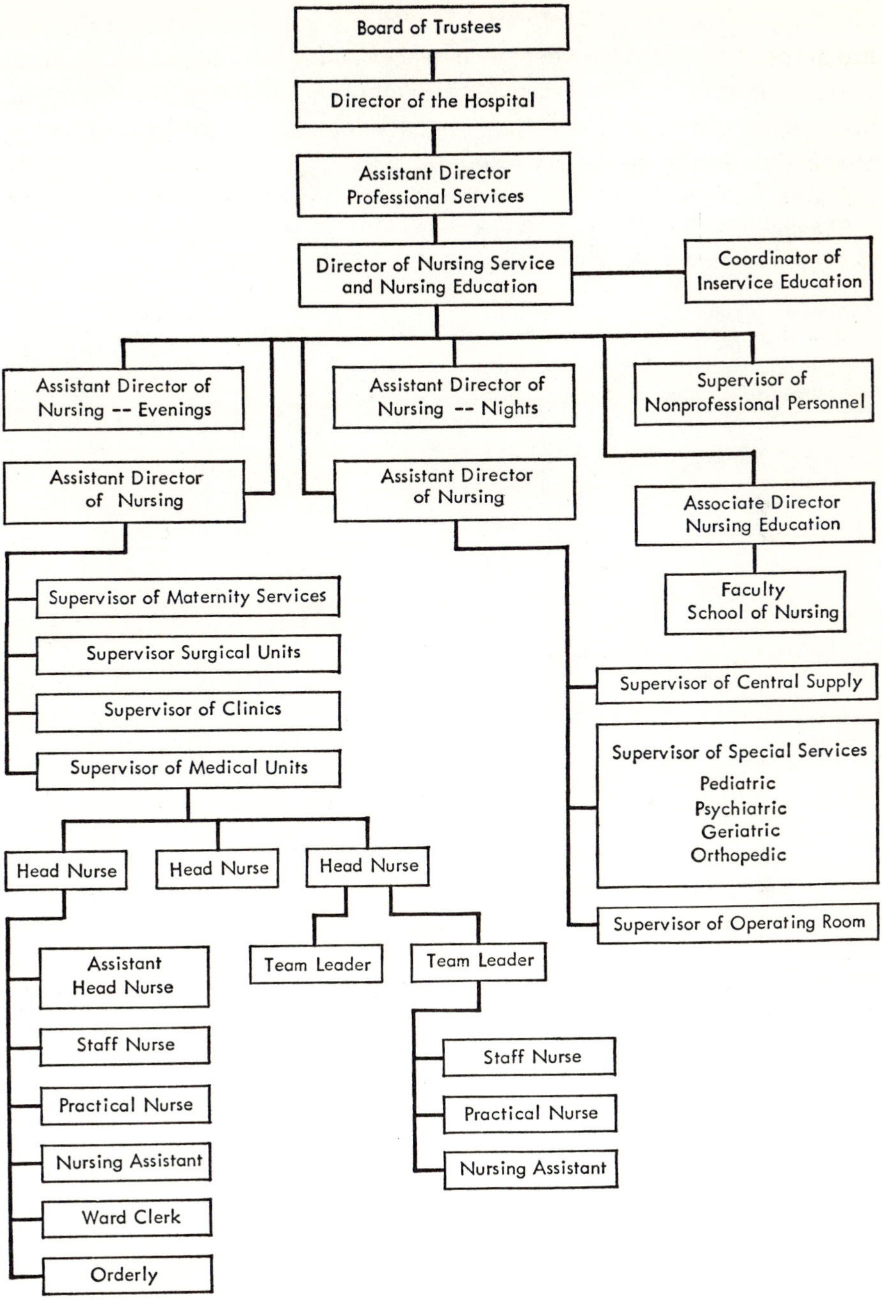

FIGURE 2. Organization chart, Department of Nursing Service and Nursing Education, Charles Evans Memorial Hospital.

hensive program of medical care.[2] It is also a social institution in which intricate relationships between personnel exist. In the course of the ensuing discussions of the case reports many aspects of the human relationships will be revealed. It is in this setting that the practice of administration in nursing and its ramifications will be examined.

[2] Donald M. Rosenberger, "A New Look at Hospital Organization," *Hospitals, J.A.H.A.*, vol. 36, p. 43, February 1, 1962.

case 1

The Staff Nurse and the Patient

Case Data	*Case Notes*
Jane Emery accepted a position as staff nurse at the Charles Evans Memorial Hospital one month following graduation from a baccalaureate degree program in nursing. She had applied for the position because she wanted to work in a teaching hospital in her home state.	Staff nurse position. New graduate. Desired work in a teaching hospital.
She was assigned to Division 5 East after expressing a preference for caring for medical patients. The unit, a medical unit with private and semiprivate accommodations for 25 adult patients, was under the direction of the head nurse, Mrs. Eloise Anderson.	Preferred assignment granted.
This assignment pleased Miss Emery because she had learned from other staff nurses that Mrs. Anderson "runs a good ward" and "lets staff nurses do something on their own." In a conference with Mrs. Anderson at the end of the first three months on 5 East, Miss Emery stated that she found her assignments interesting and stimulating.	Head nurse identified in advance by others as a "good" head nurse who encouraged staff development.
At times she was eager to make suggestions, but remarked to her roommate that she hesitated to do so because she was afraid the other staff members would think she disapproved of present practices.	Reluctant to offer suggestions for fear of being considered critical of the status quo.
On Tuesday, August 12, Miss Emery reported to the division for morning report at 8 A.M.	Time of report, 8 A.M.
She was assigned to a new group of patients, as it was Mrs. Anderson's custom to change assignments every week.	New group of patients. Groups rotated weekly.
Following the report, Miss Emery visited each patient in her new group. When she entered Mrs. Davis' room, she saw a woman who looked older than her age of fifty-five years, lying in bed, apparently staring at the ceiling.	Visited patients first.
A diabetic for fifteen years, Mrs. Davis had been admitted to the hospital six days previously, in a diabetic coma. The night nurse had indicated in her report that Mrs. Davis had responded rapidly	Patient admitted six days previously.

Case Data

to treatment and would probably be discharged from the hospital in a few days. As Miss Emery approached the bed, Mrs. Davis looked at her and asked this nurse what she wanted her to do now. When Miss Emery asked the patient for suggestions, Mrs. Davis replied that she would like to run her own tests and give herself injections of insulin, as she had at home, but that no one would allow her to do so.

At this point, Dr. Johanson, an intern, entered to do a venipuncture to obtain blood from Mrs. Davis for some special studies. Miss Emery remained at the bedside while Dr. Johanson made several unsuccessful attempts before locating a site from which he was able to withdraw an adequate blood sample. As soon as the intern left the room, Miss Emery told Mrs. Davis that she would return shortly to bring her equipment for her insulin injection.

Miss Emery rechecked the order sheet in Mrs. Davis' chart to make certain that there was no contradiction to the patient's resuming the routine followed at home. She also noted that the nurse's notes of the previous two days recorded that Mrs. Davis was anxious to resume self-care. There was no notation that Mrs. Davis had been encouraged to do so. Miss Emery asked Mrs. Anderson if this would be permissible, and she secured approval of the plan.

She then went to the supply room on the division for medication and the necessary equipment. Miss Williams, another staff nurse, entered the supply room and, upon seeing Miss Emery, asked why she seemed so disturbed. Miss Emery replied that she had found Mrs. Davis upset because no one had responded to her request to resume her own injections and that a new intern had made three unsuccessful attempts at venipuncture before obtaining a blood sample from this patient. Miss Emery then left the supply room to return to Mrs. Davis.

Case Notes

Discharge of patient imminent.

Encouraged the patient to participate in planning for care.

Other nurse apparently had ignored patient's request.

Remained with patient.

Gave patient a reason for leaving room.

Rechecked order sheet.

Read nurse's notes of previous two days.

Sought approval from head nurse.

Equipment available on division.

Miss Emery's distress visible to another nurse.

Two reasons for distress verbalized: (1) the ignoring of a patient's request, and (2) the ineptness of an intern.

DISCUSSION

Situations similar to the one described in Case 1 occur daily in hospitals and health agencies everywhere. These situations are ones in which the staff nurse encounters an unmet need of a patient and is required to assume administrative functions. The needs of the patients may differ, the actual incidents may vary in kind, but staff nurses will immediately identify with Miss Emery. Head nurses will recall similar incidents. Nursing service supervisors will recognize the similarity between this case report and their own observations of happenings on nursing units. Some may be tempted to propose immediate answers, but this must be forestalled if there is any validity to the theory that the administrative process is a scientific process.

What does this case report relate about the individual performing the administrative functions, Miss Emery, and the setting, Division 5 East of the Charles Evans Memorial Hospital? What questions may be raised about the person and the place?

Miss Emery had been a staff nurse approximately three months. This was her first experience as a graduate professional nurse. She had elected to work in this particular institution because it was a teaching hospital. Why she wanted to work in a teaching hospital is not disclosed. Could it be that as a student she had had satisfying clinical laboratory experiences in a teaching hospital? Could it be that her learning experiences were in small community hospitals only; therefore she was interested in broadening her experience? What was her concept of a teaching hospital?

Jane Emery had recently expressed satisfaction with her work assignment. It seems reasonable to assume that she was predisposed to liking the head nurse because of the favorable reports about her. Why then was she reluctant to offer suggestions? Was it more important to her to be accepted as a member of her peer group than to take advantage of the opportunity to make suggestions? Did she not feel knowledgeable enough to make suggestions? Had something happened to cause her to disbelieve the favorable reports about the head nurse?

Miss Emery was visibly disturbed by the apparent ineptness of the intern, so upset that at least one person noticed. Is this the reaction of one neophyte, a new staff nurse, to another neophyte, an intern who in all likelihood had just begun his internship? Is this reaction a manifestation of a lack of understanding of the realities of a teaching hospital, or is it the result of being placed in the equivocal position of supporting the philosophy of an agency and yet trying to protect the patient? Or is this reaction an opportunity to project her feelings on a member of another profession about the care rendered by members of her own profession? One cannot, of course, truly know why Miss Emery was disturbed, but experiences with staff nurses seem to indicate that probably several of these factors were operating in this situation.

This is a partial image of a particular person. But what can be elicited from the case concerning Miss Emery as a professional nurse? She visited all her patients immediately after morning report. It seems logical to assume that her purpose in so doing was to make personal observations of each patient and to coordinate these observations with the information learned at report in formulating her plan of care for each patient.

Her initial approach to the patient, Mrs. Davis, is an indication of the respect she held for patients as individuals. She explained to the patient why she was leaving the room and when she would return—further indication of her concept of the nurse-patient relationship. She was alert to the rehabilitative aspects of the care for the patient. She sought available sources of information and direction, the physician's order sheet and the nurse's notes, before seeking approval of her plan of care from the head nurse. Her performance to date apparently was satisfactory enough to warrant being retained in the position. This then is Miss Emery as perceived through the case description.

Of interest at this point in the case analysis is the concept of Miss Emery held by each reader. How alike are they? How dissimilar? Are they usually stereotyped, i.e., based on position, educational preparation, and status? Or does he usually identify a new person with someone he has known in the past in a similar position? Or does he look upon each person as objectively as possible? Such questions should encourage the reader to develop awareness of his own reactions to individuals.

The locale for this incident was Division 5 East of the Charles Evans Memorial Hospital, a nursing unit with accommodations for twenty-five medical patients in private and semiprivate rooms. The supply room was available on the division, hence it can be assumed that delays in obtaining equipment were minimal. The case method of assignment was used in support of the philosophy of nursing care held by the nursing service department. The staff nurse was apparently directly responsible to the head nurse, as indicated by Miss Emery's consultation with Mrs. Anderson before proceeding with her plans. The morning report was held at 8 A.M. This is later than the time established for this report in many hospitals and may be an indication of the philosophy of patient care of the Charles Evans

Memorial Hospital—a belief that this later time for the start of a new day is more like the day of the person before he became a patient. On the other hand, this may have been an attempt on the part of the hospital administration to create for the employee a work day that is more in line with the work day of persons in other occupations. Perhaps this pattern was necessitated by the schedules of the transit lines used by hospital employees.

While some of the above information may not be essential to the immediate problem of facilitating care for Mrs. Davis, it is vital to the "thinking" step in the blueprint in planning a major administrative change and thus is vital to the approach of the staff nurse in the giving of care and in the performance of administrative functions. Is a twenty-five-bed nursing unit an ideal size? Some may say that it is ideal, others that it is too large, still others that it is too small for optimal utilization of nursing personnel. Such responses would undoubtedly be based on purely personal observations. There is no ideal size for a hospital unit because optimal size can be determined only in relation to factors such as type of care to be provided, arrangement of equipment and service areas, provisions for flexibility in usage, and distance between patient areas and supply rooms.

Single rooms may enhance the possibility of dynamic interpersonal relationships between the nurse and the patient but at the same time impede communication and restrict supervision of patients and personnel. Increasingly attention is being given to the physical components of a therapeutic environment. Experimental design and study of intensive care units, round units, and wedge-shaped units should increase one's awareness of the relationship between the place, the nursing unit, and the facilitation of nursing care. It is not enough to say, "We are doing the best we can under the circumstances." Nursing can and must effect changes. In order to do this, nurses must constantly analyze the setting and its relationship to their functions as well as to the care of patients.

In many situations decisions must be made while questions such as those raised thus far remain unanswered. The administrator must weigh indefinite and intangible elements against known facts and then arrive at a decision. There are additional clues to be drawn from this case report, however, if one pauses to consider the activities described, the relationships existing between the persons in the case and the attitudes, feelings, and beliefs revealed by the behavior of the participants. In reviewing the events in the incident, further information about the person, the staff nurse, may be found. While Dr. Johanson was making the venipuncture Miss Emery remained with the patient. Since this procedure usually can be performed without assistance on an adult patient, it is conceivable that Miss Emery stayed to support the patient rather than to aid the intern. Another interpreter may suggest that in this particular hospital the staff nurse is expected to act as handmaiden to any member of the medical staff. One would hope that the need of the patient for support is the determinant for Miss Emery's action. The intent at this point, however, is not to judge her action but to explore the situation fully so that when an administrative decision is reached, the cause, not just the symptom of the difficulty, is treated.

Miss Emery did not mention the apparent ineptness of the intern to the head nurse, but she did to a fellow staff nurse. Is this indicative of Miss Emery's feelings about praise and blame? Was this because of the camaraderie that so often exists between persons in the lower echelons of the status system of an organization or a profession? Did Miss Emery consider the staff nurse but not the head nurse to be a peer? Did she feel that she had no right to evaluate the performance of the intern? These questions are based on the assumption that Miss Emery perceived the situation correctly by considering the repeated attempts at venipuncture as an indication of lack of skill instead of the presence of veins that would be difficult for anyone to penetrate with a needle. It is possible that her suspicions are without foundation.

Why, when Miss Emery approached, did not the head nurse notice that Miss Emery was upset? Was it because Mrs. Anderson was so preoccupied that she listened to but did not look at Miss Emery? Perhaps she realized Miss Emery was upset but decided to ignore that aspect of the situation. Then again, Miss Emery may have masked her feelings while talking with the head nurse.

The case report reveals that Miss Emery expressed a preference for working with medical patients and that this request was honored when her assignment was made. These facts would lead one to believe that the person in the nursing service department responsible for assigning nursing personnel to the various nursing units respected the inclinations of the individual nurse. This may have been a reflection of the philosophy of the nursing service department, or only of the individual making the assignments. Again, one would hope it is the former.

Mrs. Anderson was described as a head nurse who "runs a good ward" and "lets staff nurses do something on their own." There is no way of knowing what criteria served as the basis for evaluation. Does "good" mean satisfactory in the eyes of the patients, of nursing personnel, of both?

Does "lets staff nurses do something on their own" mean she encourages staff nurses to be creative, to display initiative? Does it mean she is permissive and yet supportive? Does it mean she is permissive to the extent of being laissez-faire?

The cataloguing of the activities, relationships, and attitudes revealed by the case report, and the suggesting of alternative interpretations, may seem laborious. To verbalize the dimensions of a process as dynamic as the administrative process, however, is not accomplished without time and effort. Remember that John VanderWaal advised (Chapter 4) that "Thinking always requires effort and expenditure of energy and it rarely becomes habitual." In actual practice one would have already acquired much of this information. This is not to say that one would not have to raise questions about the person, the place, the activities, and relationships, but that it would be possible to find many of the answers immediately at hand.

When Miss Emery returned to her patient, what was her action to be? Would she allow Mrs. Davis to give herself insulin injections, thus considering that she would be fulfilling her responsibility for meeting the needs of the patient? How may Miss Emery have used the *administrative blueprint* in the performance of her functions of planning for and directing patient care? The authors have an advantage over the reader because they observed Miss Emery in action and are familiar with her use of the blueprint. To assist the reader in comprehending fully the use of this design for action by a staff nurse in the performance of the administrative functions of planning and directing the care of an individual patient, Miss Emery's thoughts and actions are detailed below.

As Miss Emery left Mrs. Davis' room, after her initial visit, she was consciously thinking about Mrs. Davis' unmet needs and at the same time less consciously analyzing the total situation. She recognized that the immediate problem was an unmet need of a patient. She had been a staff nurse at the Charles Evans Memorial Hospital for more than three months and had given thoughtful consideration to the place, i.e., the community, the hospital, and the nursing unit—including the persons with whom she was in daily contact. Before attempting even a tentative proposal for meeting the needs of her patient, Miss Emery had subjected these factors and ideas to careful scrutiny.

Miss Emery realized that she had to explore her personal feelings about the situation and that self-understanding is an essential aspect of the process. She was dismayed to find that for two days Mrs. Davis had been asking for permission to give herself injections but that no one had heeded her requests. Jane Emery was disturbed that the staff nurses who had cared for this patient had neglected her request. She felt that this reflected on the competence of all professional nurses. Yet she forced herself to admit that perhaps there were valid reasons why the staff nurses had not complied with Mrs. Davis' request. She realized that she may be unjustly accusing her colleagues.

The intern's lack of skill in performing the venipuncture was disturbing to Miss Emery. Her immediate reaction was to lend support to her patient during the procedure. She was tempted to report the incident to the head nurse but decided not to. Why? Remembrance of her own experiences as a student in performing new procedures influenced her action, as did her rethinking on the commitment of a teaching hospital to provide learning experiences in various disciplines. In spite of her decision not to mention this at the time, she did vent her feelings to another staff nurse, with the intent of finding out whether others had observed this intern's lack of skill and of subtly alerting colleagues to the desirability of evaluating the performance of the intern.

This analysis of self brought to Miss Emery the realization that she herself was reluctant to offer suggestions for the improvement of patient care. Although she had accepted theoretically the need for sharing ideas it optimum patient care is to be achieved, she personally had failed to exhibit evidence of this acceptance. This forced her to examine intensively the responsibility and obligations of a staff nurse in a situation like this one. She concluded that she must plan to meet the immediate need of Mrs. Davis to resume some aspects of self-care, that she must evaluate the response of the patient to the plan, and above all, that she must continue to think beyond the immediate plan to the implications of a broader plan for the care of patients. Obviously this reflection was not limited to the time consumed in walking from the patient's room to the nurses station, but was in process throughout and even beyond the time spanned by the case report.

Even before becoming consciously involved in this situation, Miss Emery was utilizing Step 3 in the blueprint, communicating the proposal. She responded to the initial question of the patient, "What do you want me to do now?," with the question, "What do you want to do?" By eliciting the participation of the patient in planning her own care, she was increasing the possibility that the patient would be receptive to the final plan. She further communicated the proposal when she voiced to Miss Williams the request of the patient without disclosing what she planned to do. Miss Emery hoped that this would have a threefold effect: that it would predispose Miss Williams to be receptive toward the undisclosed tentative plan; stimulate her to think about the needs of Mrs. Davis and, consequently, of the needs of her own patients; and encourage Miss Williams to offer suggestions.

With a tentative plan formulated to permit the patient to give herself insulin injections and to test urine specimens, Miss Emery approached the head nurse to communicate this proposal. Some may question why she did not proceed without consulting the head nurse. There is no known reason why she could not have done so, but Miss Emery was interested in eliciting from Mrs. Anderson, the head nurse, additional information about the patient as well as suggestions that Mrs. Anderson may have been able to contribute from her experience with similar nursing situations. Miss Emery was not consciously thinking beyond the immediate situation when she sought approval of her plan. She realized, in retrospect, that she was thinking about another proposal and was, in fact, with this conference with Mrs. Anderson, laying the groundwork for communicating the subsequent proposal.

In planning for the performance of her administrative functions in this situation, Miss Emery thought about where she could obtain the information necessary for a decision and about whom to involve in the eventual plan. Her thinking was based on her knowledge of the principles of organization, of the organization of the hospital, and of the organization of the nursing service department. In her orientation to the Charles Evans Memorial Hospital, the organization charts of the hospital and of the nursing service department had been explained. Miss Emery knew that she was directly responsible to the head nurse, that authority to plan nursing care for certain patients was delegated to her by the head nurse, and that her functions were detailed in the job description for the position she held. Within the framework of the chart she began to formulate the plan of care for Mrs. Davis. Teaching the patient was a function of staff nurses. If teaching diabetic patients were a function of the rehabilitation department at this hospital her proposal would, of necessity, have to be different. If her plan were going to involve another department in the hospital, she would need to follow the formal line of communication shown on the chart—to the head nurse who would then either forward the communication up the line through the nursing service department and across to strategic personnel in the other department, or secure permission for Miss Emery to make the contacts. Miss Emery also knew that both the formal structural relationships established between personnel and the informal organizational relationships had to be considered in the performance of administrative functions. For this reason she realized the importance of communicating with another staff nurse.

No mention is made in the case report of the other patients assigned to Miss Emery. It will have to be assumed that Miss Emery was planning to propose a change in the approach to the nursing care of Mrs. Davis and was considering the timing required to carry out this proposal in relation to the needs of her other patients. Plans proposed for the care of a patient should be formulated in light of the philosophy of the institution and of the nursing service department. This was a teaching hospital. The definition accepted by the Charles Evans Memorial Hospital of the descriptive title, teaching hospital, was presented in the orientation of Miss Emery to the hospital. As soon as a tentative proposal had been formulated she began to consider the activation of the plan for care in relation to materials needed and actual procedures to be followed.

In this incident, the group involved was not large. The primary persons involved were the patient, Miss Emery, and Mrs. Anderson. This simplified the securing of group acceptance of the immediate plan. Acceptance by the patient is assumed because she had made the request. It is to be hoped that even if the patient had not made the request, Miss Emery would have recognized that this patient would have to be prepared for discharge from the hospital and for resumption of self-care. Miss Emery may have proceeded without consulting the head nurse, but she recognized the value of the head nurse's support if this plan were to be carried out by other tours of duty.

The case method of assignment to patient care had been established for this hospital by the nursing service department. It was not necessary for Miss Emery to establish a pattern of organization for the execution of the plan for Mrs. Davis because, in the case method, the nurse gives complete care to the group of patients assigned to her for a particular tour of duty. This includes physical care, medications, and treatments as well as diversional and educational needs of the patient. This method, also referred to as the "patient method," is no longer widely used because a large complement of the nursing staff in many nursing units consists of practical nurses and nurse aides who are not prepared to assume complete care.

If, on the other hand, the functional method of patient assignment were being used, Miss Emery would have to consider whether she or the "medicine nurse" should supervise the patient in giving herself injections of insulin since personnel in the functional method are assigned specific functions, such as taking temperatures, administering treatments, giving baths, etc. It is conceivable, then, that she would have to coordinate the plan with the activities of a treatment nurse responsible for testing urine specimens. If this so-called efficiency method had been in use, the organizing and delegating for the execution for the plan would have to be done in consultation with the head nurse.

Regardless of the method of assignment used, it was essential for Miss Emery to recognize and understand the limits of her authority in the execution of the plan. She had the authority to carry out this plan herself, but she did not have the authority to insist that other staff nurses do the same.

Again, as Miss Emery alone was involved in the execution of the plan, the need for Step 7, guiding for the execution of the plan, was limited. She did, however, guide in that she set an example for other nurses to follow. Through her recordings on the nurses' notes and through oral reports she demonstrated the leadership role of the nurse administrator.

The response of the patient to the actual execution of the plan enabled Miss Emery to evaluate the plan. Because the nurse formulated the plan in light of the patient's request, one would assume that the plan was successful. Only critical observation may indicate whether this was what the patient really wanted, or whether, even then, the plan was successful.

Evaluation of each step in the blueprint would seem to compel the staff nurse, Jane Emery, to plan beyond the immediate care she rendered to Mrs. Davis and to consider what contribution she could make toward the continuing care of this patient as well as toward more comprehensive nursing care for all patients.

This is but one analysis of Case 1. Others may suggest the formulation of another plan, or may conclude that the head nurse is the person to formulate the long-range plans. There is no one best analysis or answer.

In this case analysis, the detailing of every step of the blueprint may make the design seem unwieldy, particularly if the reader stops to realize that this particular case report concerned a minute segment of the care of a single patient. The reader is asked to recall the first demonstration of a bed bath she witnessed as a student. Was that not a seemingly endless procedure composed of "thousands" of intricate steps? And yet, with practice, how readily mastered.

Repeated conscious attempts to use the *administrative blueprint* can lead to improved performance of nursing functions at every level, and constant, consistent use of the blueprint in the performance of administrative functions will indicate the plan most suitable for the situation at the time.

SUPPLEMENTARY READING LIST

Brodt, Dagmar E.: "Obstacles to Individualized Patient Care," *Nursing Outlook,* vol. 14, p. 35, December, 1966.

Brown, Esther Lucile: *Newer Dimensions of Patient Care. Part I: The Use of the Physical and Social Environment of the General Hospital for Therapeutic Purposes,* Russell Sage Foundation, New York, 1961, pp. 18–25, 31–36.

Erickson, Janet L.: "How Nurses Feel About Their First Work Experience," *Nursing Outlook,* vol. 12, pp. 62–65, May, 1964.

Florentine, Helen Goodale: "Organization Chart: Yes? No? Why?," *Nursing Outlook,* vol. 8, pp. 262–264, May, 1960.

Frank, Sister Charles Marie: "Satisfactions in Nursing Practice," *Nursing Outlook,* vol. 10, pp. 302–304, May, 1962.

Johnson, Dorothy E.: "Consequences for Patients and Personnel," *American Journal of Nursing,* vol. 62, pp. 96–100, May, 1962.

Lambertsen, Eleanor C.: *Education for Nursing Leadership,* J. B. Lippincott Company, Philadelphia, 1958, pp. 94–104.

Larson, Richard J.: "How to Define Administrative Problems," *Harvard Business Review,* vol. 40. pp. 68–80, January-February, 1962.

Miller, Doris I.: "Administration for the Patient," *American Journal of Nursing,* vol. 65, pp. 114–116, July, 1965.

Simmons, Leo W.: "What is the Potential Role of the Nurse in Patient Care?," *Nursing Outlook,* vol. 10, pp. 103–105, February, 1962.

Simon, Richard J., and Marian E. Olson: "Assessing Job Attitudes of Nursing Service Personnel," *Nursing Outlook,* vol. 8, pp. 424–427, August, 1960.

Walker, Virginia H., and James L. Hawkins: "Management: A Factor in Clinical Nursing," *Nursing Outlook,* vol. 13, pp. 57–58, February, 1965.

Whitaker, Judith G.: "The Changing Role of the Professional Nurse in the Hospital," *American Journal of Nursing,* vol. 62, pp. 65–69, February, 1962.

Winters, Margaret C., and Lee Gilmer: "The Nurse's Judgment and the Patient's Understanding," *American Journal of Nursing,* vol. 61, pp. 50–54, December, 1961.

Wooden, Howard E.: "The Hospital's Purpose Is the Patient, But–" *The Modern Hospital,* vol. 92, pp. 90–96, January, 1959.

case **2**

The Staff Nurse and the Head Nurse

Case Data | *Case Notes*

On Tuesday, August 12, after completing the morning care for Mrs. Davis and other patients in her group, Jane Emery went to lunch. The assistant head nurse on Division 5 East, Carol Barclay, happened to be going to lunch at the same time and accompanied Miss Emery to the hospital cafeteria. They joined a group of six nurses from other medical divisions. After a few minutes of conversation about a dinner dance to be given by the medical staff for the students graduating from the Charles Evans Memorial Hospital School of Nursing, the nurses discussed the morning's activities on the various medical wards.

As they were leaving the dining room to return to the ward, Miss Emery mentioned to Miss Barclay the episode with Mrs. Davis. She also revealed that she was so upset about it that she almost mentioned it at the lunch table. Miss Barclay expressed understanding of her concern over the failure of the nursing staff to meet the needs of the patient and suggested that she discuss the situation with the head nurse. Several times that afternoon Jane considered telling Mrs. Anderson, but she did not.

That evening, as Jane recounted the day's events, her roommate asked, "What did Mrs. Anderson say when you told her?" Jane replied that she had not informed the head nurse but had assisted the patient in giving herself an injection of insulin and would do so again tomorrow.

"If that is as far as you intend to go, why did you tell Miss Williams, Miss Barclay, and now me? Why didn't you just carry out your responsibility to Mrs. Davis and be quiet?"

Case Data *Case Notes*

In responding to these questions, Jane acknowledged that her responsibility did not end with the one patient. She also admitted that her reluctance to discuss the situation with the head nurse was based on a fear of being considered critical of other staff members. Jane and her roommate then rehearsed the approach she might use to convey concern rather than criticism.

When she approached Mrs. Anderson after report the next morning, Jane found her receptive and concerned for Mrs. Davis. As they discussed the situation in detail, Mrs. Anderson questioned whether the incident was an isolated one or whether it might be an indication of a widespread lack of communication. Jane did not comment on this supposition. When Mrs. Anderson asked Jane if she had any suggestions regarding the prevention of similar occurrences, Jane recalled several recent articles on the use of a nursing care plan as a means of communication for continuity. The head nurse requested Jane to investigate these plans and arranged for her to be free of patient care assignment on Thursday afternoon so that she could review the literature for possible solutions. She also made an appointment with Jane for a conference on the following Monday morning, after asking her if it would be all right to have the assistant head nurse attend the conference too.

DISCUSSION

The closing statements in the discussion of Case 1 express the belief that the use and evaluation of the steps in the *administrative blueprint* will lead the staff nurse to plan beyond the situation described. This sequel to the first case was included in order to demonstrate that one staff nurse, Jane Emery, was concerned enough to continue to think about the situation and to identify some of the positive and negative factors that may affect the ability of a staff nurse to perform administrative functions. This case also is an example of the performance of administrative functions on two different levels: (1) the staff nurse level and (2) the head nurse level.

The format for the discussion of Case 2, which follows, is based on the assumption that a certain amount of repetition is conducive to learning and to habit formation. Thus, repeated conscious attempts to use the blueprint lead to improved performance of administrative functions. Once again the reader is asked to subject the case to close scrutiny, to raise his own questions, and to propose his own solutions before reading the case discussion.

It is conceivable and even highly probable that some of the following questions may have been raised as the first two paragraphs were read:

Why did the staff nurse and the assistant head nurse join nurses from other medical divisions at lunch? Is this behavior typical of nurses?

Why did Miss Emery feel free to mention the incident to the assistant head nurse when she did not mention it to the head nurse?

Why didn't she mention the incident when others were discussing ward activities at lunch?

Why did Miss Barclay refer the staff nurse to the head nurse instead of assuming responsibility for further action?

Why didn't Miss Emery follow the assistant head nurse's suggestion to discuss the incident with the head nurse?

Perhaps not all these questions have immediate relevance to the case. For example, if it were known why the two nurses joined, at lunch, nurses who worked in the same clinical specialty, would the knowledge contribute to the solution of the problem at hand? Probably not. Raising the question, however, may lead one to investigate whether this was a persistent pattern of behavior of nurses in the Charles Evans Memorial Hospital, and if so, supporting the behavior may contribute to job satisfaction for staff nurses. Just as the intense curiosity of the preschool child helps him to discover the world around him, the persistent "why" of the administrator contributes to effective administration.

Most of the questions raised thus far refer to Miss Emery and to Miss Barclay. To the information gleaned from the first case about the staff nurse can be added the fact that Jane Emery did not reveal the incident at the lunch table. If she had not discussed it later with Miss Barclay one may have assumed that her concern was only temporary and had abated during the morning's activities. Why, then, did she discuss her concern with the assistant head nurse? Was there something about Miss Barclay's personality that invited the confidence, or did Miss Emery think this was the line of communication she should follow? The latter supposition would be correct in many organizations where an assistant serves as an intermediary between an employee's immediate superior and employees below him in the line of organization. In nursing, however, the person who holds the title of assistant head nurse seldom serves as a true assistant. In actual practice she is both a part-time head nurse and a part-time staff nurse or team leader, serving primarily to relieve persons in either position on their days off. So equivocal is the position that some nursing service departments have discontinued the use of the title, and, instead, designate a staff nurse as "charge nurse," when the head nurse is not on the division. In others the value of this position is reflected occasionally by the statement, "She performs satisfactorily as an assistant head nurse but should never be promoted to head nurse."

The organization chart of the Nursing Service Department of the Charles Evans Memorial Hospital (page 147) shows that in the formal chain of command the assistant head nurse occupies the same position as the staff nurse, the practical nurse, and other members of the nursing staff under the direction of the head nurse. On the one hand this factor rules out the possibility that Miss Emery considered Miss Barclay the person with the authority to remedy the situation. On the other hand Miss Emery may have perceived that the informal organization within the nursing unit accorded more authority to the assistant head nurse than did the formal organization. For this reason, she may have decided that the informal chain of command was the one to follow to achieve her goal of improving patient care through the use of a nursing care plan. Whatever the reason, the assistant head nurse recognized the limits of her authority and referred the staff nurse to the head nurse, the person who had the authority and responsibility to take action should any be warranted. And since Miss Emery eventually followed her suggestion, it is not necessary at this point to speculate whether Miss Barclay would have assumed the responsibility of reporting the plan to the head nurse if the staff nurse had not.

Once again one is forced to speculate on why the staff nurse did not talk about the incident with the head nurse. It was conjectured earlier that the reluctance of a newcomer to offer suggestions may be the reason. In addition, several studies have concluded that there is a transitional period for the graduate between the completion of the program in a school of nursing and the achievement of the ability to function more independently than she did as a student. Recent graduates need the support that fosters this independence.

The vital part that the approval or disapproval of a peer plays in the behavior of an individual is demonstrated in the exchange between Miss

Emery and her roommate. A peer often serves as the sounding board, or the antagonist, that facilitates the thinking process. This need, rather than a need for physical respite, has fostered the "coffee break" to the point that it has become a necessity for employer and employee alike. Provision for sharing ideas is provided on some nursing units by daily patient care conferences, team conferences, or change-of-tour conferences, that include more than a review of orders recorded on the Kardex and notes already transcribed on the chart.

Up to this point Jane Emery, the staff nurse, had reported what she interpreted as an omission in patient care to three persons: another staff nurse, the assistant head nurse, and her roommate. This seems to evidence the intensity of her concern and her use of the thinking step in the *administrative blueprint*. For the experienced administrator much of the thinking can and should be done in solitude. The novice may need the support she can derive from discussing thoughts with others. This thought-sharing must have reaffirmed Miss Emery's belief that her responsibility in the situation went beyond the immediate needs of Mrs. Davis.

In the planning phase for offering a proposal she would have to evaluate the tentative proposal in terms of the philosophy of the nursing service department. The following statements from the philosophy of the nursing department of the Charles Evans Memorial Hospital seem to dictate some proposal: [1]

> Nursing care encompasses health promotion, the care and prevention of disease, and rehabilitation, and involves teaching, counseling and emotional support as well as the care of illness.
>
> The patient has a right to expect:
>
> . . . the patient and his family will be taught . . . .

In utilizing the planning step and the advice obtained from Miss Barclay in the thinking step, Miss Emery must have realized that although the philosophy and organization of the nursing department authorized her to act in personally giving care to the patient, she did not have the authority to insist that others do the same. In this instance the planning dictated that she communicate the proposal to the person with the authority to make a decision—the head nurse.

The case data give some information on the use of the blueprint at the

[1] National League for Nursing, "What People Can Expect of Modern Nursing Service," National League for Nursing, New York, 1959.

head nurse level. It is conceivable that Mrs. Anderson entered into the thinking phase when, in the earlier incident, Jane Emery first approached her for permission to allow the patient to give herself an injection of insulin. If not then, she certainly gave evidence of thinking when she questioned whether the situation may be a signal of a broader problem. When she questioned Miss Emery, however, she demonstrated behavior that can hinder instead of help an administrator. The staff nurse could have interpreted the question as probing, and it could have stifled her ideas. It seems that in this instance the head nurse should have listened intently rather than question the nurse. The administrator who is accustomed to making decisions and giving orders enters into the thinking process more readily and with more assurance than the novice. She is often able to project more quickly beyond a symptom to the major problem, and by verbalizing this observation she may suppress the initiative of a subordinate.

Much has been written about ferreting out messages masked by conventional approaches. Many persons become so involved in finding the "real" meaning in what others say that they fail to hear what is said. Dow and Posz of Michigan State University conducted a study to answer the question: "What listening behavior actually irritates the person speaking?" Listed below are the sixteen habits of listening identified by subjects as the most irritating listening habits among their administrators or supervisors:[2]

1. He interrupts me when I talk.
2. He asks questions that demand agreement with him; for example, he makes a statement and then says, "Don't you think so?" or "Don't you agree?"
3. Whenever I make a suggestion, he always throws cold water on it. I've quit trying to give him suggestions.
4. He is always rushed for time.
5. He gives me the feeling that I'm wasting his time.
6. He acts as if he is just waiting for me to get through talking so he can interject something of his own.
7. He puts me on the defensive when I ask a question or make a suggestion about improving things.
8. He is always trying to get ahead of my story—and guess what my point is.
9. He asks questions as if he doubted everything I say.

[2] A. Conrad Posz, Ed. D., "Do You Irritate Others When You Listen?" *Journal of the American Dietetic Association,* vol. 34, pp. 730-732, July, 1958. Quoted by permission of the author.

10. He has such a poker face and manner that I never know whether he's listening or whether he understands me.
11. He rephrases what I say as if I hadn't said it right, "Oh, do you mean . . . ?"
12. He always gets me off the subject with his questions and comments.
13. He says he has to go to another meeting.
14. He fails to get down to the basis of the argument or problem.
15. He frequently looks at his watch or the clock while I am talking.
16. He passes the buck on problems.

An awareness of the habits of listening that irritate others and the conscientious application of the principles of active listening will add to the effectiveness of the administrator at every level. Adherence to the following guides to empathic listening will assist the administrator in developing this skill:[3]

1. Listen patiently to what the other person has to say even though you may believe it is wrong and irrevelant. Indicate simple acceptance (not necessarily agreement) by nodding, . . . or perhaps interjecting an occasional "Um-hm" or "I see."
2. Try to understand the feeling the person is expressing, as well as the intellectual content . . .
3. Restate the person's feeling, briefly but accurately. At this stage, you simply serve as a mirror, and encourage the other person to continue talking. Occasionally, make summary responses . . . but in doing so, keep your tone neutral and try not to lead the person to your pet conclusions.
4. Allow time for the discussion to continue without interruption . . .
5. Avoid direct questions and arguments . . . You may want to review evidence later, but a review is irrelevant to how the person feels now.
6. When the other person does touch on a point you do want to know more about, simply repeat his statement as a question . . . With this encouragement he will probably expand on his previous statement.
7. Listen for what *is not* [italics author's] said—evasions of pertinent points or perhaps too ready agreement with common cliches. Such an omission may be a clue to a bothersome fact the person wishes were not true.
8. If the other person appears genuinely to want your viewpoint, be honest in your reply. But in the listening stage, try to limit the expression of your views since these may condition or repress what the other person says.
9. Don't get emotionally involved yourself. Try simply to understand first, and defer evaluation until later.

[3] William H. Newman and Charles E. Summer, Jr., *The Process of Management: Concepts, Behavior, and Practice,* Prentice-Hall, Inc., Englewood Cliffs, New Jersey, 1961, pp. 522–523.

The plan which finally evolved for facilitating communication in the continuity of care is not among the data for Case 2, but there is further evidence of the use of the *administrative blueprint* by the head nurse. Through thinking and planning, the need to improve communications was identified, and the proposal of the staff nurse for a nursing care plan was accepted as the tentative plan—tentative because the plan had not been formulated sufficiently to be communicated to other members of the staff; tentative because further thinking and planning may indicate that an alternate proposal may be more satisfactory.

The case data delineate the head nurse's understanding of the skill of delegating authority to coworkers. Mrs. Anderson used the following principles of delegation:

1. The person to whom a task is delegated must have the potential to perform the assignment.
2. The person to whom a task is delegated must have the capacity for assuming the responsibility.
3. The delegator must define the limits of the authority and responsibility being delegated.
4. The authority delegated must be sufficient to permit discharge of the responsibility assigned.
5. The person who delegates the task is the person to whom the report of accomplishment should be submitted and from whom any necessary criticism should come.
6. The delegator must be responsible for establishing time limits (when applicable) and the means by which the report is to be submitted.

When Miss Emery offered the suggestion, Mrs. Anderson had three choices: (1) to disregard the suggestion completely; (2) to assume responsibility for the investigation; or (3) to delegate to the staff nurse the authority to pursue the possibility further and to make recommendations. She chose the last course—perhaps because she recognized that this was the first indication Miss Emery had given of contributing to the overall functioning of the division and wanted to capitalize on this interest. It is assumed, however, that she would not have selected Miss Emery for the investigation if she did not think Miss Emery was capable of performing the assignment. In making the assignment, Mrs. Anderson defined the limits of the responsibility and authority delegated by arranging for the staff nurse to report her findings to the head nurse. In other words, she did not grant the staff nurse the authority to propose a tentative plan to the staff. She granted limited authority. In setting a definite time limit and in arranging for time to make the survey, she conveyed to the staff nurse an obligation to complete the assignment. Since Mrs. Anderson was the one to delegate the authority and responsibility, Miss Emery should be accountable only to the head nurse. This must have been the reason Mrs. Anderson asked whether the assistant head nurse may be present. This would undoubtedly conserve time for all concerned should Miss Emery's findings lead to a tentative proposal. The head nurse would generally want to discuss the proposition with the assistant head nurse before taking it to other members of the division staff.

When one thinks of the time involved for Mrs. Anderson to delegate the responsibility for the survey to the staff nurse, to assist her to use authority effectively, and to arrange for her to have time to assume the responsibility, one may say it would be easier and less costly in time for Mrs. Anderson herself to investigate the situation. It is true that it is not easy to delegate a task or a responsibility. In fact, delegating has often been identified as the most difficult task of an administrator. Why should this be true if one follows the principles apparently utilized above?

A major consideration in delegating responsibility is that the person who delegates the assignment is held accountable for the satisfactory completion of the assignment. A head nurse cannot dismiss the complaint of a physician about the care his patient received by saying, "Talk to Miss Jones, the patient was assigned to her." The head nurse, in accepting her position, accepts the responsibility for the care received by all patients on her division; and although she delegates this care to others, she is accountable. As one administrator has stated: "An administrator can never delegate accountability. If things go well, everyone gets the credit. If things go bad, he is still accountable."[4]

Too often a delegator fails to give an individual the authority commensurate with the responsibility, or he may expect the individual to have a feeling of responsibility that exceeds his authority. Suppose, for example, Mrs. Anderson had assigned Miss Emery to review the literature and to report her findings in six days and yet did not provide any time for Miss Emery to accomplish this during her working day. Under a misunderstood concept of dedication to service, nursing repeatedly violates this principle of balance between authority and responsibility. Nurses are expected to assume the obligation to achieve an objective without being given commensurate authority to use necessary resources.

Another commonly held misconception is that authority is based on

[4] Ralph L. Perkins, "The Do's and Don'ts of Delegation," *Hospitals,* vol. 36, pp. 40–42, September 1, 1962.

status and is bestowed on a person by an organization chart. In actual practice the only authority a person has is that which those serving under him will accept from him. One cannot delegate if the person being delegated is not willing to do the job. One may, of course, use pressures such as salary, promotion, or other benefits to exact compliance.

In this case the head nurse had the authority to delegate to Miss Emery the responsibility for investigating a possible solution to the communication problem. Thinking and planning had led the staff nurse to propose a nursing care plan. Such a plan is a tool for emphasizing the *nursing* needs of the individual patient, for promoting a continuity of approach to meet these needs, and for evaluating nursing practice. It is a plan formulated by the professional nurse based on clinical knowledge and on assessments made in her initial contact with a patient and revised by subsequent assessments of the nurse and other members of the nursing staff.

The important aspect of the concept of nursing care planning is not the type of form used to record the plan but the provision made for assessing each patient and for formulating a plan of *nursing* care based on his physical, psychosocial, and medical needs. Nursing takes care to make the physician's orders available for the guidance of all personnel, even persons who have no responsibility in relation to most of the orders such as aides or volunteers. Seldom is equal importance given to nursing "orders." It should be noted that this concept of the nursing care plan bears almost no relationship to the current widespread practice of listing on a Kardex card information about a patient's age, diagnosis, physician, medication orders, treatments, and diagnostic procedures. Such information may be essential to the medical care of the patient, but it does not reflect systematic planning of nursing care. The concept does not rule out the use of a standard form for the plan or even of a form as a component of the Kardex system. It remains for professional nurses in each health care setting to devise the specific means by which a nursing care plan for each patient can be made available to the persons giving care so that the nursing needs of the patient can be met and nursing practice evaluated.

Suppose that as a result of her investigations Miss Emery brought three sample care plan forms to her conference with the head nurse and assistant head nurse and each agreed that the use of one or more of the forms would facilitate communication. This issue is broader than the development of a new printed form, however. It could mean a new approach to the functions of the staff nurse on this nursing unit and, perhaps, throughout the hospital. At this point the head nurse has to engage in the thinking and planning steps of the blueprint. If it is decided that a means to facilitate communication is the only goal being sought in this situation, Mrs. Anderson may identify alternative proposals with which to compare the merits of the development of a new form. She may suggest that the emphasis in oral change-of-tour reports could be changed from relaying facts already on the chart or Kardex to a discussion of the nursing problems of patients. She may propose that each nurse report directly to the next tour instead of reporting to the charge nurse who, in turn, reports to the staff for the subsequent tour. Or she may decide that it is more advantageous to hold a daily conference of division personnel to share nursing orders.

If the review of alternative proposals indicates that the development of a nursing care plan form provides the more suitable answer to the problem, the next logical step would be to communicate to the rest of the division staff the proposal to use a nursing care plan form and to elicit their opinions and suggestions. But does a head nurse have the authority to propose the use of a new form, even for her own ward? In most nursing situations, no. She must function within the framework for recording as decreed by hospital or nursing service policy. A suggestion for the use of a new form, even on a trial basis, often must be cleared by a procedures or policy committee before it can be used. Such a practice is based on the need for agency objectives, policies, and procedures in order to achieve a united rather than haphazard effort of employees toward the goal of the organization.

Not until a decision about the form has been reached can the next step in the blueprint be activated. Nor can a technique or tool of administration be lifted from one administrative setting and transplanted to another and still be expected to bring about the same results. Either the technique must be adapted to the new situation, or the organization must be adjusted to accommodate the new tool. Utilization of the *administrative blueprint* can facilitate this approximation.

It is possible that the head nurse, the assistant head nurse, and Miss Emery may discover, in the course of the conference, that communication is not the major factor involved but that the lack of any systematic plan of nursing care is the real issue at hand. Once again the thinking and planning steps of the blueprint are activated to facilitate consideration of this broader problem in providing the nursing services needed by patients.

SUPPLEMENTARY READING LIST

Babnew, David, Jr.: "The 'Whys' of Wise Delegation," *Hospitals, J.A.H.A.*, vol. 39, pp. 62–64, July 16, 1965.

Bain, Barbara, and Jane Bailey: "How a Communication Tool Led to the Development of a Nursing Care Plan," *Nursing Outlook*, vol. 15, pp. 48–51, October, 1967.

Butler, Joan E., et al.: "Evolution of a Form," *Nursing Outlook*, vol. 9, pp. 42–43, January, 1961.

Cherescavich, Gertrude: "A Shared Nursing Care Plan," *American Journal of Nursing*, vol. 59, p. 202, February, 1959.

Ewing, John S.: "Patterns of Delegation," *Harvard Business Review*, vol. 39, p. 32, July–August, 1961.

Frazier, L. M., Jr.: "Accountability: Third Essential in the Process of Delegation," *Hospital Topics*, vol. 44, pp. 81–82, June, 1966.

Hospital Continuing Education Project: *Nursing Care Plans: Study Program in Nursing Management*, Hospital Research and Educational Trust, Chicago, 1966.

Johnson, Dorothy E.: "Consequences for Patients and Personnel," *American Journal of Nursing*, vol. 62, pp. 96–100, May, 1962.

Kelly, Nancy Cardinal: "Nursing Care Plans," *Nursing Outlook*, vol. 14, pp. 61–64, May, 1966.

Lambertsen, Eleanor C.: *Education for Nursing Leadership*, J. B. Lippincott Company, Philadelphia, 1958, pp. 141–164.

Lambertsen, Eleanor C.: "Toward a Clearer Definition of the Nurse's Function," *Hospitals, J.A.H.A.*, vol. 35, pp. 51–52, 54, 96, July 16, 1961.

Little, Dolores E., and Doris L. Carnevali: *Nursing Care Planning*, J. B. Lippincott Company, Philadelphia, 1969.

Mauksch, Hans O.: "Nursing Dilemmas in the Organization of Patient Care," *Nursing Outlook*, vol. 5, pp. 31–33, January, 1957.

Newman, William H., and Charles E. Summer, Jr.: *The Process of Management: Concepts, Behavior and Practice*, Prentice-Hall, Inc., Englewood Cliffs, N.J., 1961, pp. 512–529.

Pellegrino, E. D.: "Better Patient Care—Better Physician-Nurse Communication," in *Blueprint for Progress in Hospital Nursing*, National League for Nursing, New York, 1963.

Perkins, Ralph L.: "The Do's and Don'ts of Delegation," *Hospitals, J.A.H.A.*, vol. 36, pp. 40–42, 115, 116, September 1, 1962.

Posz, A. Conrad: "Do You Irritate Others When You Listen?" *Journal of the American Dietetic Association*, vol. 34, pp. 730–732, July, 1958.

Smith, Dorothy M.: "A Clinical Nursing Tool," *American Journal of Nursing*, vol. 68, pp. 2384–2388, November, 1968.

Spillane, Edward J.: "Improved Management Can Result from the Anatomy of a Decision," *Hospital Progress*, vol. 50, pp. 47–50, 68, April, 1969.

Wang, Mamie Kwoh: "The Intramural Nursing Referral," *Nursing Outlook*, vol. 7, pp. 346–347, June, 1959.

Wright, Marion J.: "The Precise Art of Delegation," *Hospitals, J.A.H.A.*, vol. 34, pp. 85–89, July 16, 1960.

case 3

The Staff Nurse and Her Coworkers

The nursing divisions of the Charles Evans Memorial Hospital had been using the case method of assignment to patient care for several years on the assumption that this method supported the philosophy of patient care held by the nursing service department. At their last semiannual evaluation conference, several supervisors proposed experimentation with the team method of assignment. Two head nurses agreed to implement the team method of assignment on their divisions and to report on the trial at the next evaluation conference.

Case Data | *Case Notes*

Division 4 West, a thirty-bed medical unit for private adult patients, was one of the units using the team method. Miss Shirley Allen, a staff nurse, was assigned to this division three months after the change had been initiated. She had had no previous experience in participating on a nursing care team. In her orientation to the division, information about the team method was presented. For the first two months she served as a member of teams under the leadership of two other staff nurses, Miss Lois Duncan and Mrs. Jean Broderick.

She was then assigned the responsibility of leadership for a team. At the end of the first week, in a conference with the head nurse, Mrs. Ruth Snyder, she remarked that the transition to team leader had not been difficult. She added, "Of course, I am not sure I'm really leading. Maybe the practical nurse and the nursing assistants are just following because that is what they are used to doing."

Throughout the second week the team functioned smoothly under Miss Allen's leadership. She assumed the care of five or six patients daily,

Case Data *Case Notes*

assigning the nursing assistants to help the senior nursing student and the practical nurse with their patients. The head nurse observed that the patients seemed to be comfortable, and their needs seemed to be met. Several patients commented on the "interest and enthusiasm" manifested by Miss Allen. These impressions were conveyed to the team leader by Mrs. Snyder during a conference at the end of the second week. At this time Miss Allen requested guidance in planning the assignments for the junior nursing student who was to be assigned to her team the following week. Mrs. Snyder referred her to the clinical instructor.

Assigned to Miss Allen's team at the beginning of the third week was Lois Duncan, one of the staff nurses under whom Miss Allen had served as a team member. At the team conference following morning report, Miss Duncan sat on the fringe of the group and was silent. Miss Allen asked her which patients she would like to take care of and then assigned the remaining patients to the student, the practical nurse, and the two nursing assistants on the team. Miss Allen assigned herself to the administration of medications and to supervising closely one of the nursing assistants who had been employed at the hospital just three months. Several times throughout the day she offered Miss Duncan assistance. Miss Duncan rejected the offers, saying that she was "almost finished." When the team met in conference at the end of the day, Miss Duncan reported briefly on her patients. She did not raise any questions; nor did she add any comments to the discussion. The second day on the team Miss Duncan's behavior was the same. Miss Allen noticed several times that Miss Duncan reported to the head nurse information that should have been reported to the team leader. As the week progressed, Miss Allen reduced the time spent in team conferences. At the end of the week, she suggested to Mrs. Snyder that perhaps she was not "ready" to be a team leader.

DISCUSSION

The introduction of the concept of *team nursing* in the late 1940s was looked upon by hospital and nursing service administrators with favor and acclaim. Team nursing was offered as an ideal technique for utilizing to the maximum the limited number of available professional nurses, for absorbing and using efficiently nonprofessional workers for the care of the patient, and for providing more comprehensive care for the patient. In the intervening years the concept has been implemented satisfactorily in a number of institutions, and descriptions of the favorable experiences have been recorded in the literature.[1-6] Unfortunately, the abortive attempts of some nursing departments at implementing the concept of team nursing, and the practice of others of accepting the technique without accepting the underlying philosophy as well, have resulted in the dissemination of much misinformation about this means of utilizing personnel for the provision of patient care. The application of the *administrative blueprint* to the function implied in Case 3, the provision of personnel for nursing care of patients, must start with intensive thinking about what team nursing really is.

The concept of team nursing is founded on the philosophy that various levels of nursing personnel, working together harmoniously in a group and under the direction of a staff nurse as team leader, can provide a patient with individualized care. The nursing team should not be confused with the health team mentioned so frequently in discussions of comprehensive health care. The term *health team* refers to the group of members of the many disciplines that contribute to preventive, therapeutic, and rehabilitative care: the physician, the nurse, the physiotherapist, the social worker, the nutritionist, the clergyman, the occupational therapist, and other professional workers whose services may be required in meeting the

[1] Helen G. Beltran, et al., *Guide for Leadership in Team Nursing*, The League Exchange, no. 54, National League for Nursing, New York, 1961.

[2] Janet Bozenhard and Wilhemina Fitt, "The Staff Nurse Speaks for the Nursing Team," *American Journal of Nursing*, vol. 53, pp. 425-426, April, 1953.

[3] Mary E. Brackett and Joan R. Fogt, "Developing the Nursing Team Through Workshops," *American Journal of Nursing*, vol. 53, pp. 680-682, June, 1953.

[4] Ethel A. Brooks, "Team Nursing—1961," *American Journal of Nursing*, vol. 61, pp. 87-91, April, 1961.

[5] Russell C. Swansburg, "An Experiment in Team Nursing, *Nursing Outlook*, vol. 16, pp. 45–47, August, and pp. 42–43, September, 1968.

[6] Mildred A. Vogel and Carmen F. Ross, "Team Nursing . . . An Actuality!" *Nursing World*, vol. 129, pp. 10–12, February, 1955.

needs of an individual patient. The physician serves as the leader of the health team, and the team may function in a home, in a hospital, or in a health agency.

The *nursing team* is the group that assumes responsibility for the independent nursing functions needed by an individual patient, and for the functions delegated to the group by the health team. The professional nurse serves as leader of the nursing team. This team may also function in a home, in a hospital, or in a health agency, although it is most frequently used in the hospital setting.

The phrase *working together harmoniously* is a key phrase in the team concept. Just as the football team must work together and utilize the separate talents of the players for maneuvers and plays, with the captain calling the plays and the coach supervising from the sidelines, so must the nursing team work together, with the head nurse coaching and the staff nurse directing and extending her judgment and skill through the practical nurse, the nursing assistant, and the orderly to each patient being cared for by the nursing team. Through this decentralization of control, the team leader is given the responsibility for a segment of the supervision of patient care and personnel performance that previously was under the direct control of the head nurse. The team leader can extend her particular professional skills to a greater number of patients by performing only those skills for which the other members of her team are not prepared. The diagrams in Figure 3 contrast the assignment of personnel under the team and functional methods. Under the functional method the professional nurse is assigned to total care of "acutely ill" patients or to distribute medications. The criterion for acuteness of illness is as frequently the presence at the bedside of elaborate treatment equipment as it is the severity of the physical or emotional state of the patient. In the team method a coordinated group gives patient care; the patient's individual needs dictate whose skills are needed. Under the close supervision of a staff nurse the practical nurse may give care to the patient who requires treatment with elaborate apparatus whereas the staff nurse may support an ambulatory and emotionally disturbed patient.

In the situation demonstrated in Figure 3 the judgment and skills of the two staff nurses have been extended from six patients to thirteen or fifteen. The number of persons reporting to the head nurse has been reduced from seven to three. This permits the head nurse to concentrate her skills on the development of the team leaders and on the overall supervision of patient care. The head nurse assigns the team leaders and the

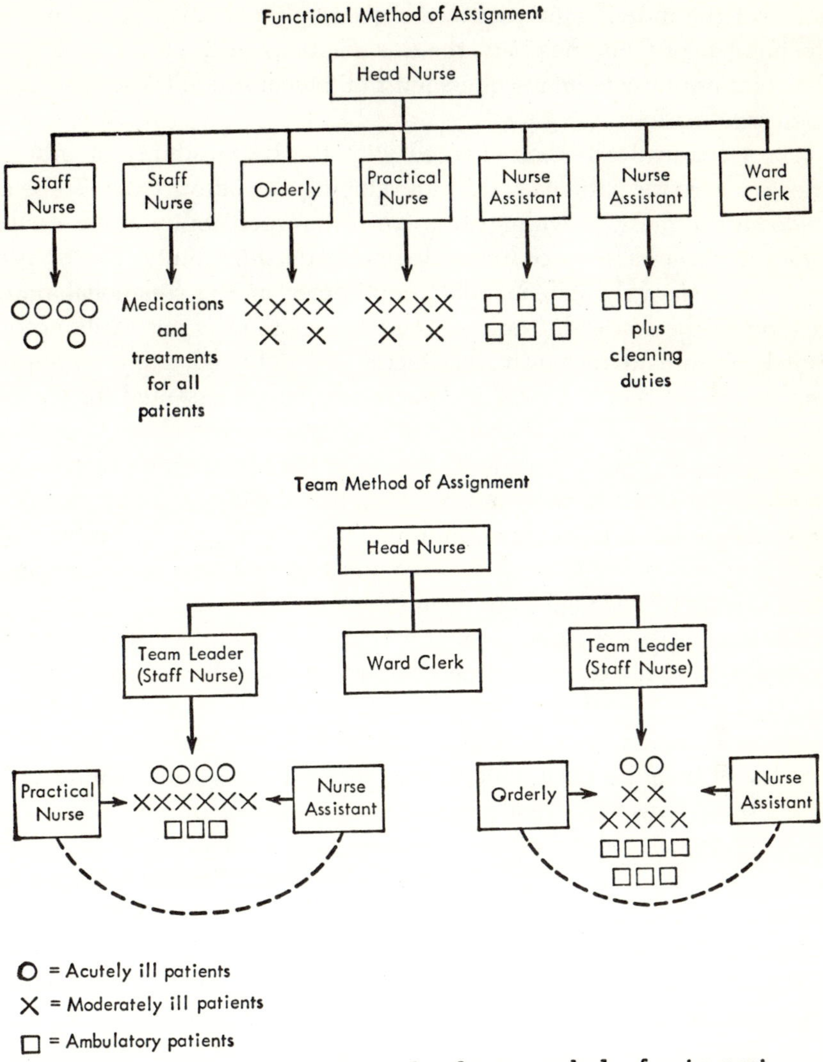

FIGURE 3. A comparison of the functional and team methods of assignment.

personnel who are to comprise the team. She then selects the patients to be cared for by the team. The diagram also depicts the distribution of patients to the two teams. Distribution need not always be equal. The needs of the individual patients, the geographic location of the patients, the number of team members, the qualifications of the team leaders, and the abilities of the team members must all be considered when the assignments are made.

The team leader is then charged with the responsibility of providing effective care for patients and for developing a cohesive team. To be able to do so she must be willing to accept the responsibility and be able to seek and accept assistance in developing leadership ability. The transition from the relatively independent practitioner in the functional or case method to the leadership role in the team method is not easily accomplished. Failure to recognize this factor has defeated many attempts to implement the method. Skill in human relations is essential for the team leader. Professional competence is prerequisite for one who is to teach and direct others in patient care, and respect for the contribution each member can make to patient care and to team functioning is indispensable. In order to use her own skills to the utmost, the team leader, before undertaking an assignment, must develop the habit of saying, "Who on my team can do this as well as or even better than I?"

The team leader must be familiar with the job descriptions of the personnel assigned to the team. She must know, for example, what functions the practical nurse is prepared for and permitted to perform in this hospital that the nurse assistant cannot. It may seem unnecessary to specify that job descriptions be up-to-date, but experience forces the issuing of two precautions, however. Frequently when an in-service training program has extended the skills or functions of a category of personnel, the team leader is advised at the time but the job description is not changed, nor are subsequent team leaders apprised of the change. It is also not infrequent that nonprofessional personnel assigned to a specific division are trained to perform functions which are not included routinely in the job description. For example, practical nurses on the post-partum unit may be prepared to catheterize patients in the presence of bladder distention; yet for patients on other divisions this function must be performed by the professional nurse. Therefore these exceptions to usual policy must be included in job descriptions.

The team leader must also know the extent of the capabilities of the individual members of her team. Not all nurse assistants perform at the same level, any more than do all staff or head nurses. When the head nurse assigns a member to a nursing team, she must identify for the team leader the strengths and weaknesses of the member. In turn, the team leader has a responsibility to supervise, to evaluate, and to inform the head nurse of each member's progress.

In addition to this knowledge about team members, the team leader must have sufficient personal contact with the patients assigned to her team in order to have an understanding of the needs of the patient. It is upon these needs that the assignment of team members is based. In the traditional method, patient care assignments are usually made by the head nurse, and a drastic change in the physical condition of the patient is usually behind any change in the daily assignment. Because the extent of the team leader's supervision of patient care is less than that of the head nurse, the team leader has a greater opportunity to observe changes in the physical or emotional condition of the patient and easily can make adjustments in assignment. Perhaps a few minutes spent by the team leader with the patient will meet the needs of the patient to the extent that the assignment of a team member need not be changed.

If the team leader is responsible for supervising patient care and the personnel assigned to her team, she must be available for consultation with and the guidance of team members. Her contact with the personnel should not be limited to delegating assignments at the beginning of the tour and receiving reports at the end. There should be a written form of communication, a record of the plan of care for the patient, such as the plan suggested in the discussion of Case 2. This plan should be developed by the professional nurse who is serving as the team leader at the time the patient is admitted to the unit. Following her assessment of the needs of the patient based on a nursing history, direct observation of and interaction with the patient, and a review of the plan of medical care, the preliminary nursing care plan is discussed with the head nurse. The plan, with any modifications prompted by consultation with the head nurse, is then communicated to the members of the nursing team. Team members are encouraged to contribute to changes in the plan as they obtain data in their contacts with the patient which suggest alterations in the patient's needs, in approaches to needs, or in changes in goals. The team leader then validates the team members' observations in her reappraisal of the patient.

The team conference has proved to be an invaluable tool for communicating plans, sharing ideas, teaching, and evaluating both patient care and personal performance.[7]

> The conference is the nucleus of the in-service nursing program. At the conference there spring up spontaneously many teaching opportunities which are invaluable in terms of the applications to specific group problems. Techniques of group process and principles of interpersonal relationship are an integral part of the procedure. Observations made during a nursing team conference offer unique opportunities for guidance of nursing service personnel.

After receiving the report from the preceding tour, the team usually meets briefly to discuss assignments and to raise any questions precipitated by the report. At a later time they meet in a conference to discuss the care given and the problems identified. The nursing objectives and nursing care plans are revised as necessary. This conference is frequently held after lunch on the day tour; after the patients have been prepared for sleep on the evening tour; and midway through the night tour of duty. During the discussion of patient care, the team leader may be called upon for impromptu teaching. She also may recognize a need for a consultation with the head nurse.

This method of organizing nursing personnel to give care to a group of patients requires the head nurse to devote her skills to stimulating and developing leadership potential in others. She is still responsible for the total environment of her unit. It is to the head nurse the team directs the problems of the patient that are beyond the province of the nursing team. It is the head nurse who then coordinates the contributions of other groups concerned with comprehensive patient care. She is still the keystone for the provision of nursing care to patients on her unit. Her leadership role is magnified. Her need to attend to minutiae diminishes as a result of the liaison work of the team leader.

The development of coordination in planning, performing, and evaluating is not accomplished rapidly. Some of the newer findings about the group process may contribute toward effecting team rapport and group cohesiveness. But, perhaps the greatest assistance can come from acknowledgement of the value of slow, steady progress toward implementing the concept over initially rapid, rising enthusiasm followed by diminishing returns. Not many head nurses or supervisors have the patience or the

[7] Eleanor C. Lambertsen, *Nursing Team Organization and Functioning*, Bureau of Publications, Teachers College, Columbia University, New York, 1953, p. 35.

perseverance exemplified by the following words of a director of nursing service and a school of nursing.[8]

> Starting with the first two units, it was not until the completion of the decade in 1960, that the system was established on all 31 bedside nursing units; and still there are variations in the strength of team relationship on different units.

An effective team leader is the core of the team plan. Because of the lack of effective leaders, progress has been halted many times in attempts to utilize the team nursing method. Some of the problems encountered can be identified in the description of Miss Allen's first experience as a team leader.

From the case data it is learned that team nursing was introduced five months ago on Division 4 West. No information is given as to the preparation of division personnel for this change, or about the knowledge and acceptance of the head nurse of the concept of team nursing. It is known that the head nurse, Mrs. Snyder, agreed to the experiment, but it is not known whether she volunteered or was prevailed upon to agree. It is to be hoped that she was sincerely interested in the concept and willing to strive continuously to implement the process. The fact that the trial has continued for five months may be considered an indication that this was her attitude. The attitudes of the other members are not identified, but it is doubtful that a head nurse could continue an effort in the face of prolonged opposition. Some degree of cooperation must have been extended.

The level of Miss Allen's performance as a team *member* is not revealed by the case data. One would have to speculate on the amount of orientation the staff nurse had had for this new role of team *leader.* Serving as a team member is not sufficient preparation for assuming the leadership role. In addition to knowing what functions the members of her team are prepared to perform, and the individual levels of their performance, the team leader must be able to identify the nursing problems of the patient and to distinguish which needs can be met by the various members of her team. She must be able to elicit from team members their observations of the needs of the patient and their suggestions for the plan for his nursing care. She must be able to delegate responsibility and authority to team members, and to respect the contribution each member can make to the care of the patient. She, herself, must also be able to render competent care, to teach others, and to evaluate the care given and

[8] Ethel A. Brooks, "Team Nursing—1961," *The American Journal of Nursing*, vol. 61, p. 88, April, 1961.

the performance of individual team members. Some of this preparation may be obtained through reading theoretical discussions and orientation programs. This preparation must be followed closely by direct day-to-day supervision, ideally by the head nurse, but, of necessity, at times by the nursing service supervisor, or by the supervisor of in-service education. The two areas in which the new team leader needs the most assistance are in determining assignments for team members and in delegating duties to others. Miss Allen seemed to be expressing some doubts about her ability to delegate when she said, "Maybe the practical nurse and the nursing assistants are just following because that is what they are used to doing." Perhaps she felt they were actually showing her what she should be directing them to do. That she assigned herself to administering medications for the team indicates that she did not fully appreciate one principle of the team concept—each member of the nursing team should be assigned to perform all the functions he is prepared to perform. The other staff nurse on the team, Miss Duncan, should have been assigned to give complete care, including medications, to some of the patients. The head nurse can provide direct assistance to the new leader in making assignments. She should, at first, discuss with the team leader the assignments in detail and, after eliciting from the leader the reasons behind a choice, help her to develop an objective approach to the matching of personnel skills with patient needs. The head nurse should also follow this planning with close surveillance of the plans in activation to give the team leader guidance in making adaptations ordained by changes in the conditions of or needs of patients, or by the responses of personnel to patients.

In addition to the principles (page 168) of what, when, and to whom to delegate are principles related to issuing directions and instructions that can be useful tools for the team leader—tools she undoubtedly has used less consciously many times in the past. One of the frequent mistakes made is the issuance of unnecessary directions or orders. The leader is anxious to make certain that something is done and gives a team member directions that are implicit in the overall assignment. For example, if a team member is assigned to take the temperatures of the patients, it would usually be redundant to add, "and record them." A new team leader may also be tempted to say still more, "Report any elevations to me." Team members may look upon this suggestion as a lack of respect or faith in their abilities. These two aspects of recording and reporting are invariably written into procedures for taking temperatures.

At least two individuals are involved in any instruction—the person issuing and the person receiving. The individual who has conceived the order knows what he thinks should be done, but do his words convey this same picture to the receiver? Encouraging the receiver to ask questions will help to clarify the order when he is in doubt. Asking him to tell how he plans to carry out the order may help to identify any misunderstanding. Acceptance of an assignment may be facilitated by encouraging the assignee to participate in the formulation of the instructions. The team member who contributes to a nursing care plan will be greatly interested in working toward the objectives of the plan, and will have a better understanding of the reasons behind the instructions or nursing orders in the plan. If it should be necessary to issue an order which, to the receiver, may not seem to be derived from the situation, every attempt must be made to explain the "why" when the assignment is made. Also, what the measure is intended to accomplish, why it must be done within a certain time limit, and how it fits into the plan for the patient should be stated. Suppose, for example, that a team leader asks a practical nurse on the team to obtain a urine specimen from a patient, and when the completion of the assignment is not reported in thirty minutes, says, "Why didn't you tell me you couldn't obtain the specimen? The doctor is waiting for the report to order medication for the patient." Had the team member known this, she conceivably would have tried to obtain results promptly, if at all possible, and undoubtedly would have reported if unable to do so. Knowledge of the reason for an order can enable an individual to act intelligently should something unforeseen occur. It is important also for the person to know *why* a task is delegated to *him*. The words used in delegating can convey approval of an individual's performance and may also set the standard for performance—"I know you will not only do this correctly, but with the facility and speed this situation demands." If the delegator can accept the principle that the situation and not the person determines an order, the questions in the mind of the receiver will be minimal and will be raised only when he needs more information about the situation.

The team leader can increase her skill in directing others if she constantly raises the searching question, "Is this order really necessary?" If she can reach the point of answering Yes 95 per cent of the times she queries herself, she can be relatively sure that when she issues an order in an emergency the response will be immediate and the order will be followed respectfully.

The head nurse cannot possibly be on hand to guide the team leader every time a new team leader must give a direction to a team member. She must plan to spend some time daily with a new team leader, however, to give her the opportunity to discuss recognized problems, to identify covert problems, and to evaluate her own progress. The head nurse must take the initiative in setting up these conferences. Too often the new team leader overestimates the performance expected of her and is reluctant to seek help until the point of complete frustration is reached. Miss Allen's statement to the head nurse at the end of the first week—that the transition from team member to team leader had not been difficult—may well have been a plea for indications from the head nurse of ways in which her performance could be improved, ways in which she could really lead. Since notation was made in the case description of weekly conferences between Mrs. Snyder and the new team leader, it seems reasonable to assume that daily meetings were not held.

On the other hand, if attendance of the head nurse at the team conferences had been mentioned, one could have assumed that Mrs. Snyder elected this alternative method of supervising a new team leader or that the head nurse was attending team conferences to keep informed about patients and to serve, when needed, as a resource person for the team. If she attends the team conference of a new team leader, she must take care not to usurp the position of leader of the group and negate the efforts of the novice to develop a cohesive group. This rapport is built on mutual respect between leader and team members, and the head nurse can, by her presence, destroy or foster it.

The incidents described in the second week seem to reveal that Miss Allen was having difficulty in delegating, that perhaps she was reluctant to assign more patients to others than to herself, that she assigned the nurse assistants to other team members and not to herself. Although the true meaning of the phrase "functioned smoothly" cannot be interpreted further, it seems to indicate, at least, that no complaints were expressed about the care rendered or the overt behavior of the group.

The patients' remarks to the head nurse about Miss Allen's enthusiasm may have been indicative of a growing feeling of security on the part of the staff nurse or of the empathy of patients for someone they recognize as struggling to learn a new skill. That Miss Allen sought the help of the head nurse in planning assignments may be a reflection of this same interest. It may have been precipitated by a feeling of security evoked when Mrs. Snyder reported the favorable comments of patients.

From the fact that the head nurse referred the team leader to the clinical instructor several points can be learned about the philosophy of team nursing held by the nursing department of the Charles Evans Memorial Hospital. First, the junior and senior nursing students were accorded a place on the nursing team. This is a hopeful sign. In some hospitals the student functions independently of the team, because of a belief that the service needs of the patients may outweigh the educational needs of the student, since the assignment of team members is in the hands of nursing service personnel. In other institutions the senior nursing student serves as a team leader, with the nursing instructor assuming the direct guidance of the student. On Division 4 West, the junior and senior nursing students apparently serve as team members and the clinical instructor orients the team leader to the needs and capabilities of the individual student, just as the head nurse does for other members assigned to the team. One may anticipate that the team leader may call upon the clinical instructor to supervise the student in new skills, just as she may have to require the assistance of the head nurse with other team members. There is no reason why the educational needs of the student cannot be met through serving as a team member as well as they would be if she were assigned to a group of patients under the case method in the same institution. In both situations there must be coordination and cooperation between nursing service and nursing education in addition to acceptance of the educational philosophy.

It would be interesting, at this point, to be able to poll the reactions of the readers to Miss Duncan's change of assignment from team leader to team member. A frequent reaction from individuals whose knowledge of the team concept is limited has been to consider this a demotion for the staff nurse who had previously been a team leader. On the other hand, individuals who have had experience in team nursing recognize that the exigencies of staffing a nursing unit with two teams for seven days a week, twenty-four hours a day with personnel who work five days a week, eight hours a day demand that there be more than six qualified team leaders for the unit. Actually nine (8.4) team leaders would be needed. This means that if a team leader were to serve in this role whenever on duty, on some days an extra team would have to be formed. This practice would seem to violate the principle of making every effort to promote continuity of care by utilizing continuity of assignment to the greatest extent possible. It seems then that there are two alternatives to establishing a group for a team leader to have someone to lead. The professional nurse could serve as a team member on the over-lapping days, or she could be given an independent assignment. Most persons would agree that to assign a former team leader to serve as a team member under the leadership of a neophyte may be threatening to the new team leader because of her lack of skill, and threatening to the former team leader if she thinks others may consider this a demotion. Unfortunately the concept of rank is a part of our culture, and this fact must be recognized. That Miss Duncan did not participate in the conference or accept the assistance offered may have been interpreted as her way of trying to take a "back seat" so that she would not be vying with Miss Allen for leadership of the team. This would not explain her lack of regard for the channels of communication established for the team method, however. These two facts then may lead one to assume that Miss Duncan was deliberately attempting to discredit Miss Allen's ability to lead.

In the third week of her leadership, Miss Allen gave evidence of being able to delegate more responsibility to team members. It is interesting to note that she did not assign patients to her peer until she had elicited her preference. As leader of the team, Miss Allen had information about patients and personnel upon which to base assignments. It is doubtful that Miss Duncan was as well informed about the total needs of the patients and personnel on the team. A team leader abdicates her leadership role if she does not assume control when the situation dictates.

Miss Allen's reaction to Miss Duncan's behavior is described in the case data by two facts: the reduction of time spent in team conference, and her comment to Mrs. Snyder at the end of the week. For a new team leader, the balance needed in a team conference between consultation, direction, and reception is not achieved easily. When frustration reaches a peak, a common defense mechanism used is that of avoidance. Miss Allen may have been reducing the duration of the conference in order to withdraw from the uncomfortable situation with Miss Duncan. This is unfortunate. This does not correct the situation, nor does it fulfill the purpose of the conference—communication for the promotion of dynamic patient care. Experience with team nursing has led to the empirical conclusion that there is a direct relationship between the time spent in group planning and the quality of patient care rendered. For example, when a nursing unit is fully occupied and the staff feels the pressure to produce, there may be a tendency to "postpone"—actually cancel—the team conference in the mistaken opinion that this time could be spent to greater advantage at the bedside. When this happens, a head nurse can support the team leader and the team by assuming the care of patients in order to free members for the conference. This practice should reinforce the importance of the conference and emphasize the relationship between conference and care, planning and performance. In the situation on Division 4 West the head nurse seems to have two alternatives: remove Miss Duncan from the team, or support Miss Allen by attending the team conference. It may be that both of these actions are required at this point. The response of the head nurse to the staff nurse's expression of unreadiness may have an enduring effect on the future development of Miss Allen as a professional nurse and as a team leader.

This case contains aspects related to the functioning of two levels of nursing personnel—the staff nurse and head nurse—in providing personnel for patient care. Although the steps in the application of the *administrative blueprint* have not been identified as such, this discussion is an *evaluation* of the care plans of the staff nurse and the head nurse and, at the same time, a part of the *thinking* phase of a plan for subsequent action.

SUPPLEMENTARY READING LIST

American Nurses' Association: "Auxiliary Personnel in Nursing Service," *American Journal of Nursing*, vol. 62, pp. 72–73, July, 1962.

Barrett, Jean: *The Head Nurse: Her Changing Role*, 2d ed., Appleton-Century-Crofts, Inc., New York, 1968.

Bauer, Annabel B.: *An Experimental In-Service Program for Implementing Team Nursing*, National League for Nursing, New York, 1966.

Beltran, Helen G., et al.: *Guide for Leadership in Team Nursing*, League Exchange No. 54, National League for Nursing, New York, 1961.

Bennett, Addison C.: "Communication and Administration," *Hospital Topics*, vol. 46, pp. 44–46, May, 1968.

Bennett, Addison C.: "Improving Downward Communication," *Hospital Topics*, vol. 46, 58–61, June, 1968.

Brooks, Ethel A.: "Team Nursing—1961," *American Journal of Nursing*, vol. 61, pp. 87–91, April, 1961.

Brown, Elaine, and John Roche: "Methods Study Shaped Team Nursing Plan," *Modern Hospital*, vol. 107, pp. 121–123, September, 1966.

Festog, Eleanor J., and Billie Cook: "Two Head Nurses Talk About Team Nursing," *American Journal of Nursing*, vol. 63, p. 93, November, 1963.

Frey, Mary: "A Look at Job Descriptions," *American Journal of Nursing*, vol. 60, pp. 1782–1783, December, 1960.

Jones, Edna M.: "Who Supports the Nurse?" *Nursing Outlook*, vol. 10, pp. 476–478, July, 1962.

Kriegel, Julia: *The Head Nurse: Thoughts and Decisions*, The Macmillan Company, New York, 1968.

Kron, Thora: *Nursing Team Leadership*, 2d ed., W. B. Saunders Company, Philadelphia, 1966.

Lambertsen, Eleanor C.: *Education for Nursing Leadership*, J. B. Lippincott Company, Philadelphia, 1958, pp. 141–164.

Lambertsen, Eleanor C.: *Nursing Team Organization and Functioning*, Bureau of Publications, Teachers College, Columbia University, 1953.

Melody, Mary, and Genevieve Clark: "Walking-Planning Rounds," *American Journal of Nursing*, vol. 67, pp. 771–773, April, 1967.

Mercy Hospital (Pittsburgh, Pennsylvania): *A Manual for Team Nursing*, Catholic Hospital Association, St. Louis, 1968.

Roth, Julius A.: "How Nurses' Aides Learn Their Jobs," *American Journal of Nursing*, vol. 62, pp. 54–57, August, 1962.

Swansburg, Russell C.: "An Experiment in Team Nursing," *Nursing Outlook*, vol. 16, pp. 45–47, August, and pp. 42–43, September, 1968.

Uris, Auren, and Betty Shapin: *Working with People*, The Macmillan Company, New York, 1953, pp. 263–273.

Wood, M. Marian: "From General Duty Nurse to Team Leader," *American Journal of Nursing*, vol. 63, pp. 104–105, January, 1963.

Wyatt, Lalla J., and Helen D. Hannah: "Does Team Nursing Work in a Psychiatric Hospital?" *American Journal of Nursing*, vol. 64, pp. 132–134, June, 1964.

case **4**

The Staff Nurse and the Evaluation Process

The following incident occurred on Division 5 South of the Charles Evans Memorial Hospital. This unit has a capacity for thirty adult patients recommended for admission to the medical service by the medical clinic. The medical care for these patients is provided by interns and assistant residents on the medical service under the direction of the chief resident and the clinical faculty of the medical school.

Case Data

Case Notes

Miss Suzanne Wood joined the nursing staff of the Charles Evans Memorial Hospital two years ago and was assigned as a staff nurse to a medical division for private patients. Six months ago, to meet a staffing need, she was asked to transfer to Division 5 South. On this division she worked two month-long tours of evening duty and one tour of night duty. Prior to her first experience on each tour she had an informal conference with the head nurse, Miss Jane Alexander, at which time her performance to date was discussed and the job description for the evening or night staff nurse was reviewed.

One afternoon Miss Wood was sitting in the ward office reporting to the head nurse about the patients for whom she had cared that day. At the completion of the report, Miss Alexander informed Miss Wood that she was writing an evaluation of Miss Wood's performance and would like to discuss it with her the following week. She gave Miss Wood a copy of the evaluation form for review and commented, "Of course, you are familiar with the form from your evaluation conferences with the head nurse on 4 South." Miss Wood said, "Thank you," took the form, and left the office.

Case Data *Case Notes*

Five days later, Miss Alexander asked Miss Wood to plan the care for her patients so that she could be free for a conference at 2 P.M. At 1:30 P.M. an acutely ill patient was admitted to the division. His immediate care required the attention of the entire professional nursing staff on the division. Consequently, the evaluation conference had to be postponed until the following day.

At the start of the conference the following day, the head nurse said that she enjoyed having Miss Wood on her division and hoped the assignment would be permanent, as Miss Wood was an asset to the staff. To this statement Miss Wood made no response. When asked whether she had any questions to ask about the purpose and use of the performance evaluations Miss Wood replied, "No." Miss Alexander then reviewed the period of time the written evaluation covered as well as the opportunities she had had to observe Miss Wood's performance. She related the areas in which Miss Wood's performance was equal to or above the performance of the other staff nurses. She emphasized the progress the staff nurse had made in the past six months. The head nurse suggested that Miss Wood now knew the division personnel and routines well enough to take more initiative in contributing to the development of the nursing assistants assigned to the division. Miss Wood appeared to listen intently to these comments. She did not question any statements, however, nor ask for elaboration on any point. She kept her hands tightly clenched and seemed to be anxious for the conference to end. Miss Alexander gave her the written evaluation to read. Miss Wood spent ten minutes reading the comments and suggestions before she signed the form to signify that it had been discussed with her. She said, "Thank you," as she returned the form to Miss Alexander. The head nurse then asked, "Does this evaluation concur with the ones you were given on 4 South?" Miss Wood replied quickly, "I have not had any written performance evaluations since I was a student. I was worried

Case Data | *Case Notes*

that I was doing something wrong when you told me that you were writing one. The policy for written evaluations was explained in my orientation to the hospital, but that was 2½ years ago. She then picked up the completed form and discussed two of the comments with Miss Alexander. As she left the head nurse's office she commented, "Thank you for the opportunity to discuss ways in which I can contribute further to the care of patients on this unit."

DISCUSSION

The prime requisite for every organization is a goal, a purpose. And as soon as a goal has been established someone, somewhere, begins to evaluate the progress of the organization toward the achievement of the goal. This evaluation may not be submitted in written form; it may be evidenced in other ways—by the bank which grants a loan to an organization, by the customer who agrees to purchase a product, by a patient who makes an elective choice of a hospital, by the ability to recruit and retain personnel.

Every organization, in turn, evaluates itself. It uses various objective and subjective measures and formal and informal approaches in appraising its progress in the achievement of implicit and explicit goals. The performance of employees in the pursuit of these goals is an integral part of the evaluation process. Some readers may deny the validity of the preceding statement by saying, "It shouldn't be considered necessary. There is no evaluation of employees in our institution and we get along." To this one would have to answer that although there may not be a systematic evaluation program, employees *are* being evaluated continuously. If the question were raised, "Which employee contributes the most?" or "Why was Sam Jones promoted instead of Richard Barker?," the answers would signify that appraisals are being made even if they are not being identified as such.

Herman Finer notes in a discussion of performance evaluation:[1]

> The earliest objective of efficiency ratings was to possess an instrument which might have a disciplinary value—which would be the criterion of promotions, demotions, salary increases or decreases, suspensions, and dis-

[1] Herman Finer, *Administration and the Nursing Services,* The Macmillan Company, New York, 1952, p. 260.

> missals. . . . The disciplinary idea cannot be abandoned, but it is one of the several objectives of the evaluation of performance.

Unfortunately, this concept of performance evaluation as an instrument for reprehension has persisted much longer in practice that it has in theory, and more apprehension than anticipation is evoked in the hearts of many when apprised of a forthcoming evaluation. The case data seem to reveal that apprehension was responsible for the behavior of the staff nurse, Miss Wood.

Evaluation is a function of the staff nurse as a part of her participation in nursing care and in administration in nursing. If a staff nurse has accepted this as a function, what are some of the possible reasons for the tension that is apt to arise when her own performance is to be evaluated?

Through the many experiences an individual has with evaluations—report cards from grade school, tests in school, tests for a driver's license or admission to a program in nursing, references from teachers, friends, employees—he develops certain reactions to evaluation. Viewed from any angle, a performance rating is certain to arouse emotions in an individual. In his book, *Managerial Psychology,* Harold J. Leavitt makes the following comments about reactions to appraisal:[2]

> . . . we can predict that they (people) will have mixed feelings about assessment, both resenting and seeking it out. We should expect resentment because assessment is a threat to independence and autonomy. But we should also expect people to "want to know where they stand," to want to know whether they are loved and thought well of by those on whom they depend.

Forewarned by these predictions, what precautions should be practiced, what principles should be applied to the function of evaluation of personnel? An analysis of the case situation may reveal some of the positive and negative components of the process. From the facts that an evaluation form was available, that Miss Alexander assumed Miss Wood had received written evaluations in her position on another division, and that the policy on evaluations had been discussed in the orientation of the staff nurse to the hospital one can postulate that the nursing department of the Charles Evans Memorial Hospital had established an evaluation program. It is not disclosed whether a definite schedule for evaluations was stipu-

[2] Harold J. Leavitt, *Managerial Psychology,* The University of Chicago Press, Chicago, 1958, p. 104.

lated, but from the fact that Miss Alexander prepared an evaluation of Miss Wood six months after her transfer to the division, it seems logical to assume, at least, that there were some recommendations regarding time intervals and that the head nurse on 4 South had not followed these recommendations. This may have been a reflection of her lack of acceptance of a philosophy of evaluation in general, of staff nurses, or of Miss Wood, in particular.

If for no reason other than to combat the destructive aspects of evaluation that seem to overshadow the constructive ones in an informal or covert system of appraisal, an organization should have a well-defined program for the evaluation of personnel. To progress rather than regress an organization must motivate its personnel to continuous development. A systematic appraisal program can serve as a tool for this objective. It can also provide a basis for administrative decisions—whom to promote, what to pay, whom to single out for additional education or training, whom to demote or transfer. In addition, an evaluation may serve to meet the ever-present, if unvoiced, need of an individual to know what progress he is making. In a service organization such as a hospital, one can also add to the service rendered patients through an evaluation of the performance of personnel. A satisfactory evaluation system can serve the patient, the hospital, and the employee.

The initiation and continuation of an effective program must be based on a philosophy of forecasting the future rather than simply recording the past. It is not enough to evaluate the past performance of an employee. One must assist this same employee to see how he can improve in the future. Even when the evaluation has disclosed eligibility for promotion, it is necessary to help the individual identify what talents he brings to the new position and what skills he will need to function effectively in the new situation.

Because accepting the value of an evaluation system is easier than implementing a program, continuous support for the program must be given by all levels of administration. Most persons undertake the rendering of a judgment with extreme reluctance. The establishment of governing policies can facilitate the process. Establishing and adhering to a definite schedule for the completion of evaluation on each employee lessens the possibility that an individual will regard the evaluation as a disciplinary tool. Miss Wood's reaction was understandable when she was suddenly faced with a recorded rating after 2½ years on the staff. Providing for the evaluation of employees at all levels, i.e., nursing assistant, practical nurse, head nurse, and supervisor, emphasizes the expectations of everyone to progress in his position, be it at the top, bottom, or middle of the organization chart. Standards must be established for evaluating performance. Unless there is a standard, neither supervisor nor employee can measure and evaluate performance. Well-written, detailed job descriptions can serve as standards. The employee, however, must be familiar with and accept the job description from the beginning if it is to serve effectively as a standard. The job description, the evaluation form, and the evaluation program should be included in the content of the employee's orientation to the position.

Selection of the form to be used for recording the data and the evaluation should be made on the basis of the established purposes and standards. There is considerable controversy about the use of the same form for all levels of personnel. Some say this is a more democratic approach; others that it is not possible to recognize the specific contributions of a head nurse, staff nurse, and nurse assistant on the same type of form. Since there are so many types of forms, the only definitive statement that can be made is that each organization must analyze published forms or original forms in relation to its own objectives or beliefs. Persons who promote the use of the same form for all levels of personnel as a more democratic technique than another must be careful to avoid the inclusion of items to which exceptions must be made for various levels. Persons who advocate the use of more than one form must consider the number of levels a supervisor is called upon to evaluate and whether the use of several different forms will help or hinder the task. These two sides of the question may be answered by the use of a relatively blank form, for all levels, based upon a guide devised for the use of the form with each classification of employee. This, incidentally, would lower printing costs.

There are many different techniques for rating the employee. Whatever the technique, the following areas should be included:

1. The aspects of the employee's performance that are outstanding and satisfactory
2. The areas in which improvement should be achieved
3. The areas into which the employee is now prepared to expand

These areas may be identified on a graphic rating scale on which certain traits are identified. The employee may then be rated within the limits listed for each trait, or against the performance of other staff members in the same situation.

Alternative ways of listing these traits are shown in Figures 4 and 5. Of these examples, the scale in Figure 4 is more descriptive; yet, an employee may well be rated, for instance, under these two limitations simultaneously: "volunteers when assignment completed" and "makes maximum use of available time." The rating "loafs unless closely super-

Utilization of time	Loafs unless closely supervised.	Volunteers when assignment completed.	Keeps busy but not always with essential tasks.	Needs direction in using time to advantage.	Makes maximum use of available time.
Ability to work with others	Shows respect for everyone on the team.	Seems to work best alone.	Works well with some but not all of team.	Able to give or take whatever necessary for effective functioning of team.	Assists others only when own work is completed.

FIGURE 4. Graphic rating scale with limitations listed.

Utilization of time	Excellent	Poor	Average	Above average	Below average
Ability to work with others	Poor	Above average	Excellent	Below average	Average

FIGURE 5. Graphic rating scale based on comparisons with the performance of other employees.

vised," however, certainly tells more about the employee's *utilization of time* than does the rating *poor* (Figure 5). In both scales the values are placed horizontally in random order rather than in ascending or descending degrees of achievement. This arrangement forces the rater to read each item to select a value, instead of deciding in advance that a person is average and automatically checking the "average" column throughout the form. This type of rating scale identifies the traits to be observed and judged and is convenient to use. This convenience is also one of its drawbacks. The speed with which it can be checked tends to defeat the careful analysis an employee's performance deserves. Too often, also, the traits are not sufficiently defined to avert a wide range of interpretations by various raters.

Figure 6 is an excerpt from a rating scale used in the past at University Hospitals of Cleveland. This form provides a definition of the factor being appraised, and it gives somewhat more detailed descriptions of behavior than do the rating scales shown previously. By means of

	☐ ☐	☐ ☐	☐ ☐
Loyalty The employee's awareness and support of the policies and goals of the hospital: 1. quality patient care 2. research goal 3. teaching goal 4. safety	Does the individual actively support and interpret hospital policies and goals, offering constructive criticism when appropriate?	Does the individual passively support hospital policies and goals?	Is the individual consistent in giving support to hospital policies and goals?
Empathy The employee's ability to objectively appreciate the behavior and feelings of patients and their families	☐ ☐ Does the individual consistently appreciate the behavior and feelings of patients and their families and respond accordingly?	☐ ☐ Does the individual usually appreciate the behavior and feelings of patients and their families and respond accordingly?	☐ ☐ Does the individual appreciate the behavior and feelings of patients and their families only when they coincide with the worker's?

FIGURE 6. Excerpt from *Progress Report—Nursing Service Personnel,* University Hospitals of Cleveland, Cleveland, Ohio, 1958.

the square above each of the three specifications for the factor, the rater has six decisions. If the specification describes the usual behavior of the individual a check mark is placed in the left square. If it does not describe the employee accurately, but more nearly than the next lower specification, a check mark is placed in the right square. In addition to rating the individual on these factors, the rater is required to write a summary of his appraisal of the worker's performance in a statement that emphasizes the individual strengths and weaknesses of the employee.

The critical incident method of rating, which has been used in schools of nursing for some time, is being used increasingly in business—perhaps because of the growing emphasis on the employee as an individual rather than as a number on a payroll card or perhaps in an effort to discard the printed rating scales, which are reminiscent of disciplinary tools.

The term *anecdotal record* is familiar to many in nursing. The critical incident rating method is based on the collection of anecdotes that describe an individual's behavior in various components of the job. These anecdotes should describe what was actually said or done and the setting in which the action took place. No attempt should be made to evaluate the behavior at the time. Two examples of anecdotes are shown in Figure 7.

Suzanne Wood, April 1, 1963

Miss Wood was walking down the corridor carrying a medicine tray. Dr. Jones stopped her and asked, "Can you tell me how Mrs. Hopkin's IV is running?" Miss Wood replied, "I do not know, but Mrs. Carlson has been caring for her. The ward clerk can locate her for you." She then proceeded down the hall, entered Mrs. Hopkin's room to administer a preoperative medication.

Suzanne Wood, April 10, 1963

Miss Wood was sitting at the charting desk. Dr. Overholtz approached to ask how much Mrs. Randall's oral intake had been in the last 24 hours. Miss Wood handed him Mrs. Randall's chart and then left the station to locate Mrs. Carlson, who was assigned to the patient. She returned in a few minutes and advised Dr. Overholtz of the amount taken but not yet recorded.

FIGURE 7. Anecdotal records.

From the anecdotes in Figure 7 one may begin to identify Miss Wood's cooperation with members of the health team, but more recordings in similar situations are needed before one can formulate a conclusion that bespeaks the subject's usual behavior in such situations. If the incidents are recorded accurately and if enough of them are collected to represent an individual's usual behavior, they can provide a factual approach to the evaluation of performance. But this requires much time and effort. The failure to collect anecdotes at frequent intervals may find the supervisor with an evaluation to make and not enough critical incidents upon which to formulate a judgment.

Many organizations use some type of free-form evaluation record. These forms usually contain a list of the attributes to consider, such as level of energy, reliability, poise, etc. Space is provided opposite each trait for the rater to describe the subject's achievement of the particular attribute. These relatively unstructured forms are usually accompanied by a guide sheet which enumerates in greater detail the behavior related to each attribute. This type of form usually individualizes the evaluation and permits greater flexibility. It is more time consuming than the rating scale; less than the critical incident method. The value of the material recorded, to the employee and to others, depends to a great extent on the ability of the rater to express observations perceptively. To write a concise, meaningful, descriptive statement of another's behavior is exceedingly difficult for many and impossible for some. For this reason, a recent trend in education and in nursing education may offer some valuable assistance to those responsible for evaluating the performance of others.

Educators have found that clearly defined goals are essential to the evaluation of the progress of the learner and to the selection of appropriate instructional content, materials, and methods. Without descriptive statements of the specific observable behaviors to be acquired by the learner through the instructional process, the educators cannot measure student attainment of educational objectives. Clearly defined goals also enable the student to evaluate his own progress.

With clear objectives in view, the student knows which activities on his part are relevant to his success, and it is no longer necessary for him to "psych out" the instructor.[3]

The same principles are relevant to the evaluation of the performance of nursing personnel. Nursing departments have stated goals for patient care in broad terms. For these goals to be useful in the guidance direction, and development of staff, additional steps are required. The goals are defined further by specifying the behaviors which are indicative of the attainment of objectives. The degree to which a supervisor, staff nurse, licensed practical nurse, and other members of the nursing staff may be expected to manifest each stated behavior are delineated next. These behavioral statements then become the criteria against which performance is measured and from which staff development efforts are derived. The initial task of stating objectives in behavioral terms is time consuming and demanding. The benefits that accrue to patients and to

[3] Robert F. Mager, *Preparing Objectives for Programmed Instruction*, Fearon Publishers, Inc., San Francisco, 1962, p. 4.

personnel are ample compensation for the effort. Grace Fivars and Doris Gosnell present many examples of behavioral statements of nursing performance in *Nursing Evaluation: The Problem and the Process.*[4] Although the statements were prepared for use in the evaluation of the performance of students in the clinical laboratory, they are relevant to the assessment of nursing personnel employed by hospitals and other health agencies. The ideal method of evaluation has not been devised. This new approach offers a challenge to more traditional methods and may provide a solution to the problems in the evaluation process.

The case data do not describe the type of evaluation form used at the Charles Evans Memorial Hospital. It is evident, however, that a form was used to provide evidence of Miss Wood's performance in the permanent record of her employment at the hospital.

Regardless of the form used, the success of an evaluation program depends upon the person or persons doing the assessing. The rater must keep in mind that he cannot be subjective; he must be objective. Granted that some tools will facilitate objectivity, it is impossible to remove the subjective element from the evaluation process. Human beings cannot disregard their personal feelings and ingrained biases. The sooner this fact is recognized the sooner progress may be made in this area. Several authorities on evaluation have proposed that having more than one individual rate the employee will reduce the degree of subjectivity. This may prove to be true if the several raters are given equal opportunity to observe the worker in similar situations. Suppose, however, the head nurse and the evening supervisor meet to discuss the performance of a staff nurse. The head nurse may be considering the staff nurse's behavior as a team member, the supervisor as a charge nurse with whom she has contact once or twice in an evening. Suppose, also, that the head nurse and the supervisor differ on judgments. Is it not possible the rank of the supervisor may influence the head nurse's final decision?

The rater must be aware of the weaknesses in any evaluation process and must strive to evaluate an individual's performance as nearly as possible on his merits, by prescribed standards, and on facts. If the rater concentrates on one trait at a time, the human tendency to react favorably or unfavorably to the individual as a whole because of the approval or dis-

[4] Grace Fivars and Doris Gosnell, *Nursing Evaluation: The Problem and the Process,* The Macmillan Company, New York, 1966, pp. 145–199.

approval of one trait will be minimal. The nurse who is not neatly dressed may be extremely accurate and orderly in recording and transcribing vital information. A recent event should not outweigh accumulated evidence. Nor should the past stand in the way of recent progress. The rater should consider the employee's performance since the last evaluation or over the period the rater, personally, has observed the employee. Also, the employee's performance, not potential, should be considered. The anticipated progress should be discussed and included in recommendations, but not in the resume of performance to date. The final caution relates to the primary objective of any evaluation—encouragement and support of the continued development of an individual. Every consideration in an evaluation should have this aim in mind. To avoid commenting on weaknesses is to deny the purpose of an evaluation. On the other hand, to criticize without offering constructive suggestions serves no beneficial purpose. The likelihood that the evaluation will be as objective as humanly possible will be enhanced if the rater is more interested in helping the employee than in justifying the appraisal.

Miss Alexander honored many of these principles and reviewed them with Miss Wood in the evaluation conference. Since the review of the evaluation with the subject is the crucial point in the whole process, it is unfortunate that the original appointment had to be canceled. If Miss Alexander had been aware of Miss Wood's anxiety, perhaps she would have arranged with the supervisor for assistance with the emergency so that the conference could have been held. The appraisal interview serves as an excellent tool for recognizing the employee as an individual rather than as just a person needed to do a job. It should be a person-to-person meeting, not an across-the-desk contact of superior and subordinate. It should be an elicitation of the employee's suggestions, attitudes, and insights; not simply a recital of faults. During the interview, the employee must be given an opportunity to express his opinion of the evaluation and to correct any misinformation. It seems unnecessary to add that the person who writes the appraisal should be the one to conduct the conference, but not infrequently, at some later date, an evaluation made by a head nurse is revealed to the employee by the supervisor.

Because of the anxiety that may be aroused when an employee is advised that a rating has been done and a discussion of it is forthcoming, some supervisors have attempted to initiate a conference without forewarning. While this may preclude apprehension, it seldom achieves satisfactory results. The anxiety is created suddenly. The employee does not have an opportunity to build up his defenses, nor to attempt to evaluate his own performance. In this instance, the "conference" may be over before the individual has had an opportunity to recover. He has not had the advantage of time in which to formulate questions, and he may thereafter distrust spontaneous conferences. The rater always has the advantage of knowing what is written. The employee should at least be told what is to be discussed. It should not be assumed, as it was in the case situation, that the individual comes to the conference with the same objectives as does the rater. During orientation, the information given about an evaluation program does not necessarily convince the employee of its need or value to him. Harold J. Leavitt issues this advice about the evaluation conference:[5]

> Such personal, face-to-face evaluation always means that information about the other person filters through the screen of the judge's own needs and prejudices. . . . The alternative for the judge is to recognize the characteristics of his own filters and then to pay attention to what comes through these filters.
>
> For whether one tries to or not, he listens to another person at two levels: at the level of the speaker's words and the information they carry, and at the level of the listener's own feelings about the speaker's words and the feelings these words convey. For example, most people can decide quickly whether or not another person seems to be afraid of them, or angry at them, or comfortable or uncomfortable with them, whether he talks too much for their liking, whether he has what they consider a good sense of humor, etc. And yet, in most formal evaluation situations, we often try consciously to block out and ignore this fundamental source of information, preferring to deal with what we like to think of as "the facts."

It is possible that Miss Alexander was so tense about holding an evaluation conference that she was unable to see Miss Wood's manifestations of anxiety—the clenched hands, the lack of response. Perhaps Miss Wood was not usually communicative. But if this were so, why did Miss Alexander persist in trying to evoke a response from her? It requires skill to convey to an individual his right, responsibility, and obligation to correct any misstatements and his freedom to express an opinion of the evaluation. It brings little satisfaction to either participant to have the employee write in the comment section, "I agree completely with this evaluation and I will try to improve."

The head nurse did suggest that Miss Wood was now familiar enough

[5] Harold J. Leavitt, *Managerial Psychology*, The University of Chicago Press, Chicago, 1958, pp. 101–102.

with the division to take initiative in the development of the nurse assistants. In other words, she was apparently attempting to motivate the staff nurse to utilize her potential and to continue to expand her realm of competence. It is to be hoped that Miss Alexander offered some clues as to how Miss Wood could do this and that the suggestions were recorded. After suggestions have been made, it is essential that they be followed up by direct observation and support. It serves no purpose if the only reference to a suggestion is made at the time of a subsequent evaluation, when a determination is made as to whether or not an employee followed a suggestion.

Some persons may feel tempted to say that the staff nurse demonstrated a lack of initiative when she did not question the head nurse on 4 South about the failure to receive an evaluation. Realistically, however, one must accept the premise that previous experience with report cards, ratings, and efficiency reports conditions an individual to avoid evaluation, whenever possible. Without guidance, an individual cannot appreciate that the purpose of an evaluation in his adult work situation is development, not faultfinding.

No discussion of evaluation would be complete without some comments on self-evaluation—a magic, meritorious, but often misunderstood term. If, by *self-evaluation,* one means "self-criticism," the term is understood correctly. It is possible for an individual to identify for himself areas of weakness and areas of strength; it is not possible for him to place a value judgment on himself. He can, however, participate in establishing the standards by which he can evaluate himself and can expect to be evaluated. To do so is a departure from the traditional approach to the evaluation process, but it offers a possible solution to a persistent problem in administration.

It is recommended that when an employee assumes a new position, he and the person to whom he is responsible, his *immediate* supervisor, discuss not only the requirements of the job but the objectives the employee can hope to achieve in the first two months of duty. These objectives should be observable and specific. For a staff nurse the objectives may be to familiarize herself with the hospital's methods of charting, requisitioning, and administering medications and admitting and discharging patients and to give direct care to the patients. At the end of the two-month period the staff nurse and her immediate supervisor, the head nurse, would review the staff nurse's knowledge of these considerations. The review may establish a new set of objectives for the next time interval, two or three months in duration. The interval between the evaluation sessions may well be lengthened each time. It is anticipated that the objectives would become either greater in number or broader in scope with each successive conference. Whenever new goals are set, these would be the employee's goals for himslf, not the employer's objectives imposed upon him. The role of the supervisor is to provide the assistance needed and requested by the employee in his efforts to achieve self-determined goals. The employee takes the initiative, the supervisor lends the support.

The above approach may eliminate some of the anxiety that occurs in relation to being evaluated. The employee knows the limits set on evaluation; the supervisor knows what the individual expects. The element of "will he be hurt or helped by what I have to say" is minimal. In nursing service, this approach may facilitate the absorption of a new staff member into the nursing team on the unit by limiting her perspective to a few specific objectives before expecting her to become oriented to the entire hospital. It would enable the staff nurse to concentrate on patient care before she is expected to assume "desk duties." And above all, this approach may serve to emphasize the adjustment and continued development of the individual.

The evaluation step of the blueprint has once again led into the thinking step of a proposed plan for action.

SUPPLEMENTARY READING LIST

Alexander, Edythe, et al.: *Nursing Service Administration: Principles and Practice,* The C. V. Mosby Company, St. Louis, 1962, pp. 52–53, 191–193.

Barrett, Jean: *The Head Nurse: Her Changing Role,* 2d ed., Appleton-Century-Crofts, Inc., New York, 1968.

Beach, Lester R., and Elon L. Clark: *Psychology in Business,* McGraw-Hill Book Company, New York, 1959, pp. 210–225.

Bloom, Benjamin S., et al.: *Taxonomy of Educational Objectives. Handbook I, Cognitive Domain,* David McKay Company, Inc., New York, 1956.

Broderick, Thomas J.: "How to Help Supervisors Evaluate Employees," *The Modern Hospital,* vol. 95, pp. 89–93, September, 1960.

Chernushin, Mary, and James Galvin: "Evaluation That Is Frankly Subjective," *American Journal of Nursing,* vol. 62, pp. 92–93, February, 1962.

Clissold, Grace K., and Edith A. Metz: "Evaluation—A Tangible Process," *Nursing Outlook,* vol. 14, pp. 41–45, March, 1966.

Cochran, Thelma C., and Paul J. Hansen: "Developing an Evaluation Tool by Group Action," *American Journal of Nursing,* vol. 62, pp. 94–97, March, 1962.

Cochran, Thelma C., and Paul J. Hansen: "A Nurse-Devised Evaluation System for Nurses," *Hospitals, J.A.H.A.*, vol. 36, pp. 100, 102, 104, March 1, 1962.

Conta, A. Lionne, et al.: "Professional Performance Committees," *American Journal of Nursing*, vol. 68, pp. 2601–2607, December, 1968.

Finer, Herman: *Administration and the Nursing Services*, The Macmillan Company, New York, 1952, p. 28, 259–263.

Fivars, Grace, and Doris Gosnell: *Nursing Evaluation: The Problem and the Process*, The Macmillan Company, New York, 1966, pp. 145–199.

Gordon, Phoebe: "Evaluation: A Tool in Nursing Service," *American Journal of Nursing*, vol. 60, pp. 364–366, March, 1961.

Jennings, Muriel: "On-the-Job Counseling—A Precious Charge," *American Journal of Nursing*, vol. 61, pp. 67–70, March, 1961.

Leavitt, Harold J.: *Managerial Psychology*, The University of Chicago Press, Chicago, 1958, pp. 81–105.

Mager, Robert F.: *Preparing Objectives for Programmed Instruction*, Fearon Publishers, Inc., San Francisco, 1962.

Mayfield, Harold: "In Defense of Performance Appraisal," *Harvard Business Review*, vol. 38, pp. 81–87, March–April, 1960.

Mitchell, Margaret L.: "Performance Review of the Executive," *Journal of the American Dietetic Association*, vol. 46, pp. 361–363, May, 1965.

Newman, William H., and Charles E. Summer, Jr.: *The Process of Management: Concepts, Behavior and Practice*, Prentice-Hall, Inc., Englewood Cliffs, N.J., 1961, pp. 537–542.

case 5

The Head Nurse and Decision Making

The pediatric department of the Charles Evans Memorial Hospital consists of two divisions for patients: Division 3 East, a thirty-five-bed unit for infants and toddlers and Division 3 West, a thirty-bed unit for children aged three to thirteen. Supervision of the patient care and nursing activities on these two units is the responsibility of Miss Helen Robertson, Supervisor of Specialty Services (pediatric, psychiatric, geriatric, and orthopedic). At the time of the following incident, Mrs. Rosalie Glenn had been the head nurse on the infant's division for two years.

Case Data

Case Notes

Four students in the Charles Evans Memorial Hospital School of Nursing invited Mrs. Glenn to serve as a guest panelist for a discussion of visiting hours for pediatric units. In the discussion period following the presentation, the students asked Mrs. Glenn why the pediatric units of the hospital had not followed the trend toward rooming-in for mothers of infants and young children. Mrs. Glenn replied that such a change had been mentioned several times by staff nurses and physicians but had never really been studied.

The following week, in the nursing staff conference on 3 East, one of the nurses presented the nursing care plan for Sue Ellen Wilson, a nineteen-month-old infant admitted the previous week with severe burns. She described the difficulties she and other staff members had encountered in encouraging Sue to drink fluids and the mother's concern about Sue's apparent withdrawal from her parents when they visited her. Several suggestions were offered as means of increasing the infant's fluid intake. These were added to the nursing care plan. It was also proposed that special arrangements be made so that Sue's mother could stay with her. All agreed that Sue needed more frequent contact with her parents than the regular visiting

Case Data *Case Notes*

hours permitted. Mrs. Glenn stated that she would notify the reception desk of the special arrangements for Mrs. Wilson. One of the new staff nurses recounted her experiences on a pediatric unit with rooming-in and asked why this arrangement did not exist on Divisions 3 East and West. Mrs. Glenn laughed and said, "The only reason I can think of offhand is the standard one—'We have always done it that way!' " This comment drew smiles from some and a proposal from one member—"Perhaps we should think seriously about this practice." The head nurse suggested that the question be raised again at the following week's conference.

When Miss Robertson came to 3 East the next day, Mrs. Glenn mentioned the discussion about visiting hours. Their conversation was interrupted by Robert Janeway, a staff nurse, who reported that Jimmy Elliott (age 14 months) had suddenly developed acute respiratory distress. Mrs. Glenn dispatched Mr. Janeway to stay with the patient while she summoned medical assistance. She then visited the patient's bedside. After observing the infant's condition, she decided that constant nursing observation and attendance would be required for a minimum of several hours. She reviewed the staffing for the division and the needs of the patients, and then revised the patient assignment to free Mr. Janeway to remain with Jimmy throughout the day. She and Miss Robertson agreed that further evaluation of the infant's condition would have to be made to determine whether additional staff would be needed for the evening tour.

As they resumed the discussion of rooming-in arrangements, Mrs. Glenn commented, "Since several members of the staff have now evidenced interest in considering the issue, I think the present policy should be scrutinized." Miss Robertson suggested that Mrs. Glenn and her staff first consider the policy in relation to the needs of the patients on 3 East and then submit recommendations to the Nursing Service Planning Committee for consideration of the broader

Case Data | *Case Notes*

implications of any change. She mentioned several areas that would be affected by any change—laundry, cafeteria, parking lot, reception and information desk, elevators. Miss Robertson also suggested that the staff on 3 West be included in the discussions because they would be directly involved in any change. She asked Mrs. Glenn to keep her informed of the progress of the discussions and to call upon her for help as needed. As Miss Robertson was leaving Mrs. Glenn commented, "I should thank Sue Ellen for precipitating a discussion of this problem at last."

DISCUSSION

The use of the phrase *decision making* in the title of this case may seem redundant to the reader who has accepted the statements (Chapter 9) that the administrative process, the decision-making process, and the scientific process are essentially the same process. If these statements are valid, then the activities of the head nurse are decision-making activities. Although it is generally accepted that the head nurse holds an administrative position, few would say that her role is primarily that of decision making. Herbert A. Simon offers an explanation which seems to reflect the opinions currently held in nursing.[1] He suggests that the concept of decision making is confined to the formulation of overall policy. For this reason the importance of decision making at every level of an organization has not been recognized. Simon emphasizes, however, that the task of deciding is as necessary to the entire administrative organization as is the task of doing.

Current concepts of administration in nursing may lead many nursing administrators to say that this case involves the staffing and planning or policy-determining functions of the head nurse; in other words, emphasizing the doing rather than the deciding. While these concepts may have served well in the earlier authoritarian atmosphere in nursing service situations, reliance on such functional concepts seems to narrow perspectives and to restrict solutions. The newer concept of decision making as the core of the administrative process is more com-

[1] Herbert Alexander Simon, *Administrative Behavior,* 2d ed., The Macmillan Company, 1957, p. 1.

patible with a democratic approach to administration in any organization.

The ability to make decisions has become the prime requisite for success in administration. The rapid advance of knowledge, the increase in specialization, and the very pace of activities preclude the possibility of establishing routine approaches to problems. The administrator in any organization has to be able to make decisions; he cannot rely on procedures alone. This requisite would seem to be self-evident to present-day nursing, but too frequently emphasis is placed on procedures rather than on principles, on techniques rather than on thinking, on doing rather than on deciding.

The term *decision* is not limited to what shall be done, but is expanded to include the who, why, where, and when of the proposed action. It is used in the context delineated by Daniel E. Griffiths in his theory of administration as decision making.[2] He applied the term not only to the initial judgment but to all subsequent steps required to effect action based on that judgment.

The steps, or facets, of the decision-making process are outlined differently by authorities in administration. Edward H. Litchfield divided the activity of decision making into five subactivities.[3] Griffiths identifies six components.[4] Newman and Summer describe four elements of rational decision making.[5] Still another writer specifies three phases.[6] All evidence indicates essential agreement in the intent and content of the decision-making process, which includes the following activities:

1. Recognition and definition of the problem
2. Analysis of the situation
3. Proposal of several possible solutions
4. Comparison of the several solutions
5. Selection of the preferred solution

[2] Daniel E. Griffiths, *Administrative Theory,* Appleton-Century-Crofts, Inc., New York, 1959, p. 76.

[3] Edward H. Litchfield, "Notes on a General Theory of Administration," *Administrative Science Quarterly,* vol. 1, pp. 13–14, June, 1956.

[4] Daniel E. Griffiths, *Administrative Theory,* Appleton-Century-Crofts, Inc., New York, 1959, p. 94.

[5] William H. Newman and Charles E. Summer, Jr., *The Process of Management: Concepts, Behavior and Practice,* Prentice-Hall, Inc., Englewood Cliffs, N. J., 1961, p. 261.

[6] Leonard Silk, *The Education of Businessmen,* supplementary paper no. 11, Committee for Economic Development, Washington, D.C., December, 1960, p. 19.

Two of these writers, Griffiths and Silk, extend the process beyond the plan to activation by including in the process the activities of execution and subsequent evaluation of the solution selected. Silk intimates that all decisions need not be provoked by problems, by suggesting that the first step in the process be the "spotting up [of] problems or opportunities." [7] Although the actual difference is undoubtedly only semantic, it is refreshing to find someone who views any aspect of administration as an opportunity instead of as a problem.

The decision-making process is usually described as a series of actions. It is seldom, however, that the process proceeds step-by-step as delineated. For example, four alternative solutions to a problem may be proposed, but in the analysis and comparison of the relative merits of each solution, a fifth and sixth alternative may become apparent. The problem itself may need to be redefined in light of the evidence accumulated. Decision making is a process, a cycle of events; it is not a standard operating procedure that can be reproduced in a policy manual.

In this case situation the head nurse, Mrs. Glenn, was faced with having to make two decisions. Although both decisions related to immediate needs of patients, one situation required that a decision be reached quickly. The other allowed time for joint consideration and served to set in motion a chain of decisions. An on-the-spot decision is frequently known as a tactical decision—a decision of relative urgency, a decision dictated more or less by the authority of the situation, a decision related primarily to the utilization of known resources. When Mr. Janeway reported to the head nurse that Jimmy had suddenly developed acute respiratory distress, the situation not only commanded that a decision be made but also established the objective the decision should meet—adequate care for Jimmy. In this instance, the decision maker, Mrs. Glenn, actually perceived the problem through the eyes of the staff nurse. The head nurse summoned medical assistance without first observing the patient. Some may say that this was a "snap" decision, a decision made without forethought. On the other hand it is conceivable that this was a rational decision, a decision based upon a split-second analysis, upon knowledge acquired from experience in similar situations, and upon confidence that the staff nurse was able to evaluate correctly the patient's condition.

It should be noted that this one decision was not sufficient to meet the

[7] *Ibid.*, p. 19

objective of adequate care for the patient. As she observed the infant's condition, Mrs. Glenn realized that some decision regarding nursing care was needed. At the same time she was forced to recognize the limitations the situation placed upon the decision-making process. The patient's condition restricted the time available for reaching a decision. It also prescribed the level of nursing care needed. Within this narrow framework the head nurse had to formulate possible approaches to meeting the objective of adequate care for Jimmy.

Almost instantaneously Mrs. Glenn began to consider several possible approaches to the situation. She appraised the nursing staff on duty on the division, their numbers and their qualifications. She considered the needs of the other patients on the division as she undoubtedly asked herself, "Can adequate care be provided for the other patients if one nurse is assigned to intensive care for Jimmy?" That an affirmative answer resulted from her survey may be assumed from her assignment of a staff nurse from the division, Mr. Janeway, to "special" Jimmy for the next few hours. The case description does not disclose the alternative solutions that apparently were deemed less satisfactory. One can only assume that the head nurse considered the advantages and disadvantages of the other possibilities, and after weighing the relative merits, reached a decision and activated it. That this decision was to be evaluated is apparent from the disclosure that another decision regarding care for Jimmy, during the evening, would be made later in the day. The evaluation of one decision serves to perpetuate the decision-making process. So sequential become the decisions that it is often difficult to identify the original decision in the series of decisions most situations provoke.

With the emergency situation under control, Mrs. Glenn was able to return to a consideration of the question concerning rooming-in on the infant division. Again, she was involved in a decision precipitated by an earlier decision. If she had not sanctioned the suggestion of rooming-in for the mother of Sue Ellen, it is doubtful the staff would have proposed that consideration be given to a change in policy. In this instance, a tactical decision precipitated decision-making of a more strategic nature. Whereas tactical decisions are provoked by less complex situations—situations that in and of themselves delineate solutions—strategic decisions have broader implications and frequently involve changes in policy, in objectives, and in broad goals.

It is interesting to speculate why Mrs. Glenn seemed to be receptive to some consideration of change in policy when earlier suggestions apparently had been ignored. Much credence is still accorded the concept of sudden change of mind, yet authorities have concluded that this happens rarely, if ever. The change of mind probably is not sudden but rather is a result of the gradual perception that manifests after a problem has been defined clearly. The case identifies several factors that may have contributed to the head nurse's awareness of a need. Mrs. Glenn admitted to the students that consideration of a change to rooming-in had been mentioned several times earlier. One can assume that these suggestions were stored in the head nurse's memory as the first of many similar clues that would accumulate to the point of provoking conscious awareness of the situation. The challenge of the students, the presentation by the staff nurse of one explicit need for a change, and the response of the staff to the proposed solution for Sue Ellen's need all contributed, undoubtedly, to Mrs. Glenn's recognition that herein lay an opportunity for improvement.

The steps detailed above seem to indicate that if clues or suggestions arise regularly, or even intermittently, in the mind of an administrator, the "dawn will break" and the existence of a problem will be perceived. Unfortunately, such is not the case. Individuals have many built-in defenses or barriers against perception. It is well recognized that cultural and environmental factors limit the ability of the individual to perceive. Situations that threaten the security of the individual are perceived with reluctance, if at all (the phenomenon of perceptual defense). For example, the failure to identify potential leaders can often be traced to present leaders who are "blind" to the qualifications of subordinates for leadership training because of the possible threat to their own position. Persons who are familiar with the literature regarding children in the hospital will recall that in some instances the reluctance of staffs to institute rooming-in for mothers may be attributed to the fact that mothers represent an unconscious threat to the authority of pediatric nursing personnel.

The culture of the organization itself may restrict the perceptions of an individual. For many years hospitals looked upon patients as helpless individuals for whom treatment was provided with little thought to the ability of the patient to participate in the process. There also are examples in which the perceptions of nurses have been limited by the culture of the hospital, which conceived of nurses solely as handmaidens to the physician.

Mrs. Glenn also suggested a very real block to perception when she said, "We have always done it that way." Habit not only limits the individual's ability to envision different approaches to a solution but also interferes with his ability to recognize the existence of a need for action.

The tendency of many individuals to look upon most situations as dilemmas also tends to suppress fleeting perceptions. In this case, if the head nurse had perceived the question as one of specified visiting hours versus limitless rooming-in for both parents, she may have discarded any consideration of the suggestion to investigate.

At this point it may seem surprising that perceptions can penetrate the barriers in the mind of the decision maker. Many researchers hypothesize that a distinguishing characteristic of an effective administrator is the ability to perceive extensively, discriminately, and yet creatively. Widespread perception should be accompanied by the ability to distinguish accurately that which is perceived. The decision maker must be able to look beyond the symptoms of the problem to the problem itself. Many examples of failure to do this in nursing service can be found in the attempts to solve staffing problems by increasing the number of personnel when, frequently, the problem was actually precipitated by factors unrelated to the number of personnel. Time spent in diagnosing the situation can serve the decision maker well. A clearly defined problem will facilitate activation of the other elements of the process.

Creative perception refers to the recognition of an opportunity to make a decision when no real problem exists. It is a form of prediction in that a future need is sensed before the first symptoms appear. It is also a form of preventive intervention, of moving up a rung on the ladder before the present rung has begun to show signs of wear.

Once the problem or the fortuitous situation has been perceived, it must be subjected to intensive analysis. The administrator should ask himself: What are the critical factors involved? What objectives should the solution meet? What one factor, if changed, would allow the objectives to be met? Is this a decision that I should make, or should it be referred to either a superior or a subordinate? What are the limitations within which I must operate in formulating this decision? What obstacles may stand in the way of a satisfactory solution? And, if the problem is complex, which aspect should be considered first?

At the first reading of the case, it may have seemed to the reader, as indeed it must have to her staff, that Mrs. Glenn was remiss in dismissing the proposal of the staff nurse and suggesting that the question be raised again in conference the following week. Without the information concerning the subsequent discussion with the supervisor, one would have been predisposed to assume the head nurse anticipated that the proposal would be forgotten before the next conference. With the information, however, it seems more reasonable to conjecture that she postponed the discussion for one or more of several reasons: (1) Time prevented further discussion; (2) She wanted to be certain that the staff was sincerely interested in the matter; (3) She was not certain she had the authority to encourage the staff to propose a change; (4) She needed time to ferret out obstacles and limitations in order to be able to guide the staff in proposing solutions. Regardless of the reason or reasons, the delay permitted her to elicit from the conference with the supervisor information that would contribute toward the proposal of a solution and reassurance of her authority to formulate a recommendation to be forwarded to the Nursing Service Planning Committee.

The outcome of this particular case in decision-making is a matter of speculation. As disclosed by the discussion, however, there is sufficient consensus on the elements in the process to make it possible to identify some of the administrative or decision-making steps were additional case information available.

The crucial factors identified in the analysis of the problem indicated the data needed so that several approaches could be formulated. The case discloses that Mrs. Glenn had already been exposed to some information about alternative approaches to rooming-in for pediatric units. She had attended the nursing students' discussion, and she had listened to the staff nurse relate previous experiences with rooming-in. The literature on pediatric nursing is replete with discussions concerning the need of hospitalized children for parental contact as well as with suggestions for ways of surmounting difficulties encountered in attempts to meet the need. Additional information could be obtained from visits to, or correspondence with, other institutions. All the above would provide pertinent information of a general nature.

As a prelude to proposing solutions, relevant data concerning this situation would have to be collected. Questions relating to the actual needs of the patient population should be raised. Do all hospitalized children have an equal need? Is the need greater for one age group than for another? If so, what is the usual distribution of ages in the patient census? What space is actually needed by parents on the division? What facilities are presently used by parents? These are just a few of the questions for which data should be sought. The data will serve as the basis for the possible solutions. It is important, however, to recognize that new insights into a problem may arise at any time, that the need for perception does not cease with the analysis of the problem. The data may well disclose the desirability of scrutinizing the problem again and perhaps even redefining it.

Armed with a completed diagnosis and with information concerning the present situation and similar situations, the decision maker is prepared to consider alternative solutions to the problem. Once again the administrator must suppress the tendency to consider a solution from an either-or approach, a right-or-wrong way, or a radical-versus-conservative standpoint. Concentrated effort will invariably disclose several approaches to the solution. Some approaches may come from the past personal experience of the administrator; others from the experiences of other organizations in similar situations. It is essential that the decision maker scrutinize these experiences in an attempt to identify dissimilar elements and to adapt the solutions accordingly. It is wise to remember that although the physical characteristics of two situations may approximate one another, it is highly probable that the personal or personnel factors are dissimilar.

Imitation need not be the only approach to solutions although, admittedly, it is used frequently. The alternative to imitation and adaptation is creation—the formulation of unique, novel proposals. Not everyone has the ability to look beyond the known to ferret out an uncharted path. Seldom does a decision maker approach a solution alone. In many instances someone else may suggest a distinctive or seemingly unique approach for which a less creative administrator can supply the elements to convert the proposal into a creative yet practical solution.

Eventually a halt must be called to cogitation. A decision must be reached. The alternative solutions should be enumerated on a "balance sheet," with the advantages and disadvantages of each possible solution stated clearly. The merit and the probability of the successful activation of each proposal should be considered. It is conceivable that the proposal with greater advantages and fewer disadvantages than another proposal may be, at the same time, the one least likely to succeed at this time.

After the comparisons have been made, the preferred solution becomes evident. This solution actually is a decision resulting from many earlier decisions made throughout the decision-making process; decisions relative to the definition of the problem, to the collection of data, and to the choice of possible solutions. It is also a decision made, of necessity, on incomplete data, for it is always possible for one to conceive of another item of information that may contribute to a more effective decision. Yet the realities of the situation must be faced. Just as the young child pleads for "just one more story," the decision maker has to "turn out the light," not, as in the case of the child, to go to sleep, but to put his decision to work.

Although some authorities terminate their outlines of the process with the formulation of the final decision, one cannot evaluate the decision without activation. Evaluation is necessary for two reasons: (1) to test the decision and make any necessary corrections, and (2) to increase the ability of the decision maker to make decisions by identifying facets that need further consideration before the decision is activated. It is possible to engage in recapitulation without activation; however, it would be no more than a theoretical self-evaluation. Activation is the true test of a decision and may be done as a frankly acknowledged trial run. If it is not, the decision maker must be willing to follow the activation closely and to admit readily any indication that the objectives are not being met and to initiate the decisions necessary for corrective action.

The foregoing has been a discussion of the decision-making process as the function, primarily, of a single individual. In reality, in many situations the final decision is the responsibility of one person; yet, if decisions are to be rational, the efforts of several individuals may be needed. Griffiths makes the following point about the use of groups in decision making: [8]

> Although the literature of decisioning is quite clear on the point that individuals make better decisions than groups, it is entirely reasonable that a wider range of possible solutions could come from the use of groups. The groups should not be required to solve the problems or settle on a single solution, but they could be asked to present possible solutions.

Other authorities, however, readily agree that acceptance and activation of a decision can be accomplished more readily when the persons involved participate in the decision making and group consensus is reached. Thus the decision maker is forced to consider the relative merits of these two approaches to the use of groups in the process. Obviously, in an emergency situation, one cannot wait for group consensus. If an administrator has included his subordinates in the process when time was not a major factor, however, the group will invariably respond effectively in the face of a time restriction. The degree to which participation is utilized should be determined by the decision maker, as he has the ultimate responsibility

[8] Daniel E. Griffiths, *Administrative Theory*, Appleton-Century-Crofts, Inc., New York, 1959, p. 104.

for the consequences of the decision. He must use discretion in the amount and kind of participation elicited, and in the selection of subordinates for participation. His intent must always be to obtain the maximum effectiveness in decision making.

This approach to decision making removes all decisions from the realm of so-called "snap" decisions, "lucky breaks," or "wild guesses." It serves to channel thought in an orderly approach to rational judgment. Its objective is continuous improvement in the ability to make decisions.

The similarity between decision making and the *administrative blueprint* should now be apparent. The blueprint is a comprehensive design for the performance of any administrative function; the decision-making process is the cycle of events involved in reaching the solutions required in resolving administrative problems. Both are designed to promote the scientific approach to the performance of administrative functions.

SUPPLEMENTARY READING LIST

Argyris, Chris: "Interpersonal Barriers to Decision Making," *Harvard Business Review,* vol. 44, pp. 84–97, March–April, 1966.

Bennett, Addison C.: "Focus on Management Methods I: Setting Departmental Objectives," *Hospital Topics,* vol. 45, pp. 49–52, October, 1967.

Bennett, Addison C.: "Focus on Management Methods II: Determining Objectives," *Hospital Topics,* vol. 45, pp. 71–72, September, 1967.

Dietrich, Betty J., and Doris L. Miller: "Nursing Leadership—A Theoretical Approach," *Nursing Outlook,* vol. 14, pp. 52–53, August, 1966.

Drucker, Peter F.: "The Effective Decision," *Harvard Business Review,* vol. 45, pp. 92–98, January–February, 1967.

Griffiths, Daniel E.: *Administrative Theory,* Appleton-Century-Crofts, Inc., New York, 1959, pp. 71–113.

Johnson, Dorothy E.: "Consequences for Patients and Personnel," *American Journal of Nursing,* vol. 62, pp. 96–100, May, 1962.

Kriegel, Julia: *The Head Nurse: Thoughts and Decisions,* The Macmillan Company, New York, 1968.

Leavitt, Harold J.: *Managerial Psychology,* The University of Chicago Press, Chicago, 1958, pp. 226–229.

Litchfield, Edward H.: "Notes on a General Theory of Administration," *Administrative Science Quarterly,* vol. 1, pp. 3–29, June, 1956.

Longstreet, Victor M.: "Management R and D (Research and Development)," *Harvard Business Review,* vol. 39, pp. 125–134, July–August, 1961.

Magee, John F.: "Decision Trees for Decision Making," *Harvard Business Review,* vol. 42, pp. 126–138, July–August, 1964.

Newman, William H., and Charles E. Summer, Jr.: *The Process of Management: Concepts, Behavior and Practice,* Prentice-Hall, Inc., Englewood Cliffs, N.J., 1961, pp. 253–340.

Norris, Louis William: "Moral Hazards of an Executive," *Harvard Business Review,* vol. 38, pp. 72–79, September–October, 1960.

Silk, Leonard: *The Education of Businessmen,* Supplementary Paper No. 11, Committee for Economic Development, Washington, D.C., December, 1960.

Simon, Herbert A.: *Administrative Behavior,* 2d ed., The Macmillan Company,. 1957, pp. 1–19 and 79–109.

Tannebaum, Robert: "Limitations on Decision Making," in Robert Dubin, *Human Relations in Administration,* Prentice-Hall, Inc., Englewood Cliffs, N.J., 1951, pp. 206–211.

Viguers, Richard T.: "Building a Hospital Communications Network," *Hospitals, J.A.H.A.,* vol. 36, pp. 48–51, February 1, 1962.

Wilson, Robert N.: "Five Maxims of Decision Making," Part I, *Hospitals, J.A.H.A.,* vol. 33, p. 44, August 1, 1959.

case 6

The Staff Nurse and the Nursing Supervisor

Each year in March the personnel department of the Charles Evans Memorial Hospital sends a vacation request form to each employee. The form apprises the employee of the amount of vacation time to which he is entitled and requests that he signify a first, second, and third choice of dates. After the forms have been returned, this department prepares for each department head a list of the vacation requests, the time to which each employee is entitled, and a report of the number of positions, if any, budgeted for vacation relief. Each department head and/or his assistants prepare the vacation schedule for his department.

Case Data | *Case Notes*

The day after the vacation request forms were distributed to the nursing personnel on Division 3 East, Miss Cynthia Albright, a staff nurse, told the head nurse that she was certain an error had been made in her vacation slip.

Mrs. Rosalie Glenn, the head nurse, asked, "Didn't they allow you enough vacation?"

"Just the opposite. The slip says I am entitled to three weeks, and I thought that since I have been on the staff for only eleven months I would be entitled to just one week. I would like to have three weeks, but not if it means that when the error is discovered I would have to repay the money or the time."

"I can understand your concern. There's nothing worse than discovering you have overspent your bank account or your vacation account. Let me refer this to Miss Robertson when she makes rounds this morning. As supervisor, she knows more about personnel policies than I do."

When Miss Helen Robertson, the supervisor, came to the division later that morning, Mrs.

Case Data | *Case Notes*

Glenn related her conversation with Miss Albright. The supervisor suggested that she would be available in her office at 1:00 P.M. to talk with Miss Albright if she could be released from assignment for a short time. Mrs. Glenn replied, "Fine. It would be better to have her away for a few minutes at one o'clock than at the peak visiting time of two o'clock."

At one o'clock Miss Albright left the division and, taking her vacation request form with her, reported to Miss Robertson's office.

As she entered Miss Robertson said, "It is not often that someone thinks he has been granted too much vacation!"

"Well, I would rather find out now than have to change vacation plans later when someone found the mistake," replied Miss Albright. "Don't think I don't want a vacation! I just wouldn't feel right about being 'overpaid,' anymore than I would relish being 'short-changed'."

Miss Robertson had already opened the hospital policy manual to the pages describing vacation policies. Miss Albright pointed out the particular statement of policy she had read in her copy of the employee's handbook: "The employee who has been on the staff more than six months but less than one year is entitled to one week of vacation the first summer."

The supervisor asked Miss Albright for the date she joined the nursing staff of the hospital. When she learned that the staff nurse was employed on March 22, nearly a year ago, she realized that the staff nurse had not noticed the initial paragraph of the section on vacation policies. This stated, in part: "Every effort will be made to schedule all vacations between April 1 and November 15 of each calendar year. Exceptions will be granted to meet the needs or interests of an individual employee upon request to the Personnel Department and subsequent approval by the department head."

Miss Robertson pointed out that by the time the official vacation period started on April 1 Miss Albright would have completed one year of service;

Case Data *Case Notes*

therefore, she would be eligible for a three-week vacation. She commended the staff nurse for calling attention to the possibility of an error.

Miss Robertson devoted the remainder of the half-hour to an informal discussion of the progress and growth of the staff nurse in her first year as a member of the nursing staff on the pediatric division. Miss Albright expressed satisfaction with her present position. She added,

"I am learning and experiencing more about the nursing of children than I had anticipated. Almost every day something new happens. Just this morning one of the residents told me the pediatric department had just received a research grant for special metabolic studies relating to the nutrition of infants. He said Dr. Barbour will soon be initiating the study on 3 East. Undoubtedly the nurses will have an opportunity to assist in collecting the data."

After Miss Albright left the office, the supervisor thought about the comments on the possibility of a new research study involving the nursing staff on 3 East. She phoned Dr. Michael Barbour, Chief of Pediatrics, to confirm the report and to make arrangements to discuss with him the plan for the research study.

Dr. Barbour commented, "I should know by now that the grapevine travels faster than the written word! This morning I sent you a memo about the study through the hospital mail. You will probably get it in the morning. I will need your help in working out the nursing aspects of the study and in guiding the nursing staff in the collection of data."

DISCUSSION

If awareness of the need to question and to clarify in case analysis has been stimulated by the preceding cases, it is expected that the title of the present case has provoked the question: "What is meant by the term *supervisor*?" If one were to ask hospital, medical, and nursing personnel in health agencies large and small, in all sections of the country, to define the broad functions and responsibilities of the staff nurse, one may expect to find more similarities than dissimilarities in the definitions. It is highly probable that in their individual terms of expression, the respondents would imply that a staff nurse (1) occupies a first-level position in any area of professional nursing; (2) participates to a greater or lesser degree in giving direct care to patients; (3) works closely with auxiliary nursing personnel and has some degree of responsibility for directing their activities; and (4) works under the direct guidance and control of a professional nurse who occupies the next highest position in the organization of the nursing department in a particular agency. It is also likely that there would be a consensus among these same persons about the role of a head nurse. It is rather unlikely, however, that such unanimity would be reached in relation to the role of a supervisor in a nursing department. Some would refer to the supervisor as "a keeper of the keys" or a "carrier of the clip board." Eleanor Lambertsen described the nursing supervisor in the average hospital as ". . . the most highly qualified messenger and clerk in existence." [1] Others would define the role as that of buffer between the upper and lower echelons of the organization. A few may approximate the position more closely with that so often described in the textbooks—teacher, adviser, and counselor. Of all the traditional positions in nursing service, the position of nursing service supervisor has been the most maligned, the most equivocal, the most scorned, and the most nebulous. It may be said that when a definition is requested of the position *nursing supervisor* confusion reigns. The title "supervisor" is often used indiscriminately for purposes of increased salary or status, regardless of function. Many persons assume that the supervisor is the sole possessor of the right or ability to supervise when, in actuality, anyone who guides and directs the work of others supervises. Finer suggests that for convenience, many persons called "supervisor" might better be called "nurse executive." [2] When one reads in the professional literature about positions described as supervisor, with a capital "S," one becomes further confused by, for example, the use of the term in public health agencies to describe a position that is more similar to the position of the head nurse on a hospital unit than to the position of the supervisor in a hospital situation. One article refers to the supervisor as a key person in facilitating patient care, while another article reports a study in which

[1] Eleanor C. Lambertsen, "Toward a Clearer Definition of the Nurse's Function," *Hospitals*, vol. 35, p. 52, July 16, 1961.

[2] Herman Finer, *Administration and the Nursing Services*, The Macmillan Company, New York, 1959, p. 178.

supervisors themselves indicated that their roles were not closely related to professional nursing.[3, 4] Still another article takes particular care to distinguish between supervision and administration, implying that these titles represent a dichotomy.[5] In view of these disparities in the opinions regarding this position in nursing service, it would be difficult to analyze the present case situation and the actions of the supervisor, Miss Robertson, without some definitive information about the administrative principles that support the position of supervisor in nursing.

The title *supervisor* is used in business organizations and in nursing departments for individuals charged with overseeing the performance and functioning on one or more segments of the total enterprise. In nursing, the supervisor's range of control is less than that of the director of the nursing department, yet greater than that of the head nurse. The experiences of many kinds of businesses have shown that no leader can personally and, at the same time, effectively direct large numbers of personnel. The span of control must be narrowed to reasonable limits for the benefit and support of personnel and for the promotion of institutional aims. While many administrators disagree on what constitutes a reasonable limit, all support this principle of organization. Various factors have been identified as guides to the structural framework for organizations. Newman and Summer[6] suggested the following factors as determinants in establishing the span of control in individual situations:

1. Time devoted to supervision.
2. Variety and importance of activities being supervised.
3. Repetitiveness of activities.
4. Ability of subordinates.
5. Degree of decentralization.
6. Staff assistance provided.

[3] Helen Donovan, "What Is Supervision?" *Nursing Outlook,* vol. 5, pp. 371–374, June, 1957.

[4] Marion Pearsall, "Supervision—A Nursing Dilemma," *Nursing Outlook,* vol. 9, pp. 91–92, February, 1961.

[5] Cecilia M. Perrodin, "Principles and Practices Defined," pp. 43–47, in Edythe Alexander et al.: *Nursing Service Administration,* The C. V. Mosby Company, St. Louis, 1962.

[6] William H. Newman and Charles E. Summer, Jr., *The Process of Management: Concepts, Behavior and Practice,* Prentice-Hall, Inc., Englewood Cliffs, N.J., 1961, pp. 108–109.

A brief examination of the responsibility of the director of nursing, as viewed by Newman and Summer, establishes the need for one or more levels of supervisory personnel in the nursing department. The director necessarily and justifiably spends much of her time in planning meetings with her own staff and with directors of other departments in the organization. She must also work with directors in other community agencies. She participates in public relations activities. These activities are essential aspects of her responsibilities, although they limit the time she will have available for direct supervision of patient care.

In a small general hospital with services limited primarily to the care of acutely ill medical and surgical patients, the demands for nursing service are less complex than in a large teaching hospital used chiefly as a diagnostic center. The degree of specialization expected of nursing personnel influences the amount of orientation and subsequent supervision that must be provided. It should be obvious that the life-supporting services of the nursing department require closer supervision than do the services of employees in the accounting department of the same health agency. The services for patients are rendered primarily by human beings instead of by machines operated by human beings. Close supervision of personnel at the unit level by the chief executive of the nursing department is not possible; this responsibility must be delegated to others.

Activities that are repetitive in nature require less supervision than activities which must be adapted to a variety of patient conditions, personalities, and situations. The ratio of supervisory personnel to subordinates can generally be lower in the central supply department than on active inpatient divisions.

In situations in which the nursing care of patients is rendered almost completely by registered professional nurses the supervisory personnel can assume responsibility for overseeing, guiding, and directing the work of a greater number of staff members than when aspects of the care are divided among registered nurses, licensed practical nurses, and hospital-trained auxiliary workers. The ratio of supervisors to employees can also be affected by the tenure of the staff. New personnel require and deserve more supervision than acclimated personnel. The effectiveness of supervision is influenced by the ability of individuals to make wise decisions and to assume initiative relevant to their positions. These factors, unfortunately, are not necessarily related to preparation or training.

The supervisor who delegates authority to competent subordinates and who limits her decision-making to matters that affect a number of units is a supervisor who can usually function effectively with a wide span of control. Traditionally, however, nursing reserves major decision-making for persons somewhat removed from the bedside of the patient. Also, more emphasis has been placed, in the past, on developing followers than on developing leaders. The director has reserved too many decisions for herself. This has prevented supervisors from becoming adept at making decisions or from delegating authority to subordinates.

When a director has the services of other departments for some of the initial data gathering, record keeping, and recruiting she can supervise a greater number of subordinates than when she has these additional functions. The same would be true for descending levels of supervisory personnel. When the agency uses a time clock and the personnel or payroll department calculates and prepares the salary checks for nursing personnel, a nurse in the nursing department is freed for more direct supervision. When the housekeeping department assumes the responsibility for cleaning rooms following the discharge of patients, nursing supervisory personnel can supervise more closely the personnel engaged in direct care to patients.

There is no ideal maximum or minimum number of personnel that one person can or should supervise. Nevertheless all the factors listed above should be considered. The personality and energy of an individual supervisor will limit or extend a satisfactory span of control. It is generally recognized also that a supervisor can supervise larger numbers of personnel effectively as she gains experience. These factors must be considered in the orientation of a supervisor to a new position and in the extent of the authority given her by the next higher level of supervisory personnel.

The nursing department of the Charles Evans Memorial Hospital has 975 members serving on twenty-three inpatient divisions, outpatient clinics, and auxiliary areas such as the central supply service and the operating room. If one considers the factors relevant to span of control it is evident that the director, Miss Elliott, alone cannot provide the support or promote the coordination and communication needed at the unit level. It is these functions that administrative supervisors perform at the Charles Evans Memorial Hospital and in health agencies throughout the country. It is for these reasons that Finer refers to the supervisor as a "between woman."[7]

[7] Herman Finer, *Administration and the Nursing Services*, The Macmillan Company, New York, 1959, p. 178.

Why, then, is there controversy among administrators about this position? Why do some administrators advocate replacement of this position by persons with titles such as administrative assistant, clinical specialist, Nurse II, Coordinator? Is this a denial of the administrative principle just defined? A cursory review of articles which propose changes may seem to indicate rejection, but upon analysis it becomes evident that the principle is being upheld. The emphasis seems to be on removing the "paperwork," the desk-sitting aspect of the position in order to facilitate more active supervision for the promotion of improved care for the patient. Because the title has been so misused, a new title may be needed to clarify the service provided. Many persons who provide staff assistance in the nursing department bear the title "supervisor" (e.g., Supervisor of Equipment and Supplies, Supervisor of Central Supply) but have limited responsibility for the direction of personnel, and negligible contact with patients. Others titled supervisor have the responsibility for training personnel (e.g., Supervisor of Practical Nurse Training, Supervisor of Nonprofessional Personnel, Supervisor of In-Service) but have no direct authority over the personnel at the bedside. Still others, such as the Evening Supervisor or the Night Supervisor, often are required to devote more of their time in hospital management than in the guidance and direction of nursing service personnel. They are often responsible for carrying out certain activities in the admitting office, the pharmacy, the business office, and the dietary department in addition to serving as an assistant hospital administrator when hospital rules and regulations are involved and when the signature of a representative of administration is required on forms and permits. Persons in health agencies are accustomed to thinking of the supervisor as a guardian of rules and regulations, as a police officer for hospital management rather than a resource person or consultant on nursing care for patients.

All too frequently nurses have been promoted to the position of supervisor without adequate help in learning how to assist others on a broader scale than the self-contained nursing unit in which they were generally functioning before "advancing" to the position of supervisor. The principles of direction (or supervision) are the same, but this may not be evident to the new supervisor who considers herself an authority on nothing and who, at the same time, feels that she is expected to be an authority on everything. In her insecure state, she tends to concern herself with the paperwork details and keeps her contacts with personnel at a minimum. It is not the theory behind the position but the practice that is being challenged.

The term *administrative* was attached to the position title in an attempt to distinguish this position from that of the *clinical supervisor*, whose responsibility usually is limited to guiding nursing students in giving care to patients on hospital wards. These adjectival appendages tend to imply that the one does no teaching, while the other is not concerned with anyone except the students. As this position is conceived in nursing service today, however, the word "administrative" is redundant and promulgates further misunderstanding. The primary responsibility of the supervisor is to facilitate the work of personnel on the various units under her jurisdiction in providing effective nursing care for patients. The two major components of this charge are teaching and management. Each component is vital to the task; each is an administrative function necessary to the achievement of effective nursing care.

The entire nursing department and the other departments in a hospital operate under two commands: (1) the nontherapeutic authority of the hospital administration, which is charged with providing service and yet maintaining a sound financial condition, and (2) the therapeutic authority of the medical staff. This situation is inherent in health agencies and cannot be avoided. There are, however, violations of the principle of a single chain of command that can be avoided. The position of the supervisor is weakened frequently by her failure to respect the right of an individual to receive assignments from, and to be accountable to, one person. The division nursing staff is responsible to the head nurse or, if team assignment is used, to the team leader. It is the supervisor's obligation to respect this chain of command and to approach division personnel through, or with the sanction of, the head nurse. The director of nursing and her assistants must operate within this same chain of command and approach the head nurse through the supervisor. This does not preclude direct contacts between the assistant director and the head nurse, or between the supervisor and the staff nurse. Such person-to-person and face-to-face communication can be very valuable. The person who is to be responsible for results, however, deserves to be the person through whom a direction or charge is communicated to a subordinate. The concept of team nursing has been obscured many times because the head nurse has not been able to relinquish to the team leader the authority to command the team members.

No job description, no organization chart, and no policy manual can delineate explicitly the intricate details and subtle qualifications of the activities necessary in achieving the goals of an institution as dynamic as a health agency. In assisting the director of nursing with the responsibility for providing and improving the nursing care for patients, the supervisor must constantly evaluate the care rendered on the units under her direction and must guide the personnel in suggesting and activating the changes necessary for adaptation to the current situation and for progress toward expanded goals. The personnel in a situation need frequent encouragement and recognition for the goals they attain; but they must also be stimulated to look ahead to improved ways of action. Promotion of the search for improved nursing care for patients is the energizing role of the supervisor.

The head nurse charged with the care of 30 patients in varying degrees of illness most frequently conceives of her task as a day-to-day or, at the most, a week-to-week assignment than as a long-range mission. The rapid turnover of patients and of personnel has tended to increase this tendency. The supervisor may assist the head nurse and her staff in looking beyond the present to the future. She does this not by criticizing or commanding but by reviewing the situation with the staff and by interjecting an occasional question, suggestion, or confirmation of an idea. She also does this by assisting each head nurse to establish definite goals for the unit under her direction. For example, the head nurse in this case is in charge of the pediatric unit for infants and toddlers. If the staff decided that they could improve the care for these children by creating a home-like atmosphere, the supervisor may assist the group in establishing aims for one aspect, such as eating arrangements, rather than attempt a random approach to the changes. If realistic goals are defined and an approach is programmed, both staff and supervisor have a tangible end toward which they can strive. In order to evaluate progress one must be familiar with the starting point and must have a definite end in mind. The failure of the supervisor and her staff to establish specific goals for service for a definite period of time is a deterrent to progress. Without the time-goal factor, one cannot truly evaluate progress toward the improvement of patient care.

In order to evaluate the progress of program and personnel, the supervisor must be where patient care is being given. She cannot, from behind a desk, determine whether there is sufficient quantity and quality of personnel, equipment, and supplies to serve patients adequately. It requires more than a brief visit to a division during daily rounds to assist the head nurse in identifying the strengths and weaknesses of the personnel and to investigate the needs of the staff for further development. Some of the above information may be obtained from records, reports, conferences, and committee meetings. But these should serve only to provide preliminary data and guides to areas in the actual situation that require investigation.

"Making rounds" has long been recognized as one of the prime activities of supervisors. Often, in actual practice, however, "rounds" become "runs." The supervisor appears at the nurses station with a sheaf of papers in hand, confronts the head nurse, and in rapid-fire order, interrogates:

"What is the census?"

"How many 'ops' today?"

"Who's on the danger (critical) list?"

"Who didn't appear for work today?"

Having collected these vital statistics, she may hand the head nurse two memorandums with the comment, "These probably don't apply too much to your unit, but we have orders to post them on the bulletin board." She will then depart to collect the same data from the next unit, and eventually to relay these facts to someone in the nursing office. The head nurse may have tried to raise a question, confess a worry, or state a problem, but change-of-shift time is at hand and the supervisor must secure certain information for the central office. If the above information is vital to operations, could it not be gathered by someone other than a professional nurse?

If rounds are to be effective, the supervisor must be free to supervise. Nursing rounds are necessary for many reasons, but the major purpose should be to observe carefully and to evaluate the adherence to established standards of care. The time for making rounds should be varied so as to give a picture of the full range of division activities. If the supervisor routinely starts with Ward A, proceeds in order to Wards B, C, and D, and devotes an equal amount of time to each ward, it is doubtful that much thought has been given to the purpose and value of rounds.

Obviously, if a supervisor has six or seven units under her jurisdiction, she must allocate her time according to the best interests of the various units. The units will require varying amounts of supervision, depending upon the types of patients, the abilities of the personnel, and the activities in progress. Some staff will need more assistance than others. Some areas will need more attention, for example, during the inauguration of a new procedure or when the patient census is unusually high. A new head nurse needs more attention and support than an experienced head nurse needs. These fluctuating circumstances compel the supervisor to evaluate constantly the needs for her services.

Constant evaluation of the activities on the units under her supervision may reveal to the supervisor that Ward C, for example, needs considerable assistance at this time because of an unusually high number of patients who are isolated. She will have to determine what kind of assistance they need. There may be times when the physical presence of the supervisor will provide the staff with tangible support. If, in her judgment, such help is needed, the supervisor should plan to devote a greater portion of her time to Ward C than to the other wards. Care must be taken, however, to utilize the time in a way that will help, not hinder, the personnel already under the stress of an unusual situation. A wise supervisor will permit the charge nurse to give her an assignment rather than usurp the position of the charge nurse. In so doing she will demonstrate that she can utilize her hands as well as her head in contributing to the welfare of the patients and personnel. She will understand that this is not the time to make major changes in the customary procedures on the division. She will observe well but will, for the most part, refrain from offering suggestions until the pressure has lessened and the personnel can look beyond the daily necessities. She will also be extremely careful to adhere to the chain of command and work with personnel through the head nurse.

When a supervisor devotes more time and attention to one division, she must remain alert to the needs of other divisions and keep the lines of communication open so as to be apprised of changes that may occur on other divisions at any time. In this example (Case 6), the supervisor recognized the need and offered her services. At other times the requests may come from the head nurses. If a supervisor does not receive requests for assistance or consultation, she must examine her practices carefully. It would be false security to assume that there are no problems. It would be more realistic to recognize that the number of requests submitted to the supervisor by nurses under her supervision is usually related to the amount of response and support elicited from the supervisor. A receptive supervisor can accomplish so much more because the staff is aware of the problem; this is the first step in the process of change. For the supervisor to rebuke or to ignore, at this point, is to stifle initiative and progress.

In addition to lending assistance and to evaluating services for patients, the supervisor has a responsibility for evaluating the progress of the nursing staff for, ultimately, it is through personnel that care for patients is improved. She shares this responsibility with the head nurse and with staff nurses. They can make judgments on the development of the nursing personnel on the individual unit, and the supervisor, through her contacts with several units, can obtain a wider picture of needs for in-service education and contribute observations that are difficult for persons within the situation to make. Again, there must be standards for evaluating performance. Observations of personnel must also be planned to ensure that judgments are made on usual practices, not on isolated incidents. Should the supervisor observe behavior that is not meeting standards, this should be conveyed to the head nurse as a guide in making future observations. The supervisor should not break the chain of command, except in the infrequent instances when the safety of the patient is in jeopardy. At the request of or with the permission of the head nurse, the supervisor may contribute to the development of personnel by demonstrations, by attending ward conferences, by attending ward reports, or by direct assistance at the bedside. She may also contribute to the professional development of other nurses by setting an example that they will wish to emulate. Supervision is essentially a process of achieving goals through the efforts of other persons. Nurses and teachers seem to have difficulty in accepting that successful supervision of others can be as important and as satisfying personally as rendering direct care to patients.

For the last decade there has been growing interest in freeing the head nurse and the staff nurse of some of the tasks that can be assumed by auxiliary nursing personnel and clerical workers. Only recently has such relief been suggested for the nursing supervisor. Freed from counting equipment, signing requisitions for supplies, keeping census figures, calculating "nursing hours," and collecting daily and weekly time sheets, the supervisor can devote her talents to upgrading the quality of nursing care on the units under her supervision. In some instances the traditional positions of evening and night supervisors have been assumed in part by administrative assistants who serve on these tours and are responsible to the hospital administrator. Some nursing departments have extended the supervisor's jurisdiction over all three tours, subject to call at any time. This has been done in theory for many years. In actual practice, however, the evening and night supervisors have functioned rather independently, with only token recognition of the around-the-clock authority and responsibility of the head nurse and the service supervisor. Two conditions are necessary when a clinically oriented concept of supervision is to be promoted. First, and foremost, there must be someone to take over the managerial functions that have accrued to the position of nursing supervisor. For this purpose the position of unit manager has been created in some agencies. In other agencies, some of these functions have been assigned to other departments, such as housekeeping and payroll, or the supervisor has been assigned a secretarial assistant. The approach varies, but the principle is the same—to reserve for the supervisor functions that require the judgment and skill that cannot be provided by a person with less professional education.

The other prime requisite is that the person be willing to accept this position, which has been stripped of the protective shield of desk duties and which requires flexible, creative approaches to the directing of nursing care for patients. It is not easy to cast aside the traditional way and to embark on the new way, especially when so few qualified persons are in a position to lend support during the pioneer period. The process of learning a new approach, of discarding the familiar and easier way, can be lonely, painful, and yet exciting.

The case data reveal some of the functions of one nursing supervisor at the Charles Evans Memorial Hospital. The head nurse expected the supervisor to make rounds at least once a day and to be informed about the personnel policies of the institution. The supervisor apparently accepted these functions, as evidenced by her actions in the case situation. Miss Robertson also assumed the responsibility for discussing with the staff nurse her performance on a division under her jurisdiction. When the staff nurse revealed information that might affect the staffing and the responsibilities of the nursing personnel on the pediatric unit, the supervisor initiated contacts for securing the information needed in planning the proposed changes. If one assumes that Miss Robertson was adhering to the functions as outlined in the job description for the position of nursing supervisor, one can suggest that the following are included in the broad functions of the position:

1. To facilitate nursing care
2. To provide personnel for nursing care
3. To provide for job satisfaction of personnel through personnel policies

Undoubtedly, Miss Robertson has other functions, but these are the only ones revealed in this case situation.

It is interesting to speculate whether the head nurse would have consulted the supervisor as readily about a patient care problem as she did about the personnel problem. Her rapid referral may be interpreted as a lack of respect for, or interest in, personnel policies. On the other hand, it may reflect an understanding of the importance of personnel policies accompanied by recognition that authority to take action was in the hands of someone else. Some may say that the head nurse had an obligation to know the personnel policies. Most persons would agree that she should be aware of the general policies but need not attempt to keep abreast of the finer details. It is far more important that she know where to locate needed help. In this instance, for example, she may not have had access to the specific information that would reassure the staff nurse. Why she elected to refer the staff nurse's problem to the supervisor instead of to the personnel office is not disclosed. Perhaps she did not know that the personnel department had issued the request forms. This seems unlikely since her own request form undoubtedly came from and was returned to the personnel department. The referral may also be a reflection of her concept of the functions of the supervisor. The head nurse assured the staff nurse that the problem would be considered by the supervisor. This gesture indicates a receptive supervisor to whom she, a head nurse, did not hesitate to take problems. Regardless of the reason, her immediate response to the staff nurse's concern demonstrates a respect for the individual that must have contributed to job satisfaction for the nurse. It also seems reasonable to assume that this same respect may be conveyed to patients.

Why, when the problem of vacation time was referred to the supervisor, did she not, in turn, refer the staff nurse to the personnel department? This department has been assigned the responsibility of providing department heads with the information necessary for scheduling vacations within each department. They are providing for the nursing department a service that relieves department heads (e.g., the director of nursing) and their assistants of tasks formerly theirs but not requiring specialized education to complete. The service is provided up to the point where professional judgment is required. The personnel department is not qualified to determine who is prepared to relieve a head nurse for her vacation or which division can be operated safely with fewer personnel during vacation periods because this is not necessarily a matter of numbers but of balance between types of patients and abilities of personnel. With the basic information collected, the task of actually scheduling vacations is referred to the person who has the judgment required for making the decisions. The question raised by the staff nurse may have been answered by recorded facts interpreted in the light of stated policies. There would seem to have been no reason why the supervisor, in this instance, should have felt compelled to clarify the question instead of referring the staff nurse to the personnel department. Unfortunately, even when steps have been taken to free supervisors of tasks that can be assumed by others, many supervisors are often unable to relinquish the tasks. They are, first of all, reluctant to cast off tasks that have been in their province for many years. Secondly, many do not know how to utilize released time. They feel inadequate for assisting or supervising closely in the clinical area because many of them have not had close contact with patients and personnel for several years. Head nurses and staff nurses have learned to function with minimal guidance from the supervisor and may exhibit resentment of closer supervision. It should be noted that supervisors who more recently have attempted to revitalize the position of nursing supervisor have advocated elimination of the head nurse role and turning over to a unit manager the managerial duties and to the staff nurse the full responsibility of planning the care for a group of patients. This should enhance direct communication between staff nurse and supervisor and may prove to be a satisfactory approach.

The above factors may have been operating in this situation. However, another aspect should be considered. The supervisor may have been waiting for an opportune moment for a conference with the staff nurse. Perhaps, in her judgment, this was a less threatening approach than to request a conference for no apparent reason. This tentative assumption is based on the fact that she arranged for the nurse to come to her office even though she could have answered this question in a brief contact on the division. Perhaps she had reason to believe that the staff nurse's question was merely a prelude to another problem. If so, then her decision to talk with the staff nurse in the office may have been a decision of choice.

Several supervisory principles are exemplified in this case situation. The supervisor recognized that when a complaint is received, whenever possible, it is best to make adjustments promptly, before the complaint is magnified by discussion with persons not involved. The case data reveal that the supervisor was prepared for the conference. She had reviewed the vacation policies in order to be able to answer the staff nurse's question. She commended the staff nurse for assuming the responsibility for questioning the vacation allocation, thus recognizing the value of reinforcing desirable behavior.

One may question the wisdom of the action of the supervisor in reviewing performance with the staff nurse at this time. If the practice were repeated frequently, it could create among personnel the impression that every conference with Miss Robertson would be an "evaluation conference." Of far greater concern would be whether this conference was a review of performance that the staff nurse and the head nurse had already discussed. Miss Albright worked under the direction of Mrs. Glenn, and her performance should have been evaluated by Mrs. Glenn. It is hoped that the supervisor would contribute to this evaluation, but not to the exclusion of the head nurse. It may be that an evaluation conference had taken place between the staff nurse and the head nurse and that Miss Robertson was simply using this material as a tool for learning more about a nurse under her supervision.

Miss Robertson indicated an active rather than passive supervisory role when she utilized the grapevine information, recognizing the possible implications for the divisions under her supervision. If the supervisor can keep the goals of nursing service foremost in her mind and in the minds of the staff, if she can emphasize the positive aspects of progress while assisting the staff to identify and approach the negative aspects, and if she can look upon her role as a vital contribution to patient care, she can eliminate much of the confusion that exists about her role and can gain for her role the degree of respect accorded the role of the head nurse.

SUPPLEMENTARY READING LIST

Abbott, Ruth D.: "New Sight and Insights for Supervisors," *Nursing Outlook,* vol. 7, pp. 476–478, August, 1959.

Bennett, Addison C.: "Department Policies—Guides for Action," *Hospital Topics,* vol. 45, pp. 44–46, November, 1967.

Bennett, Addison C.: "Focus on Management Methods: Communication and Administration," *Hospital Topics,* vol. 46, pp. 44–46, May, 1968.

Carlisle, Ben: "Developing Policy and Procedure Manuals," *Hospitals, J.A.H.A.,* vol. 43, pp. 47–50, April 16, 1969.

Carner, Donald C.: "Overcoming Employee Dissatisfaction," *Personnel Journal,* vol. 39, pp. 399–403, March, 1961.

Coffey, Robert E.: "The Challenge of Modern Supervision," *Journal of the American Dietetic Association,* vol. 47, pp. 32–36, July, 1965.

Davis, Keith: "Management Communication and the Grapevine," *Harvard Business Review,* vol. 31, pp. 43–49, September–October, 1953.

Donovan, Helen M.: "Making Rounds With a Purpose," *Nursing Outlook,* vol. 8, pp. 394–395, July, 1960.

Donovan, Helen M.: "What Is Supervision?" *Nursing Outlook,* vol. 5, pp. 371–374, June, 1957.

Finer, Herman: *Administration and the Nursing Services,* The Macmillan Company, New York, 1952, pp. 178–184.

Frank, Sister Charles Marie: "The Utilization of Nursing Personnel," *Nursing Outlook,* vol. 8, pp. 202–203, April, 1960.

Hilkert, Robert N.: "Achieving Competence As the Boss," Part I, *Personnel Journal,* vol. 38, pp. 85–88, July–August, 1959.

Lambertsen, Eleanor C.: "Toward a Clearer Definition of the Nurse's Function," *Hospitals, J.A.H.A.,* vol. 35, pp. 51–52, 54, 96, July 16, 1961.

Mercadante, Lucille T.: "An Organizational Plan for Nursing Service," *Nursing Outlook,* vol. 10, pp. 305–306, May, 1962.

Mooth, Adelma M., and Miriam A. Ritvo: *Developing the Supervisory Skills of the Nurse: A Behavioral Science Approach,* The Macmillan Company, New York, 1966.

Newman, William H., and Charles E. Summer, Jr.: *The Process of Management: Concepts, Behavior and Practice,* Prentice-Hall, Inc., Englewood Cliffs, N.J., 1961, pp. 190–198.

Pearsall, Marion: "Supervision—A Nursing Dilemma," *Nursing Outlook,* vol. 9, pp. 91–92, February, 1961.

Perrodin, Cecilia M.: "Principles and Practices Defined," in Edythe Alexander et al., *Nursing Service Administration,* The C. V. Mosby Company, St. Louis, 1962, pp. 43–47.

Rosenberger, Homer T.: "A Supervisor Looks at 'Human Relations,'" *Personnel Journal,* vol. 38, pp. 292–294, January, 1960.

Stearns, Lina: "Changing Concepts in Nursing Supervision," *American Journal of Nursing,* vol. 59, pp. 63–65, January, 1959.

Towner, Alfred M.: "No More Supervisors?" *Nursing Outlook,* vol. 16, pp. 56–58, February, 1968.

Trull, Samuel G.: "Strategies of Effective Interviewing," *Harvard Business Review,* vol. 42, pp. 89–94, January–February, 1964.

Viguers, Richard T.: "What It Takes to Be a Good Supervisor," *The Modern Hospital,* vol. 91, pp. 63–66, July, 1958.

Wanuka, Maxine J.: "A Dissenting Opinion: Is Management Making 'Great Pretenders' Out of Supervisors?" *Hospitals, J.A.H.A.,* vol. 39, pp. 66–67, May 1, 1965.

Yauger, Ruth Anne, and Betty Oberlies: "A 'Do It Yourself' Program in Supervision," *Nursing Outlook,* vol. 15, pp. 75–77, April, 1967.

case 7

A Nursing Division and the Process of Change

One year ago a pilot workshop on work simplification was conducted for members of the top management group at the Charles Evans Memorial Hospital. Following the completion of the experiment, the group voted to institute a Work Simplification Program for administrative personnel in all departments. It was decided that full-time members of the professional nursing staff together with colleagues from other departments in the hospital would participate in the program. To date assistant directors of nursing, the administrative supervisors, and one-half of the head nurse and staff nurse groups had attended the workshop conferences. Each participant had worked on a problem situation from his area, applying the work simplification approach to a solution. The progress of this program was revealed to the hospital personnel in the employees' newsletter. The projects completed by the members of the professional nursing staff included an improved procedure for administering intravenous fluids to adult patients, a simplification of the form for ordering supplies from Central Service, the inauguration of a messenger service, and a change in the method of linen distribution. After trials on a single nursing unit, these time- and work-saving methods were put into effect on all nursing divisions.

Case Data	*Case Notes*
On 10 South, the orthopedic division, the head nurse, John Kilborn, conducted a weekly meeting for the division nursing staff. The purpose of these meetings was to focus on problems and proposals related to the improvement of patient care and the promotion of job satisfaction for personnel. Shortly after he began to attend the conferences, Mr. Kilborn asked his staff for suggestions concerning a project that he might consider undertaking in conjunction with the workshop. Miss Mary Jenkins, a staff nurse, suggested that something should	

Case Data *Case Notes*

be done about rearranging the storage of sterilized syringes and needles. Mr. Kilborn recalled that Miss Jenkins was scheduled to attend the next series of conferences. He suggested that she may want to wait to investigate the situation when she was a participant. One of the orderlies, Peter Henry, proposed that Mr. Kilborn devise a form that other divisions could use in requisitioning orthopedic supplies from the storage room on 10 South. Two other members suggested that the staff may have more suggestions if they could use the coming week to think about possibilities. All agreed to this suggestion.

At the staff meeting the following week the group seemed to have reached a consensus that the most pressing need was that of consolidating information related to the nursing care for each patient. They told of the difficulties they have in piecing together information from the medication list, the treatment list, and the supportive care cards, all maintained for each patient but kept in three separate books. Mr. Kilborn agreed that this would be a worthwhile project and began to elicit positive and negative comments about the established procedure and suggestions for a new method. Following this meeting he began to work on the project. There was no discussion of the progress of the project at subsequent staff meetings other than brief responses to the queries of personnel, "Are you working smarter, not harder?"

At a division staff meeting two months later, Mr. Kilborn distributed mimeographed copies of a Kardex form he proposed to substitute for the separate lists in use. He reported that the nursing supervisor and the director of nursing had approved a trial of the new form. The sample form was discussed briefly. Some staff members expressed reservations about the new form because all the information now would be in one place and would permit only one person at a time to have access to the cards. Questions were raised about the use of ink and/or pencil in recording data on the cards. After this discussion, the head nurse announced that the ward clerk would start to tran-

Case Data *Case Notes*

scribe the information from the old lists to the new forms on Monday, and that the trial period for the new form would start on Tuesday. Mr. Kilborn explained the forthcoming change to the evening staff that same day and to the night staff the next morning.

At coffee break on Tuesday, the "medicine nurse" complained that twice as much time had been required for checking medications because of interruptions from other persons seeking information from the Kardex about the treatments and supportive care for their patients. Later that morning, Dr. Donald Burroughs, the assistant resident on the orthopedic service, approached Mr. Kilborn and said that when he wanted to check the medication orders for his patients he had to wait while a staff nurse reviewed the treatments ordered for her patients. When Dr. Lloyd Wainscott, Chief of Orthopedic Service, came to the division to make rounds, he viewed the Kardex with suspicion and asked, "Was this change really necessary?" As rounds were completed he commented, "Dr. Burroughs says this change makes it more difficult for him to check on medications ordered for patients. We may have to go back to the old way if this continues."

All morning Mr. Kilborn heard comments about the relative merits of the old over the new. At lunch the nursing supervisor asked him how the new form was being accepted. He replied, "It seems as though everyone wants a change *until* a change is made." Throughout the week the number of negative comments decreased and a few favorable reactions were voiced by the nursing staff on the day tour. Dr. Burroughs continued to express dissatisfaction with the change. Dr. Wainscott told Mr. Kilborn that he would wait for the reaction of the new assistant resident to the form before approaching the nursing supervisor to suggest returning to the former method.

At the end of a four-week trial period Mr. Kilborn asked for an evaluation of the new form. The staff nurses said they had been able to resolve satisfactorily the conflicts between the needs of

Case Data | *Case Notes*

the medicine nurse and the other staff members. They suggested one or two minor changes in the trial form, and the addition of the intern's name to the information column. The consensus was that the new form should be used for the next two months on 10 South. The staff suggested that it may then be ready to be placed before the Nursing Service Planning Committee for consideration for use on all nursing divisions. As one of the practical nurses was leaving the staff meeting she said to Mr. Kilborn, "When I worked the evening tour last week, I noticed that the charge nurse makes out a medicine list and treatment list for the evening staff to use. I wonder why they don't use the new form."

DISCUSSION

It used to be said that there are only two things of which we can be certain—death and taxes. To this time-worn adage, the twentieth century has added a third component—change. Change comes occasionally slowly and almost imperceptibly, but frequently of late, the status quo is being challenged. The reverence that was previously accorded tradition has now been transferred to innovation and creativity. The individual has but two choices: (1) to sit back and be forced to adapt to the changes imposed by the environment or (2) to become an energizing force in initiating change. Unfortunately, many examples can be given of ways in which nursing has adapted to the environment; too few can be cited in which nursing has stimulated or initiated change.

Case 7 is an instance in which professional nurses were encouraged to consider a need for change and to propose a new approach to a problem. The change described in the case is not unique. It is more adaptive than creative, but it represents a springboard for other innovations.

In reading and analyzing the case, perhaps the first questions to be raised concern the term *work simplification.* Is work simplification any different from daily attempts to do things easier and faster? How does work simplification differ from methods improvement, time and motion study, operations research, and problem-solving?

From the case data one can learn that the administrative personnel in all departments of the Charles Evans Memorial Hospital are involved. Full-time staff nurses are included in the category of administrative personnel, and a series of interdepartmental conferences is involved. As a participant in the conferences each individual selects from his area a problem to which he applies a solution. Some of the projects completed by the nursing staff are given as examples. Because the program was initiated after the top management group had participated in a pilot project, one may assume that the program and the individual participants will have the support of the majority of department heads and that tangible results will be encouraged. This factor and the interdepartmental approach seem to differentiate a work simplification program from the informal attempts of isolated individuals to make changes in their work habits for the direct or indirect improvement of patient care.

Hospital and other health agencies have, in recent years, recognized the need for better organized approaches to methods improvement programs. In order to provide better patient care despite a shortage of qualified personnel, and within a framework of rising costs, it has been necessary for these agencies to find more effective approaches to serving the patients and the community. In a booklet on methods improvement programs the American Hospital Association stated: [1]

> Hospitals need a planned approach to methods improvement. The many variables of day-to-day operation lead to rapid change and increased complexity. Hospital management will be better equipped to meet these variables if sporadic and marginal improvements are replaced by an organized search for opportunities to make major shifts in the means of achieving the basic objectives. This is true of all hospitals regardless of size, location or type.

When methods improvement programs were first instituted in health agencies, nursing departments were seldom involved because of the persistent attitude of nurses and other hospital personnel that so-called efficiency approaches could not be applied to anything as individualized as patient care. In recent years, however, experience with work simplification programs has demonstrated that such programs can exert a vital influence on patient care through the development of time- and work-saving methods for nursing personnel and for personnel in ancillary departments.

A number of the "catch" phrases used to define methods improvement

[1] Committee on Methods Improvement, American Hospital Association, *Organized Methods Improvement Programs in Hospitals*, American Hospital Association, Chicago, 1958, p. vii

programs are expressions such as: "Work smarter, not harder." "Find a better way to do the job." "There is always a better way." "Organized common sense." A more explicit definition is: [2]

> Methods improvement is a study of the multitude of activities performed by persons in an organizational unit. In this study, specific techniques are employed, the complexity of which is determined by the problem.

Several of the approaches to work improvement used in hospitals and other health agencies are adaptations of two basic approaches first used in industry: (1) the "expert" approach, in which either an outside consultant or a staff specialist is assigned the responsibility of diagnosing and initiating improved techniques; (2) the "do-it-yourself" approach, in which the individual is given the responsibility and support for initiating change in work procedures. Because of the human relations problems involved in gaining acceptance of the proposals of experts, the difficulties of acquainting an outside consultant with the complexities of hospital activities, and the perpetuating aspects of employee-involved programs, many institutions are using work simplification programs like the one instituted by the Charles Evans Memorial Hospital.

Allen Mogenson, a noted methods consultant, coined the term *work simplification* and defined it as the "organized use of common sense to find easier and better ways of doing work." [3] The approach outlined by Mogenson can be applied continuously, in any area, to any job. It is based upon a philosophy that all levels of supervisory personnel are in active contact and communication at the operational level and therefore are in the most advantageous position to initiate and promote improvements. Work simplification conferences are designed to introduce the participants to techniques and attitudes that will generate improvements. Experience has shown that, once established, the methods are subsequently applied to many activities in the participant's department, thus activating an endless chain of better methods.

The primary tool of work simplification is the problem-solving process—a logical, orderly approach to a particular situation. This systematic consideration includes the following steps:

1. *The selection of a problem.* This activity may be related, for example,

[2] *Ibid.*, p. 4.

[3] Stanley A. Ferguson and Charles B. Womer, "Work Simplification Is the Worker's Job," *The Modern Hospital*, vol. 87, p. 61, August, 1956.

to an area in which errors occur, to tiresome tasks, to sources of patient or personnel complaints, or to effective yet complicated procedures; in other words, to any situation which may be improved, extended, or eliminated for the purpose of improving service for the patient.

2. *The collection of all the facts relevant to the situation.* Each step, each piece of equipment used, each person, and each department involved is listed. The activity involved may be graphically represented on the flow process chart (Figure 8). The purpose of this chart is to break down the procedure in detail. A standard flow process form uses symbols to indicate the processes that persons or products undergo in completing a job. By listing each segment of the activity and then drawing lines to the column of the symbol which describes the action taken (operation, transportation, inspection, delay, or storage), the problem areas may well be highlighted. For example, in an investigation by one of the authors [DAK] on the use of a formula requisition in a pediatric hospital, the flow chart disclosed that because of the timing of the pick-up schedule for the requisitions, the delay in many instances was so long that a telephone order had to be given to the formula laboratory. The written requisition was still completed. When it was picked up several hours later it was carried to the formula laboratory, compared with the requisition made out in the laboratory by the person receiving the telephone order, and then discarded. A waste of time and effort was revealed, and the possibility of introducing an error in the verbal transmission of the order was noted.

Several other tools have been devised to record the facts of a situation. These include:

a. Work distribution chart. This chart is a graphic representation of the work done in a single department. It shows the division of work among employees, the work performed by each employee, and the approximate amount of time each employee spent on each assigned duty. This would be of importance when, for example, consideration is being given to the transfer of certain tasks from the head nurse to a ward clerk, or to a unit manager. Can the new work load be absorbed into the present load? Do adjustments have to be made in the present assignment of the clerk? If so, who is to assume the tasks removed from her assignment?

b. Operator chart. This chart is a detailed study of the actual hand and/or foot operations of a single operator. It is used in studying the repetitive, relatively permanent activities of workers such as those in central supply or the kitchen.

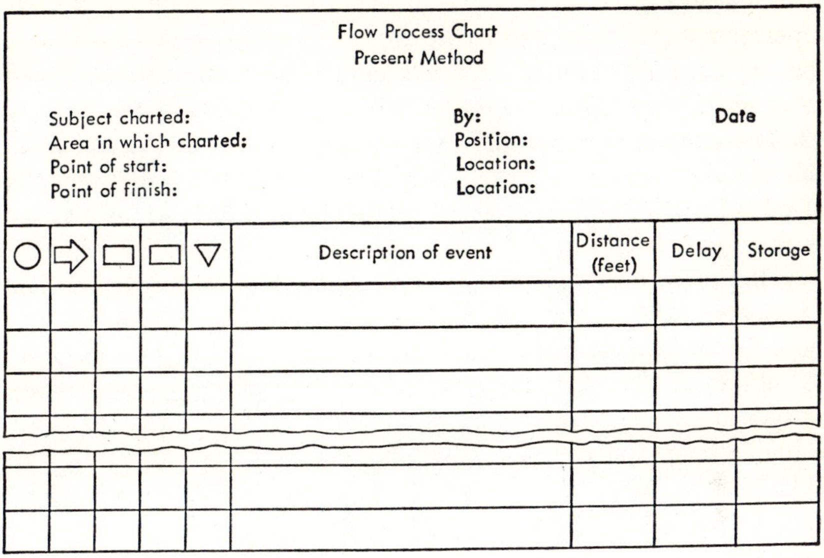

FIGURE 8. Flow process chart.

c. *Multiple activity chart.* In situations requiring the extensive use of machinery or equipment, e.g., in the laundry, this chart is used for recording the operations. It would seldom be used by members of the nursing department.

3. *The analysis of all the facts.* Each and every detail should be challenged. Questions such as the following should be raised:

What is the basic purpose of this activity?
Is this a necessary activity?
Is it duplicated by any other activity or department?
What is actually being done?
Are all the steps necessary?
What could be eliminated?
Who is doing the activity?
Could someone else do it?
Is too much time being spent on unnecessary details?
What activities take the most time? Should this be so?
Are activities arranged in logical order?
Is the activity being done in the best place at the best time?

In the study of the formula requisition mentioned above, the information requested on the form was challenged. On each requisition the following information was to be filled in: name of the patient, age, division, bed number, date, new order or change of order, name of formula, amount each feeding, number of feedings, name of physician, name of the nurse—eleven items. In reviewing the form it was found that two of the items, name of physician and bed number, were not necessary, and that two others, date and division, were the same for every patient. The net result of this aspect of the study was a new form that could be used for formula orders for all patients on the division each day.

4. *The development of a better method.* The thorough analysis in the preceding step may suggest activities that can be eliminated, combined, rearranged, or simplified to produce more effective and efficient procedures. On the other hand, it may indicate the need for a completely new approach. The replacement of reusable syringes with disposable syringes may be an example of the latter. In any case, the time for a creative approach is at hand. One should not settle for the first possibility, but should explore a wide range of approaches before narrowing the field. Once the new or revised method has been formulated in tentative form, a new flow process chart should be made. This will help to identify errors or omissions before the plan is made final, thus ensuring a smoother transition from old to new.

5. *Installation of the new method.* Before a new method can be implemented, the necessary administrative approval must be secured. The approval will stand for nought, however, if the personnel directly involved do not sanction the change. Even though personnel have contributed to the development of the better approach to the problem, it is wisest to continue to emphasize that the new procedure is being implemented on a trial basis and that subsequent modifications will be effected should they be necessary. Care must be taken, also, to explain the new method to *everyone* concerned and to observe the procedure carefully in an effort to identify any weaknesses and to make necessary adjustments.

This final step in the problem-solving process is perhaps the most difficult to accomplish. Much of its success depends upon the extent to which the human factors have been considered along with the material factors. It is for this reason that an organized methods improvement program concentrates on human relations and the methods of facilitating change as much as it does on the mechanical aspects of the work.

In this case situation, John Kilborn, the head nurse, began his project by inviting his staff to make suggestions. In so doing, he recognized one of the prime factors related to facilitating change—the desirability of involving at the outset the persons who will be affected by the change. One may question, however, whether his approach will yield the results he wanted. When Miss Jenkins made a proposal, he turned the suggestion back to her. The immediate rejection of the first suggestion will tend to stifle additional proposals. He may have considered his reason for refusal not only logical but also fair. And yet, Miss Jenkins may have interpreted it as either dictation of her future project or as lack of regard for her suggestion. No reaction was recorded of Mr. Henry's suggestion about the method for requisitioning orthopedic equipment. The staff's suggestion to take the coming week to consider possibilities may have been made to ease what seemed to them to be a tense situation, or it may have been proposed with sincerity. Experience has shown that the majority of persons involved in a situation become silent, momentarily, when given the opportunity to make suggestions. The leader who cannot tolerate this silence and hastens to make a suggestion may well lose not only an audience but the chances of a group approach as well. The group which is slow to respond may think that the leader has already made a decision and merely wait for a clue to the expected response. If assurance is given that no decision has been reached and still no response is evoked, the leader may obtain results by directing questions to individuals who are least likely to feel threatened. Involvement in the planning stage tends to overcome the employee's feeling that he is helpless in relation to organization policies and decisions.

The following week, when the staff proposed an evaluation of the methods of recording orders for patient care, Mr. Kilborn readily agreed to pursue the problem. He may have recognized a mandate from the staff and thus discarded any ideas he had, or the suggestion of the staff may have met an interest he had. One cannot exclude the possibility that he may have dropped a hint concerning the project he would like to undertake. It is to be hoped that one of the first two mentioned factors was operative in this situation. Few things can destroy respect so quickly as autocracy under the guise of democracy.

As soon as the group had concurred on the problem, the head nurse recognized that the person closest to the job is often in the best position to contribute worthwhile information to the accumulation of data and to the analysis of the facts, as well as to a possible solution. In the process of gathering information, one must be careful not to imply that the method under review is outdated or ineffective. This implies criticism of present behavior and may well arouse defensive attitudes among personnel. If the emphasis is on what is being done, by whom, where, when, and how, without challenging each statement for the why, the group will feel less threatened and will be able to realize that objective considerations, not rationalizations, are basic to the formulation of an improved method.

From the case data one may speculate that Mr. Kilborn accepted in theory the consultative approach, but that his practice evidenced only token acceptance. He did ask the group for suggestions at the outset, but, from then until the presentation of the sample form, he apparently worked alone on the project. One may interpret the query, "Are you working smarter, not harder?", as sarcasm. The slogan, "Work Smarter, Not Harder," however, has become the motto for work simplification conferences. This phrase had undoubtedly been used in the writeups in the employees' newsletter. The staff's use of it with Mr. Kilborn may have been their way of showing interest or, perhaps, concern about the progress of the project.

Any anticipated change in methods may arouse anxiety. There is security in established ways of performance. In this instance, for example, the ward clerk may have been concerned that her work load would be increased; the auxiliary nursing personnel may have assumed that in any new method they would not have access to the same information they have under the present system; some of the staff nurses may have worked with other methods of recording patient care information, methods that were no better than the present ones. If employees are not given the opportunity to voice fears, they may magnify apprehensions to the point of blocking acceptance of the new method. This risk may be minimized by keeping employees informed and by encouraging them to participate in each step of the work simplification process.

Two additional factors that operate against change are fear of losing status and fear of economic loss. Many persons associate methods improvement programs solely with the cutting of costs and reduction of the labor force. For this reason, when University Hospitals of Cleveland established a work simplification program the administration accepted and publicized the policy that no employee would lose employment as a result of the new program.[4] One must also recognize that any time it is

[4] Stanley A. Ferguson and Charles B. Womer, "Putting Work Simplification to Work," *Modern Hospital*, vol. 87, pp. 76–78, September, 1956.

suggested that an employee with less training could do the work of a more highly skilled employee, the suggestion may be interpreted as a loss of status by the more skilled employee and a very real threat to his security. Many fears of economic loss or loss of status are unjustified in the eyes of administrative personnel, but the employee needs and must be given assurance if change is to be effected successfully.

When the new form was ready Mr. Kilborn presented it to the group at staff meeting. Apparently consideration had been given to several other factors that may facilitate acceptance of change, because the new form had been mimeographed instead of printed. This fact, coupled with the announcement of a "trial period" of use probably conveyed to the personnel that the decision was not irrevocable, that there would be opportunities to criticize and to evaluate the new method. Mr. Kilborn had also given thought to the timing of the transition from the old to the new method. This permitted him to give advance notice to the entire staff. Had he announced that use of the new form would be in effect the following day, the result may have been panic at the thought of getting the necessary transcribing done. On the other hand, if he had announced that use of the new form would be instituted the following month, interest may have waned. It is to be hoped that Mr. Kilborn had discussed the assignment with the ward clerk before making the announcement to the staff.

One wonders what the reaction of the staff was to his announcement that the form had been approved by the supervisor and the director before the staff had had an opportunity to see it. Granted that administrative approval is needed prior to implementation, but so too is staff approval needed. The question is, Which should be secured when? Tentative approval of both groups is needed at the outset of the project. It would be of little value for one nursing division to devise a new form if there is no possibility of eventual acceptance of the form by all divisions, with or without modifications. It would also be of little advantage to propose a new form when the storeroom has a five-year supply of the present form, especially if, for reasons of economy, the old form has to be used before a new form may be printed. Administrative approval of the initial idea could forestall delays in implementation. Because the staff had proposed the project originally, Mr. Kilborn could assume that he had their support of the basic idea. He could not assume, however, that he had their approval of the final product any more than he could assume that the supervisor and the director would sanction it. An organized methods improvement progam implies encouragement of innovation, but it does not ensure blanket approval of all projects.

When a change is introduced, the person who introduced it must be receptive to complaints as personnel try to adjust to the change. Resistance to change does occur and should be anticipated. It may be valid or not, but the mere fact of its appearance "is by itself neither good nor bad. . . . It is always, however, an important signal calling for further inquiry by management."[5] The instigator of the change must content himself with listening instead of justifying. He will soon find that if the new method has merit, the complaints will give way first to passive and then to active acceptance. Also he should solicit criticism from the more reticent and manifest sincere interest in the comments of all.

Undoubtedly the assistant resident's resistance may have been minimal had Mr. Kilborn discussed the change with him before implementing it. If one analyzes the proposed method carefully enough, the potential trouble spots can be identified. One can then exert special efforts to ease the adjustment at these points. For instance, had Mr. Kilborn anticipated the inconvenience for the assistant resident, he may have enlisted the cooperation of the staff nurses in yielding access to the Kardex to the assistant resident until the resident had a chance to adjust to the change. This does not imply that another department should have the right to dictate methods or procedures that are in the jurisdiction of the nursing department. It does mean, however, that the proposed change must be considered in the light of its effect on the work of other personnel and departments. For example, the laundry division may decide to operate five days a week instead of six and organize its work schedule to provide adequate linen to meet the needs of the hospital. On Friday enough linen is sent to all units to last until Monday afternoon. Because, in the past, only one day's linen was issued at a time, however, there is storage space for one day's linen only. Under the new method linen is left in laundry carts, which block the corridors, create a fire hazard, and requires more time to locate a needed article. The nursing department cannot insist that the laundry return to the old schedule. A problem has been created that might have been avoided by discussion between the departments prior to the change.

Because the traditional dependency relationship between nurses and the medical staff persists, a number of nursing methods and forms serve

[5] Paul R. Lawrence, "How to Deal with Resistance to Change," *Harvard Business Review,* vol. 47, pp. 4–12, 166–176, January–February, 1969.

physicians first and nurses second. To change these forms is difficult. It can be accomplished, however, if all proposals are viewed in terms of the benefit to the patient, whom both serve.

Mr. Kilborn was able, apparently, to accept the criticisms of the new method, although his remark to the supervisor, "Everyone wants a change *until* a change is made," seems to reflect discouragement. By encouraging the staff to work together he was able, eventually, to gain support for the form and to elicit some necessary modifications. It is important that the initiator of change recognize that resistance to change is a reality and must be met with patience until the group has adjusted to the new method. The support of an immediate supervisor is extremely helpful at this point if it consists of support for the innovator, not imposition of the method on a reluctant staff.

In this situation it is not surprising that the nursing staff did not accept the new form. The case data reveal little consideration of either the evening or night staff at any step of the work simplification process. Although hospitals have always operated on a twenty-four-hour basis, they have seldom given equal recognition to the three tours of duty. This is as true of other departments as it is of nursing. The omissions in nursing are more glaring because of the number of persons involved. In many organizations differential pay is accorded persons who work evening or night tours. This, in itself, seems to identify these tours of duty as less desirable than other tours. The services provided during tours are as necessary to the patient's welfare as the services provided during the day tour. Improved methods are as needed on the later tours as on the day tour. To impose a new method without eliciting information and suggestions from the evening and night staffs is to invite disregard, and even perhaps to decrease patient care by increasing the staff's work, as it did in this instance. Had Mr. Kilborn followed-up the change on the evening tour, he may have discovered that the new form was not being used by the evening staff. He would then have to determine whether this was personal resistance, or whether there were logical reasons for the lack of regard. The task would undoubtedly have been easier if the pattern of resistance had not been built up during the four weeks since the trial had been started. If the form is to be presented for consideration by other divisions, the problems it presents must first be resolved on Division 10 South. At this point, Mr. Kilborn must face the rejection of the form by the evening staff. Since the trial is to be extended two months, he will be able to establish a firm basis for evaluation so that all personnel may know the standards on which the final decision will be based. The extended trial may be an optimum time to include personnel from the other tours in the weekly staff conferences for the purpose of an across-the-board discussion of the progress of the new method. Around-the-clock representation has been tried repeatedly with minimal success. All too frequently such meetings have been planned to necessitate the attendance of evening and night personnel during the daytime. Even when the time is repaid, this plan has not met with success. Separate meetings on each tour with one person serving as liaison seem to provide wider dissemination of information. Several institutions have used tape recorders with success, as a means of ongoing communication between the various tours. Obviously recorders cannot replace face-to-face discussion completely. Succinct, pertinent change-of-tour reports are perhaps most valuable given face-to-face. It is suggested, however, that staff discussions and in-service meetings be recorded and relayed to the individuals who were unable to attend. The absentees should then be given an opportunity to discuss their reactions with someone and to add their comments. In this situation, Mr. Kilborn should arrange to serve as liaison and establish continuity between tours. In a continuous program, the in-service coordinator may serve in this capacity.

Case 7 is an example of an administration that is reaching down from the top for new ideas that may lead to improved patient care through better work methods and increased personnel satisfaction. Rather than support a fire-fighting program of improvement which leaps from one crisis to another, the administration has planned a program which stimulates an interest in improvement and encourages questioning of the status quo. The director of nursing participated in the pilot program and recognized that this approach may be as effective in the nursing area as in any other department.

In an institution that has not yet undertaken a methods improvement program, the director of nursing may not only encourage her staff to study their methods but also promote acceptance of such a program by top management. She may also arrange to send personnel to workshops on methods improvement and to include this approach in the in-service program. Such a policy should not promote change for the sake of change but should be directed toward the improvement of work methods and the increase in job satisfaction, with the benefits accruing to the consumer, the patient.

SUPPLEMENTARY READING LIST

Adam, Antoinette: "Revise and Consent," *American Journal of Nursing,* vol. 64, pp. 85–87, January, 1964.

Bennett, Addison C.: "Improving Upward Communication," *Hospital Topics,* vol. 46, pp. 29–31, July, 1968.

Bennett, Addison C.: "Work Simplification Techniques Make Easy Methods Not So Hard to Find," *Hospitals, J.A.H.A.,* vol. 31, pp. 45–47, February 16, 1957.

Bennis, Warren G., et al. (eds.): *The Planning of Change,* 2d ed., Holt, Rinehart & Winston, New York, 1969.

Bobbitt, John C.: "Ways to Stimulate Suggestions," *Personnel Journal,* vol. 38, pp. 295–297, January, 1960.

Brown, Elaine, and John Roche: "Methods Study Shaped Team Nursing Plan," *The Modern Hospital,* vol. 107, pp. 121–123, September, 1966.

Brown, Esther Lucile: *Newer Dimensions of Patient Care, Part I, The Use of the Physical and Social Environment of the General Hospital for Therapeutic Purposes,* Russell Sage Foundation, New York, 1961, pp. 99–117.

Close, Guy: *Work Improvement,* John Wiley & Sons, Inc., New York, 1960, pp. 42–65, 117–130, 339–354.

Committee on Methods Improvement, American Hospital Association: *Organized Methods Improvement Programs in Hospitals,* American Hospital Association, Chicago, 1958.

Corson, John J.: "Innovation Challenges Conformity," *Harvard Business Review,* vol. 40, pp. 67–74, May–June, 1962.

Dubin, Robert: *The World of Work,* Prentice-Hall, Inc., Englewood Cliffs, N.J., 1958, pp. 110–123.

Ferguson, Stanley A., and Charles B. Womer: "Don't Preach Work Simplification Unless You Expect to Practice It," *The Modern Hospital,* vol. 87, pp. 71–73, October, 1956.

Ferguson, Stanley A., and Charles B. Womer: "Putting Work Simplification to Woık," *The Modern Hospital,* vol. 87, pp. 76–78, September, 1956.

Ferguson, Stanley A., and Charles B. Womer: "Work Simplification Is the Worker's Job," *The Modern Hospital,* vol. 87, pp. 60–62, August, 1956.

Ferrell, Edward S.: "Methods Improvement Workshops Teach Organized Common Sense," *Hospitals, J.A.H.A.,* vol. 36, pp. 40–43, May 1, 1962.

Gilbert, Albert F.: "Managing Change in the Hospital," *Hospital Topics,* vol. 47, pp. 40–41, July, 1969.

Kelly, Nancy Cardinal: "The Question Is Why," *American Journal of Nursing,* vol. 59, pp. 360–363, March, 1959.

Lapniewska, Janina B., and Mary O. Martinetti: "Working Smarter (Not Harder!)," *Nursing Outlook,* vol. 10, pp. 812–813, December, 1962.

Lawrence, Paul R.: "How to Deal with Resistance to Change," *Harvard Business Review,* vol. 47, pp. 4–12, 166–176, January–February, 1969.

Levy, Samuel: "Must There Be Conflict in An Organization?" *Hospitals J.A.H.A.,* vol. 37, pp. 53–57, May 16, 1963

McNulty, Matthew F.: "Annual Administrative Reviews: Methods Improvement," *Hospitals, J.A.H.A.*, vol. 35, pp. 121–123, April 16, 1961.

McWhorter, R. Clayton: "Methods Improvement Raises Quality of Care, Combats Rising Costs," *Hospital Topics*, vol. 44, pp. 48–50, 53, February, 1966.

Newman, William H., and Charles E. Summer, Jr.: *The Process of Management: Concepts, Behavior and Practice*, Prentice-Hall, Inc., Englewood Cliffs, N.J., 1961, pp. 137–154.

Silverman, Anne R.: "Work Simplification Teams," *Hospital Management*, vol. 91, pp. 42–46, April, 1961.

Stryker, Ruth P.: "Ramifications of a Procedure Investigation," *Nursing Outlook*, vol. 13, pp. 75–77, April, 1965.

case 8

The Nursing Staff and Professional Development

Ten years ago the nursing department of the Charles Evans Memorial Hospital instituted an in-service program for its professional nursing personnel. To direct the program, a Supervisor of In-service Education was appointed. Mrs Elaine Murphy, the head nurse on 6 South, was selected for this position. Two years later, the Supervisor of Nonprofessional Personnel started a formal in-service program for auxiliary nursing personnel. When the Nursing Planning Committee evaluated the separate programs last year, it decided to incorporate the two into a single program for all levels of nursing personnel. This program was placed under the direction of the Coordinator for In-service Education, a position assumed by Mrs. Murphy. When Mrs. Murphy submitted her resignation four months ago, the Director of Nursing announced the forthcoming vacancy and asked the head nurses and supervisors to suggest possible candidates for the position. When no applications were received from the staff, the position was awarded to Miss Elizabeth Flanders, a recent graduate of a graduate program in medical-surgical nursing. During Miss Flander's orientation, the In-service Education Advisory Committee conducted the program. At the completion of a three-month orientation period Miss Flanders met with Miss Anne Elliott, Director of Nursing, to discuss the future of the program.

Case Data | *Case Notes*

As a prelude to asking Miss Flanders to voice her impressions of the present in-service program, Miss Elliott stated: "Ten years ago we had no in-service tor the nursing staff. At present we have a program, but many of us feel it has become a token effort for employees rather than a vital part of our service for patients. Maybe it's time for a 'housecleaning'."

The new coordinator then reviewed with the director her evaluation of the present program and

Case Data *Case Notes*

commented that perhaps the original purpose and philosophy had been lost in the transition from a "vertical" to a "horizontal" program. She had observed several program meetings during her orientation and wanted to offer the following suggestions as an approach to the revitalization of the in-service program:

1. A meeting with the In-service Education Advisory Committee to review and restate the philosophy and objectives for the program.
2. Distribution to all nursing service personnel of a questionnaire seeking an evaluation of the present program and suggestions for changes.
3. A meeting with the nursing supervisors and head nurses to identify the needs manifested by nursing personnel.
4. A meeting with the Personnel Department to clarify the objectives and content of the orientation program for all new hospital employees.
5. A meeting with the Supervisor of Nonprofessional Personnel to clarify the objectives and content of the training programs for auxiliary nursing personnel.
6. Consideration of changes in the functions and membership of the In-service Education Advisory Committee.
7. Active participation of nursing personnel in the planning and execution of the program.
8. Formulation of some means of continuous evalution of the program.

The director expressed admiration of the proposals made by Miss Flanders and signified her approval of the preliminary approach to revitalization. She agreed with the coordinator that a review of the philosophy and objectives for the program was needed. She added, "This discussion has also made me realize that you, not I, should serve as chairman of the advisory committee. With your permission, I shall propose this change at our next meeting."

Miss Flanders indicated that she would assume the responsibility of the chairmanship if the advisory committee were in accord with the change. The conference ended with Miss Elliott's

Case Data | *Case Notes*

remark, "You have only completed your initial orientation, and your job description needs revision already!"

Miss Flanders arranged for a luncheon and extended meeting of the advisory committee. An agenda was prepared and distributed one week in advance. Each member was asked to review the stated philosophy and to be prepared to evaluate the present program. By the time the group met, Miss Flanders had prepared a tentative form for a questionnaire for the nursing staff. This was approved by the advisory committee, as was Miss Elliott's suggestion that the coordinator become chairman of the group. A lively discussion of the philosophy ensued. The members frankly admitted that the program had fallen short of the real goal of improved nursing care for the patient, and had actually been promoted as a "fringe benefit" for personnel. They also realized that the result was a segmented program instead of a comprehensive, coordinated program which would include orientation, on-the-job training, and continuing development. A tentative restatement of philosophy was formulated. The group agreed to meet again one week later to complete the revision.

At the next meeting the statement of philosophy was revised to make explicit the belief that the primary objective of an in-service program for nursing personnel is improvement in care for patients. The group identified certain basic aspects for the orientation and skill training for various levels of personnel. It was agreed that these would be considered tentative until the results of the survey questionnaire became available. Several members commented that a reorganization of the nursing department may contribute toward coordination of the program for all nursing personnel.

The results of the questionnaire indicated that the majority of nursing personnel preferred a multidisciplinary, multilevel approach to personnel development. The need for assistance in the areas of person-to-person and person-to-patient relations was the most frequently stated need. The staff nurses who were recent graduates of basic pro-

Case Data *Case Notes*

grams in nursing requested assistance in directing nonprofessional personnel. The nursing assistants and licensed practical nurses, as a group, indicated an interest in team nursing and in knowledge about the educational programs of the medical and nursing students who had clinical laboratory experiences at the hospital. Personnel in all levels expressed the belief that they could contribute to a greater extent if they knew more about the various research projects in progress on several of the divisions. These findings led to several additions to the orientation and skill-training aspects of the in-service program.

When Miss Flanders suggested that a greater number of nursing personnel be involved in planning the program for professional development, skepticism was expressed by some of the members of the advisory committee. They feared that the personnel may not select the content the supervisors and head nurses had identified as pertinent. After listening to the comments, Miss Flanders suggested that interest in the new program may be stimulated if attention is first paid to the needs expressed by the staff and then to the areas identified as vital to staff development at various levels. She added, "Studies have shown that participation promotes personnel development, whereas manipulation tends to destroy motivation."

The advisory committee planned to hold meetings to report to nursing personnel the findings based on the questionnaire and to organize planning groups within the nursing staff. Miss Elliott suggested that the next meeting of the present advisory committee be devoted to a consideration of changes in the membership and of functions of the advisory committee

DISCUSSION

The necessity for providing in-service education for hospital personnel has been widely accepted by hospital and nursing administrators. Few hospitals cannot advertise that they offer an in-service education program, at least for the nursing staff, if not for all employees. In spite of this general acceptance of the concept of in-service education, most hospitals have faced situations similar to those described at the Charles Evans Memorial Hospital. Programs have been started, but all too frequently the original purpose has been forgotten, or the initial enthusiasm has given way to grudging acceptance and token attendance of in-service program meetings. The case data is not explicit regarding the difficulties that beset the in-service program for nursing personnel, but the need for revitalization is evident from the remarks of the director of nursing, the suggestions of the newly appointed coordinator, and the lack of applicants for the position of coordinator when the opportunity was presented.

To assume the position of coordinator of an unsatisfactory or ineffective program is not easy. In some instances it is a more difficult task than inaugurating a program. Suffice it to say here that although the approach may differ slightly, the principles basic to in-service education apply both to the formulation of a new program and to the revitalization of an existing program.

One of the prime requisites for an effective in-service education program in any organization is the positive participation and support of top administrative personnel. From the case data one learns that for ten years the nursing service department has budgeted a position for someone to direct the in-service program for the professional nursing staff. This is indicative of administrative support. Further support is evidenced by the orientation period allotted to Miss Flanders. The Director of Nursing and the In-service Advisory Committee were willing to assume the responsibility for the in-service activities in the interim so that Miss Flanders would have sufficient time to investigate the existing situation without pressure to produce changes immediately. Administrative support must, however, continue beyond the initial planning. The director and the assistant directors of nursing must serve as models for the staff. They must demonstrate conviction of the need for continuing development by requiring of themselves as much as they expect of the nursing staff. This does not mean that meetings attended as a part of their job responsibilities can serve this purpose. The director who is involved in learning, or in expanding her own skills in an area directly related to patient care, can inspire the staff to follow suit. She must also show continued interest in, and support of, the person whose job it is to coordinate the in-service program. This person usually functions in a staff position and does not have direct authority over the nursing personnel. The plans for the in-service program may become entangled in the bind between the anticipated benefits of the program and the pressures of daily needs for service to patients. It is the ultimate responsibility of the director and her assistants to balance these pushes and pulls and to support the program and the coordinator in her assigned task.

The case data do not reveal whether Miss Flanders had any previous experience with in-service programs. Such programs have been utilized widely in hospitals only since 1955. It would be reasonable to speculate that she did not have experience in conducting or in participating in an in-service program prior to accepting the position. Some persons say that lack of experience need not be the handicap it may seem to be. To paraphrase a statement in *Doings, Highlights, News* of the Department of Hospital Nursing of the National League for Nursing:[1]

> Few nurses have experienced true inservice education. Those who try to give it and those who expect to receive it try to apply to it the concepts of education gained in formal schooling.

When one accepts a new position, there is a temptation to prove one's worth by acting immediately. It is far more important, however, to spend time in a thoughtful appraisal of the situation. When Miss Flanders accepted the position as Coordinator of In-service Education, she apparently recognized that much thinking and careful planning would have to precede any action if she is to fulfill her responsibility for the position. The suggestions she forwarded to the director of nursing at the end of her orientation indicate thoughtful appraisal and exemplify the use of the thinking step of the *administrative blueprint* in approaching the problem of reorganizing the in-service education program in the nursing department of the Hospital.

It seems apparent that the two areas of initial exploration centered around the questions, "What really is an in-service program?," and "What is the present status of the program in the nursing department at the Charles Evans Memorial Hospital?"

The majority of the numerous articles on in-service programs describe tools and techniques developed for particular institutions without describing the theoretical bases upon which they are based. Two primary purposes are usually stated for in-service education programs: (1) the improvement of patient care, and (2) the promotion of job satisfaction.

[1] Department of Hospital Nursing, National League for Nursing, "Stereotypes May Handicap Nurses," *Doings, Highlights, News*, vol. 7, pp. 1, 3, April, 1962.

The authors firmly believe that only one aim—the improvement of patient care—justifies the time, effort, and expense required for an in-service education program. Admittedly, an effective program will contribute to job satisfaction for the personnel involved, but this should be a means to the end, not the end itself. Reductions in the turnover of employees and in absenteeism have been claimed as benefits to be derived from an effective in-service program. But if these factors become the purpose of the in-service program, other possible causes for turnover rate may be overlooked and the services to patients may be reduced instead of improved. Employee satisfaction is not always compatible with patient needs. The outstanding example of this is, of course, the patient's need for care around the clock, whereas the majority of employees prefer to work conventional day tours. Almost every hospital claims that its primary purpose is to serve the patient. Each program that is supported financially by the hospital is expected to contribute to this major purpose. An in-service educational program should not be conducted simply as a fringe benefit for employees.

If all in-service programs have the same stated purpose, can a single program be devised for use by nursing departments throughout the country? A single program may simplify the endeavor considerably, but the dissimilarities in patient and personnel populations of different health agencies outnumber the similarities. If one accepts the improvement of care for the patient as the major purpose, one can appreciate the different approaches required, for example, in an in-service program in a Veterans Administration hospital, in a maternity hospital, in a children's hospital, in a psychiatric hospital, and in a public health agency. Such differences also exist between large general hospitals and small community hospitals. It is necessary for each nursing department to formulate the objectives of its in-service education program in light of its philosophy of nursing and nursing service, and the needs of patients and personnel. The principles will be relatively universal; the practices will vary.

In-service education is one form of adult education. It is an on-the-job approach to learning directed toward producing greater staff competence and toward expanding interest in and understanding of patients. It is a means of keeping abreast of the rapid advances in medicine, in nursing, and in the contributing disciplines. And although this discussion focuses on in-service education for persons employed in health agencies, the concept is equally applicable to any service organization. In fact, many of the ideas about in-service education have come from organizations other than health agencies.

An in-service education program has four components: orientation; skill training; continuing education; and leadership training. *Orientation* is the introduction of the employee to his job and its requirements, to his fellow workers, and to the institution as a whole. It is the phase designed to stimulate the employee to identify himself with the organization and its goals.

Skill training provides the employee with the manual, intellectual, and interpersonal skills necessary for carrying out assigned functions. For a person employed as a nurse aide, the training period may be extensive. For the graduate professional nurse assigned to a staff nurse position it may be limited to training in team leadership, in the use of electrical monitoring devices, or in the use of an automatic medication-dispensing system. Nursing service departments utilize orientation and skill-training more readily and more universally than the less-structured and less time-limited components—continuing education and leadership training. The pressures of providing service to patients have forced nursing service to adopt measures to absorb and train new personnel as rapidly as possible.

Continuing education, or staff development, is the most dynamic, flexible, fluctuating, and challenging component of in-service education. It is designed to motivate personnel to gain greater knowledge and experience. Consequently it is the most frustrating and most difficult area to organize and present. In contrast to the other phases, it is not time-limited. It must be directed toward all levels of personnel. It must strive to meet the learning needs of nurse aides, ward clerks, practical nurses, and professional nurses—all with varying backgrounds of education, experience, and length of service to the particular health agency offering the program.

The *leadership,* or *management training,* phase is generally concerned with the preparation of professional nurses for head nurse or supervisor positions. It may also be considered for other levels of nursing personnel who have demonstrated potential leadership ability. Of the four areas described, leadership training and orientation are most frequently shared, at least in part, with other departments in the hospital or health agency.

There are two divergent philosophies about in-service education. One philosophy advocates that all who work together should learn together whenever possible, that all members of the nursing team should participate together in the in-service program—the so-called horizontal approach to in-service. The other insists that the needs of personnel with such varied levels of preparation cannot be met at the same time, that a vertical approach should be planned with separate programs for the various levels of personnel. Those who hold to the latter position point out that even within the professional nursing staff a wide variety of preparation and experience may be found at any one time. Working side by side are graduates of many years ago and graduates of last year. There are graduates of diploma programs offering only the minimum experience necessary for state approval and graduates of programs enriched with college-level courses in the liberal arts and in the sciences. There are graduates of collegiate nursing programs who have had experiences in a variety of settings and who possess a broad understanding of the scientific, sociologic, and cultural implications of nursing. To plan an in-service education program to meet the needs and interests of these varied groups within the professional nursing staff would seem to be a difficult task. It remains, however, for each agency to evaluate its own situation and to reach a decision about the approach that best meets its requirements.

After studying the basic knowledge about in-service education, Miss Flanders was in a position to investigate the present status of the program at the Charles Evans Memorial Hospital. The suggestions presented by Miss Flanders upon the completion of her initial survey indicate that some of the probable "trouble spots" in the existing program were vague or outmoded philosophy and objectives; lack of coordination between the institutional program for all employees and the departmental program for nursing personnel; lack of coordination and communication within the department itself; absence of provisions for evaluation of the program; an apparent need for reorganization within the nursing department; and lack of active involvement of personnel in the program. This study demonstrates the use of the thinking phase of the *administrative blueprint* in relation to planning, organizing, and evaluating, and the assembling of basic information.

Miss Flanders had been charged with the responsibility of revitalizing the in-service education program. If she had presented a definite plan for reorganization of the existing program, it is very probable that her plan would have been accepted without much argument. She chose, however, to offer suggestions and to approach any changes through the existing channels of authority. She may have effected changes more quickly had she presented definite plans, but all findings regarding ways to produce enduring improvements seem to support the approach she chose. She merely pointed out some of the apparent trouble spots in an attempt to gain acceptance for revisions by involving the group in formulating the new plans. There are drawbacks to this method if one is working with a group that does not recognize a need for change, but the case data indicate that the nursing personnel at the Charles Evans Memorial Hospital were aware that the existing program was not satisfactory.

The first steps in the planning phase were *revision* of the philosophy and objectives and *clarification* of the relationship of the program in the nursing department to the hospital in-service program. In-service programs in most hospitals have been developed in response to departmental needs, with the nursing department usually initiating the first one, followed frequently by the establishment of a program for the dietary department or the housekeeping department. Because a great number of clerical and nonprofessional workers have been added to the hospital work force, hospitals have tended to establish in-service programs for all hospital personnel. Some have created a separate department of in-service education. The current trend indicates that it is economically possible for a hospital of 250 beds or more to have a separate training department. Few hospitals have organized such departments, but many have devised an orientation program to provide a simultaneous introduction for all employees to the hospital, its philosophy and goals, its organization, and its physical plant.

Before plans are made for in-service education for nursing employees, the plans and content of the institutional program should be reviewed. The organizational relationship between the persons responsible for each program should also be clarified. Some authorities advocate that all departmental in-service efforts be placed under the direction of a director of in-service who would hold a top-level administrative position with staff and line functions. This individual would be responsible for the personnel who conduct training programs at the departmental level. Such a plan would have the following advantages: provision for coordination; avoidance of duplication of effort; possibilities for a comprehensive evaluation program; and opportunities for training personnel to share ideas and common interests. The chief disadvantage is that persons who are responsible for performance at the departmental level have no direct control over the training given to personnel for whom they are responsible. This objection could be invalidated by a training program advisory committee composed of representatives from all departments. The need for economy of time, money, and resources will, in the future, force department heads to relinquish some autonomy and to participate in interdepartmental programs.

The case data reveal that the Personnel Department conducted an orientation for all new hospital employees but do not disclose the existence of in-service efforts outside the nursing department. As director of nursing, Miss Eliott should have been aware of any possibility of an impending extension of the institutional program. It is assumed that her approval of Miss Flanders' suggestions indicates that a broad approach was not being contemplated by the administration.

Before any further planning could be done, the basic beliefs regarding the in-service program needed to be reexamined by the nursing personnel charged with the major responsibility for supervising nursing care at the Hospital. Do they still believe, for example, that the horizontal approach to education produces better results? Do they believe that attendance at program meetings should be compulsory? Should leadership training be given to all professional nurses, or to a few identified as potential leaders? What are the obligations of the staff to the in-service program? The beliefs regarding these questions and others must be clarified before specific objectives can be stated.

From her study of in-service education Miss Flanders undoubtedly formulated a philosophy of in-service education, but to impose this philosophy upon the nursing service department certainly would have reduced the possibility of developing a program the supervisory personnel would support. Once a statement of philosophy is revised and accepted by the group, specific objectives can be established for the in-service program and for the several areas within the program. These are essential for long-range planning and for evaluation of the program. It is important also that nursing personnel know the objectives of the in-service program so that their expectations are in accord with the objectives and that they, too, have a basis for evaluating the program.

As soon as the philosophy and objectives are formulated, the organization of personnel to facilitate achievement of the objectives must be considered. Several references in the case data indicate that reorganization may be necessary. It is indicated that the supervisor of nonprofessional personnel is responsible for the training program for the auxiliary nursing personnel. Since skill-training is one of the components of the in-service program, this area should be considered within the framework of the total program, not as a separate entity. In her discussion with the director of nursing, Miss Flanders had suggested that the objectives and content of the training program be discussed with the supervisor of the auxiliary personnel. It may be that she was reluctant to suggest that the lines of authority and responsibility be clarified and that the separate program be made a part of the whole. The very title, *supervisor of nonprofessional personnel,* is confusing. One wonders what responsibilities and functions are assigned to this position. Obviously one person cannot adequately supervise all the auxiliary personnel on the nursing staff of the Charles Evans Memorial Hospital. And if it were possible, it would be a violation of the principles of organization that the person who has the responsibility for achieving a goal must have authority over the persons working toward the goal. Thus the head nurse should have authority over all nursing personnel assigned to her division. All in-service education efforts for the nursing department should be under the direction and supervision of one individual, the coordinator of in-service education. In a large hospital she may have one or more assistants. In a small hospital this may be a part-time position or one of several responsibilities assigned to a member of the nursing staff. When the members of the advisory committee suggested that a reorganization of the nursing department may contribute to coordination of the program for all nursing personnel, they may have been referring to the need for clarification of the relationship between the roles of in-service coordinator and supervisor of nonprofessional personnel.

In suggesting that a questionnaire be used to elicit opinions from the staff prior to program planning, Miss Flanders was heeding one of the principles of learning—start where the learner is. With the survey she hoped to discover the needs and interests identified by the various levels of personnel. Such a device may also indicate to personnel that their participation in the planning of the program is not only desired but expected. Many in-service programs have failed because they have been imposed on the staff without regard for interests and felt needs, and because the staff has not had a voice in the planning or a hand in the presentation. It takes more time to involve the participants, but it also reaps more benefits for all concerned. The role of the in-service coordinator should be that of motivator, not dictator; of coordinator, not coercer.

From the results of the questionnaire, from the meetings with the supervisors and head nurses, and from the meeting with the person responsible for the institution's orientation program, Miss Flanders should have had some clue to the content for the various areas of the program. Since the position of in-service education coordinator is a staff, or advisory, position and, as such, carries no direct authority over nursing service personnel, means must be provided for communication with persons in authority. The In-service Education Advisory Committee serves this purpose. Composed of representatives from the various clinical and service areas in the nursing department, this committee has among its functions broad planning and policy-making for the in-service education program for the nursing service department. It is also responsible for evaluating the program. The coordinator is chairman of the committee. Some nursing departments include representatives from the medical staff and the school of nursing on the advisory committee for the purpose of securing cooperation from these areas in presenting the program. The responsibility of developing nursing personnel is the obligation of the nursing department; other disciplines and departments should not be expected to assume this responsibility. Their advice and consultation should be sought, but care must be taken not to impose upon others responsibility that belongs to the nursing service department.

Perhaps the most crucial policy to be decided is the policy regarding attendance. Should attendance and participation be voluntary or compulsory? If the primary purpose of the program is the improvement of patient care, can one justify voluntary attendance? And yet, does mental absorption always accompany physical compliance? How receptive is a captive audience? Both approaches have been tried. Compulsory attendance may reach a few who would not attend voluntarily; yet it may well antagonize many who would have been motivated to attend voluntarily. The real challenge in in-service education is the creation of a program that will attract and hold the interest of the personnel it is designed to reach. Flexibility is the key to such a program: flexibility of content, of approach, of timing. There are some policies and practices in nursing service that must be communicated to the staff for the safety of the patient. A channel of communication other than the in-service program should be used for disseminating such information so that the personnel that must be communicated to the staff for the safety of the patient. A channel of communication other than the in-service program should be used for disseminating such information so that the personnel can think of the in-service program as a program for professional development, not indoctrination.

and in what ways the budget for in-service should be allocated. Some institutions use the advisory committee for specific program planning. This is perhaps less time consuming, but experience has shown that participants have a greater investment in programs when they participate in the planning.

Miss Flanders' approach to the planning may depend upon the philosophical decision relative to the horizontal or vertical approach to in-service education. If a horizontal approach is selected, the planning committee would be composed of representatives of the various levels of nursing personnel on the staff. If, on the other hand, the decision is to consider the needs of each level independently, then planning groups would be formed for each different level. In either approach, the role of the coordinator would be the same: to provide assistance; to serve as consultant and resource person; to facilitate arrangements; to help others teach one another; to arrange for continuity and evaluation.

In planning a new in-service program or when reorganizing an existing program, determination must be made of the area of greatest need: orientation, skill training, continuing education, or leadership training. All four areas are essential, but a concentrated effort in one area at a time has a greater chance of producing good results than does a diffuse approach to all areas simultaneously. Success in an area tends to stimulate interest when a program is initiated in a second area. It will be necessary for the advisory committee to determine which area has the priority for initial attention. If, for example, the institution has an orientation program for all new hospital employees, and if the nursing department has a training program for nursing assistants, the improvement of patient care may be approached by giving priority to the inauguration of a continuing education program. An evaluation may disclose, however, that although a training program exists, the need is greater in this area. In establishing priority the advisory committee must consider all possible approaches to the improvement of patient care. In addition, two other factors deserve consideration: staff interests and the skills of the in-service coordinator. The programs for the preparation of nurses to assume leadership positions in in-service education are few. The demand for the services of such persons is great and is increasing. Some consideration must be given to the particular ability of the individual employed to assume the direction of the in-service program. In the case of Miss Flanders, whose advanced preparation was in medical-surgical nursing, one may speculate that she would be more adept and at ease in initiating a program with clinical content than a program with emphasis on administrative content. The adage, "Nothing breeds success like success," is applicable to this situation. The new coordinator who is able to inaugurate an effective program in a familiar area is generally encouraged to venture into unknown territory with some confidence.

Staff interests must also be considered in the inauguration of a new program. A survey may disclose that the majority of the nursing staff identified a need to improve the orientation for new personnel. Participation of the staff in the total program could be stimulated through heed to expressed interest. The case data reveal that Miss Flanders was planning to elicit from the head nurses and supervisors opinions about the needs manifested by nursing personnel. Suppose this group identified improvement of observational skills as one of the major needs. Through the questionnaire survey the nursing staff had expressed an interest in the research projects being carried out on several wards. It would be possible to capitalize on the interests of the staff and the needs of the head nurses and supervisors by means of a program relating to the research projects, with emphasis on the relationship of observation to research. This may, in turn, motivate the staff to increase their own observational skills.

The content and approach to each area of in-service education must be determined by each nursing service after the needs of the patients and the staff have been evaluated. It should be remembered that orientation sets the stage for the employee's relationship with the hospital. In fact, orientation starts before the individual joins the staff. It starts with the first contact between prospective employee and employer. Every effort must be made to inform the prospective staff member of the institution's philosophy of patient care and nursing service to enable him to compare it with his own philosophy and reach a decision regarding the compatibility of the two. In planning the induction of a new employee, consideration must be given to information that is essential for her assigned position. Some of this can be presented in general sessions with employees from all departments. When this is done, however, care must be taken not to present material which is so general that it is of little interest.

Two common faults of orientation planning should be avoided. The first is the tendency to dispense too much information too fast, before the employee has a chance to estimate the value of such information. The learner needs time to assimilate new experiences and to correlate them with past experiences. The purpose of orientation is to establish identification with the people and the situation. This takes time. Perhaps the most effective way of introducing the new employee to the agency is to assign an individual to guide the new staff member. The knowledge that there is one person to whom one may turn for advice, information, and guidance provides a feeling of security. Care must be taken in the selection of the guide, however. Not everyone can or should fill this role. The guide must be a person whose beliefs are in accord with those of the institution; who is interested in helping to develop another's talents, not merely in displaying her own; whose approach is flexible; who is able to identify and respond to the needs of the new person; and who can provide assistance without creating dependence. The length of time allotted to orientation must vary with each individual. The use of a guide facilitates this adjustment to individual needs.

All too frequently the immediate need for the services of "two more hands" is allowed to interrupt or even to terminate the orientation of a new employee. This is the other common fault in orientation practices. If the in-service coordinator is expected to achieve certain objectives with the orientation program, she must be given the opportunity to carry out her plans. Some institutions believe so strongly in the value of an adequate orientation as a basis for future performance that the new employee is not made available for service until he has been released by the in-service coordinator.

Other points to consider in establishing an orientation program are:

1. The first day in a new situation, which may stimulate or destroy the interest of the new employee.
2. Definite plans, especially for the first day, should be made so that the employee will feel expected and that time is not to be wasted.
3. Written information should be presented in order to avoid burdening the new employee with detail and to give him a source of review.
4. A written job description should be presented to each person so that he will be aware of what is expected of him.
5. Information should be given as to when the employee can expect to receive his first pay check.
6. The new employee is far more interested in the specific area and the persons with whom he will be working than he is in touring the institution and meeting the heads of all departments.
7. Orientation may be needed each time an individual assumes a new position within the institution, not just prior to the initial position.

8. Orientation plans for every employee—full-time and part-time, administrative, clerical, clinical, and service—must be made.

In recent years nursing departments have established on-the-job training classes for aides, or assistants, because few formal educational programs are designed to train personnel for this position in the health field. These agency-based programs range from a few hours of instruction in the methods of taking temperatures and giving baths to more extensive programs which include content related to human relations and the emotional and physical needs of individual patients. Until there are licensed educational programs for nonprofessional nursing presonnel, hospitals will have to assume the responsibility for training the persons they employ to assist the professional nurse and the practical nurse in giving care to patients. The content of the program will be determined by the job description for the various nonprofessional or auxiliary positions. This training task must not be assigned to persons who are responsible for caring for patients at the same time. Placing untrained or partially trained workers on a nursing unit takes the time of persons who are already trained without contributing anything to the unit or to patients and is a hazard to patients. The smaller institutions admittedly have a problem of having to train so few nursing assistants when the time and expenditure needed are open to question. It is anticipated that cooperative programs will be developed among several small institutions in a given locale. In the meantime, the best solution seems to be for the in-service director to assume responsibility for the supervision of the new employee until this employee can contribute safely to the care of patients.

Several important factors must be considered in training programs for auxiliary personnel. Provision must be made for supervision following instruction, and this supervision should be by the person who gave the training, in order to ensure similarity between theory and practice.

The training period should be considered a probationary period for the new employee. The professional nurse and the licensed practical nurse have gone through numerous screening processes in their basic educational programs to determine their fitness for giving care to people. The nonprofessional person should be screened for interest, motive, and emotional stability during the training period. Not all persons who express an interest in giving care to people can or should be permitted to render such care.

The content of the training program and the performance of the trainee should be discussed with the person in charge of the unit to which the individual is assigned. The timing of the training program must be flexible enough to meet the learning needs of the trainees. The trainee should not be "graduated" from the program until he is able to meet the requirements of the job description of the position. Throughout the indoctrination period, the trainee should be kept informed of his progress.

Skill-training programs should be available also for professional nurses and practical nurses. When a new employee joins the staff, the job description for the position should be reviewed in detail with the individual, and a training plan should be devised for any area in which the employee lacks the necessary skills. For the professional nurse this may be training as a team leader; for the practical nurse it may be training in the administration of medications. This component of in-service education has all too seldom been considered for professional and practical nurses.

Leadership training, another component of in-service education, is difficult for smaller institutions to offer because of the minimal numbers of personnel involved. Some hospitals have made such a program economically feasible by using an interdepartmental or hospital-wide approach to leadership training. Others have arranged for a nearby educational institution to conduct a leadership training program for several hospitals in neighboring communities. Many have resorted to an understudy approach. Larger institutions can usually plan and conduct their own programs economically. Originally many institutions offered separate departmental programs, but the current trend seems to be toward a single program for prospective leaders in all departments. The content for such a program generally centers around problem-solving techniques and human relations skills. This approach supports the belief that administrative principles are universal.

The major difference that exists among leadership training programs offered for nursing personnel seems to be the time factor. The majority of institutions wait until a vacancy occurs or is impending before preparing someone to fill the vacancy. A few seek to identify staff members with leadership potential and to invite them to attend leadership training courses in order to have trained personnel available when the need arises. The majority group argues that the latter approach is costly because of the rate of turnover among personnel in health agencies. The authors support advance preparation on the theory that persons who attend the courses not only benefit but also contribute to the learning of others in the course. The incentives acquired through attending the course may be such that personnel who may have resigned are encouraged to remain. A broad overall approach to leadership training is more economical in the long run than separate training programs for the positions of assistant head nurse, head nurse, or supervisor.

It is the obligation of every professional person to continue to learn so long as he remains in practice. Ideally, every professional nurse would recognize her obligation and would assume the responsibility for continuing her own education. Some do; many unfortunately do not. At the same time the hospital and its nursing department have an obligation to promote continuing education in order to improve the care for patients. The area of continuing education is the most dynamic and most challenging area of in-service education. The nursing department of the Charles Evans Memorial Hospital has 975 full-time employees. A continuing education program that would interest, stimulate, and educate each staff member seems almost beyond the range of possibility, but if some of the stereotyped methods of in-service education are discarded and the advisory committee and the coordinator dream a little and dare to experiment, a comprehensive program can be devised.

First and foremost the staff must be helped to realize that nursing service personnel can learn from one another and can teach one another. It is not easy to convince personnel of this. When invited to participate in planning, the first suggestions of nursing personnel are to import someone to lecture, to demonstrate, or to give a concise answer to a specific problem. This pattern is understandable when one reviews the methods of teaching under which these same persons received much of their general and professional education. Somehow this must be changed if the continuing education program is to produce results that will contribute directly to the improvement of patient care. A lecture by a representative of a business machines company on the future use of data processing machines in hospitals may add to the general knowledge of the nursing staff, but it does not make a direct contribution to the nursing care of patients.

There are, however, many topics of interest and concern to several levels of personnel and related to the immediate care of the patient. One of these topics is *visiting hours*—the meaning to and value for the patient, and the implications for the nursing staff. Actual incidents may be acted out to provoke discussion. The nursing personnel should be responsible for planning, conducting, and participating in the program. This is just one example of the multilevel problem-solving approach, which may be applied to an endless number of areas.

Educational institutions have long recognized that it is difficult for a person who is involved in the daily activities of teaching to keep completely abreast of the advances in his field or to study a subject in depth. For this reason educational and sabbatical leaves were devised. Nursing may consider utilizing these devices as means of continuing education for professional personnel. For instance, a staff nurse could be encouraged to identify a problem of interest, then to apply for a leave of several days (with pay) to investigate the problem and to report on her findings. The time required may be no more than the time she would have spent in attending several "monthly lectures," but it may produce more benefits for patients and for other staff nurses.

Study groups offer another interesting approach to continuing education. These can be formed on any level, related to any area of patient care, and permit an intensive study of an aspect of nursing care by a relatively small group of people. The planning committee for the staff nurse group may arrange to offer six study units during the year in such areas as the nursing care of patients following thoracic surgery, or the care of patients on isotope therapy. Staff nurses are permitted to register for groups in which they are interested, and attendance is scheduled so that no division staff is seriously depleted. Resource materials and bibliographies are assembled, and participation is in seminars, not through lectures. The units are usually designed to be covered in twelve to twenty hours of study over a two- to four-week period. Tangible results have been produced by the study group approach. Many participants have been motivated to investigate further on their own. This approach need not be restricted to utilization by professional personnel. For example, a study unit on the characteristics of the newborn has been effectively used by one of the authors [DAK] for newborn nursery aides. A unit on the care of the patient following a cerebrovascular accident was of particular interest to practical nurses in the same agency.

Programs designed for an individual staff member offer still another approach to continuing development. The advent of programmed instructional materials and small portable audiovisual equipment have expanded the possibilities for individualized instruction. In fact these and other technological and educational advances may, in the future, lead to a form of institutional development program undreamed of in the past. Suppose, for example, that after a head nurse prepares and reviews a performance evaluation with a staff nurse, an appointment is made for the staff nurse with the in-service coordinator or instructor. At this time the coordinator and the nurse consider the recommendations of the head nurse for improvement and further development in the performance of the staff nurse. These recommendations then become the objectives for a program of independent study designed to meet the needs of this nurse at this time. While instituting such a program on a broad scale may be a bold venture in in-service education and a radical break from traditional methods, the possibilities for improving care for patients inherent in this approach are many and should be tested.

Regardless of the approach used to stimulate and promote continuing education, all nursing service personnel should be considered—supervisors, aides, staff nurses, and head nurses. Provision must be made, also, for continuing education for evening and night personnel.

In-service education cannot force individuals to learn, but it can emphasize the need to learn and can be the stimulus for personal and professional development. It has suffered many vicissitudes in its introductory use for nursing service, but it is now generally accepted as a necessary component in nursing service and is rapidly becoming a successful method toward improving care for patients.

SUPPLEMENTARY READING LIST

Brown, Esther Lucile: *Newer Dimensions of Patient Care, Part II, Improving Staff Motivation and Competence in the General Hospital,* Russell Sage Foundation, New York, 1962, pp. 122–136.

Brueck, Robert P.: "Employee Orientation: A Channel for Good Will," *Hospitals, J.A.H.A.*, vol. 33, pp. 46–48, August 1, 1959.

Department of Hospital Nursing, National League for Nursing: "Stereotypes May Handicap Nurses," *Department of Hospital Nursing Doings, Highlights, News,* vol. 7, pp. 1, 3, April, 1962.

Fine, Ruth B., and Catherine Vavra: "Content and Consequences of an In-service Program," *American Journal of Nursing,* vol. 62, pp. 54–56, January, 1962.

Fogt, Joan R.: "In-service Concerns Everyone," *American Journal of Nursing,* vol. 63, pp. 83–85, November, 1963.

Hall, Bernard H.: "Creating a Climate for Learning," *Nursing Outlook,* vol. 7, pp. 421–422, July, 1959.

Helvie, Carl O., et al.: "The Setting and Nursing Practice," *Nursing Outlook,* vol. 16, pp. 27–29, August, 1968.

Lindberg, H. G.: "Mental Health Concepts in In-service Education," *Nursing Outlook,* vol. 17, pp. 34–35, April, 1969.

Long, Lewis K.: "Motivating Personnel for In-service Education," *Nursing Outlook*, vol. 7, pp. 333–335, June, 1959.

McClellan, Marilyn: "Staff Development in Action," *American Journal of Nursing*, vol. 68, pp. 298–300, February, 1968.

Marshall, Minna H.: "In-service Programs Require Effective Follow-up," *Nursing Outlook*, vol. 12, pp. 42–44, August, 1964.

Metzger, Norman: "Sound Orientation Can Reduce Turnover," *Hospitals, J.A.H.A.*, vol. 41, pp. 62–64, September 1, 1967.

Miller, Mary A.: *In-service Education for Hospital Nursing Personnel*, Department of Hospital Nursing, National League for Nursing, New York, 1958.

Naber, Mary: "A Development Program for Head Nurses," *Nursing Outlook*, vol. 16, pp. 48–49, June, 1968.

Packer, Annie R.: "In-service Education: Busy Work or Basic Need?" *American Journal of Nursing*, vol. 68, pp. 2404–2407, November, 1968.

Payson, Mary R., and J. Colman Salloway: "In-service Revisited," *American Journal of Nursing*, vol. 68, pp. 812–815, April, 1968.

Pirnie, F. Anne: "Why, What, and How of In-service Education," *Nursing Outlook*, vol. 12, pp. 47–51, January, 1964.

Poole, Drusilla: "Study Units—A Means for In-service Education," *American Journal of Nursing*, vol. 54, pp. 194–196, February, 1954.

Puleo, Sister Mary P.: "Comparison of On-the-Job and At-Home Use of Programmed Instruction and Lecture Method in an In-service Education Program, *Nursing Research*, vol. 17, pp. 356–360, July–August, 1968.

Tosiello, Frank: "University-Oriented In-service Education," *Nursing Outlook*, vol. 12, pp. 40–42, April, 1964.

case **9**

Cooperation for Improved Care for Patients

Some years ago, at the suggestion of the Director of Nursing, the administrator of the Charles Evans Memorial Hospital organized a Committee for Patient-centered Care. Prior to that time many aspects related to patient care were in the hands of committees such as the Infections Committee, the Nursing Procedures Advisory Committee, the Medical Council, and the Management Committee. The nursing department had been represented on the procedures and management committees, but none of the existing committees had provided an opportunity for the medical staff, the administrative personnel of the hospital, and the members of the nursing department to consider jointly the problems related to the provision of optimum care for the patient.

When the committee was being organized by the administrator, some resistance to the idea was evident. The first time the group convened the members generally expressed approval of the announced function of the committee, suggesting that their initial reluctance stemmed from the idea of "one more committee." Through the discussions of several situations described by John Alexander, the director of the hospital, the committee members recognized that many hindrances to improved care for patients are a result of inadequate coordination and communication among the hospital administration, the nursing department, and the medical staff. The chairman of the medical staff seemed to express the consensus of the group when he said, "We have all been trying to help a patient who seems to be in the center of a triangle. Perhaps we can move him to the hub of a smoothly rolling wheel."

The group defined its major purpose as that of stimulating coordination and innovation for the continuous improvement of care for patients and of formulating recommendations for specific changes to facilitate the accomplishment of this goal. The group accepted the administrator's suggestions for the composition of the committee: the chairman of the Medical Staff; three members of the medical staff appointed by the Medical Council; the Director of Nursing Service and Nursing Education; two Assistant Directors of Nursing; the Associate Director in charge of Nursing Education; a representative of the faculty of the nursing school; a representative of the faculty of the university nursing program; a representative of the college of medicine; the administrator and two assistant administrators. The chairman of the Medical Staff was elected chairman of the committee. The monthly meetings were planned to follow the regularly scheduled meetings of the Medical Council and the Planning Committee for Nursing Service.

In the first years of its existence the committee was responsible for several major changes in policy and procedures. After attending two meetings, the new Assistant Director of Professional Services commented, "The coordination and rapport that seem to have been established between these various groups of professional people exemplify that which is described in the texts but which is too seldom seen in practice."

Case Data	*Case Notes*

When the agenda for the March meeting of the Committee for Patient-centered Care was distributed several days before the meeting, one item under "new business" was listed as "brainstorming on the concept of Progressive Patient Care (PPC)." Several members assumed that consideration of this topic was related to the fact that a neighboring hospital had just opened a new Intensive Care Unit. Others speculated that it had some relationship to the new addition proposed for the hospital.

When the item was reached on the agenda, the chairman stated, "For the last six meetings we have been involved primarily in deliberating on existing problems. We have clarified several, and have referred others to standing committees for action. It seems that we may now take some time out from subjects of immediate practicality to consider patient-centered care from a philosophical approach. A discussion of Progressive Patient Care was suggested because from time to time the concept has been mentioned, but we have never stopped to share ideas about this trend in patient care and its possible relationship to our institution."

Before the chairman completed his introductory statements, the members displayed signs of want-

Case Data | *Case Notes*

ing to express opinions. Comments such as these were made spontaneously:

"Our recovery room is really an Intensive Care Unit."

"If we just staffed the recovery room around the clock, it would save many patients the cost of private duty nurses."

"A Self-care Unit could be opened in the house officers' residence, which is sparsely occupied now that most of the interns are married and live out."

"We would have to revise our training program for interns and residents if we group patients by degree of illness rather than by clinical service."

The discussion continued for approximately thirty minutes. At that point, the chief of the medical staff exclaimed, "We seem to have shunned the proposed philosophical approach to PPC in favor of the practical aspects. Perhaps this is evidence of a lack of broad knowledge about the concept. It may be that I am generalizing from my own lack of familiarity with this innovation in patient care; but I wonder if sufficient interest hasn't been generated to warrant devoting time to another meeting to discuss this further after we have had a chance to read about the proposals and experiences of others."

The group responded to this suggestion by agreeing to a discussion at another meeting and by suggesting that a special session be devoted to the discussion. A time for an extra meeting was established. The chairman announced that he would ask the hospital librarian to compile a file of information on progressive patient care for the members to read. The director of the hospital commented that he had a number of articles he could contribute to the file.

As they left the meeting, one of the assistant directors of nursing, Louise Hollingsworth, commented to Miss Elliott that several staff nurses and one of the head nurses had had experience in hospitals organized under a PPC program. The director suggested that after the nursing representatives had had an opportunity to review the

Case Data *Case Notes*

literature on PPC it would be helpful to meet with persons who had worked in such situations to clarify the different ways in which the proposal had been implemented and to elicit the reactions of these staff members to this method of patient care. Miss Hollingsworth agreed to arrange for a meeting before the special session of the Committee for Patient-centered Care. As they separated to return to their respective offices, Miss Elliott said, "We haven't had a 'dream' session in our planning committee for a long time. This meeting today reminded me of the value of putting aside temporarily the business of the day in order to indulge in thoughts of the future."

DISCUSSION

This case report concerns one committee at the Charles Evans Memorial, the Committee for Patient-centered Care, but it also mentions five other committees. The existence of additional committees was cited in the previous cases. This hospital is not unique in its utilization of committees. As the trend moves toward involving more and more persons in decision-making, the number of committees utilized increases. In fact, so many committees have been formed in some organizations that proposals have been made to create a Committee to Abolish Committees. Nevertheless, a committee is an important administrative tool. It is a technique that has become an indispensable part of the American way of achieving communication, coordination, and efficiency.

A committee is a group of persons charged with performing certain functions conjointly and cooperatively. It may be created for a function that could be done by one person. A procedure committee is established to write procedures that could be written by one person. A small group of persons may be formed to do a special task for a larger group. The Committee on Patient-centered Care is an example of the latter type. It would be impossible for all members of the medical, nursing, and managerial staffs to sit down together to discuss problems related to patient care, but selected representatives of each group can accomplish this purpose.

Committees are organized for the purposes of (1) stimulating participation; (2) pooling skills and knowledge; and (3) communication. The committee organized for the purpose of stimulating participation is often referred to as a morale-building committee. A committee approach can facilitate a united, cooperative attack on a problem. It tends to involve all the participants in responsibility for the action decided upon in committee. A morale-building committee may be used as a means of identifying a group with a specific purpose. Suppose, for example, that an organization has worked out a new insurance plan for employees. A written report of the proposed changes could be distributed to all employees. If representatives of various employee groups are chosen to function as a committee to devise a way of informing all employees about the new program, however, they will be able to identify the aspects in which their fellow employees would be interested and inevitably will become personally involved in selling the program. The reader will recall that the preceding case (Case 8) suggested the formation of committees to stimulate participation in the in-service education program. The purpose of any committee will be defeated, however, if the committee is formed just to give rubber-stamp approval to something an administrator has already planned down to the last detail.

The skill-collecting committee is composed of members selected because they are able to contribute some special knowledge to the solution of a problem or a group of problems. The nursing procedures committee is an example of a group formed to pool skills and knowledge. It usually has representatives from various clinical areas, each of whom is expected to have special knowledge of the needs of the patients in that area and to be able to point out the factors that must be considered in devising procedures to meet their needs. In any organization composed of groups of highly specialized departments or units, committees are essential for pooling diverse approaches, for clearance of information about each other's roles, and for functional coordination.

Committees may also be used as a communication device. Representatives of various groups may be organized into a committee to receive information, to distribute information to their own groups, and to report foreseeable problems. Such a committee has a liaison function, rather than an advisory or policy-making function. Conciliation is often effected through a committee composed of representatives of two different groups and chaired by an impartial third party. In such instances, the committee members are empowered to take certain actions only. In this instance, also, the committee is no more than a communication device. The only policies the committee members may support are those prescribed in advance by the group they represent.

Careful consideration and evaluation should precede the formation of any committee. A committee is too costly in man hours to be used indiscriminately. It should never be used to accomplish a purpose that one individual, working alone, could achieve equally well. If the purpose for which a committee is organized can be fulfilled within a certain period of time, the committee should be designated as a temporary or special committee, and it should be disbanded when it has accomplished its purpose. Far too many committees persist long after a need exists for group participation or group judgment.

Most organizations, however, will find times when the use of a standing committee seems clearly indicated. For the nursing service department, the need for the continuous surveillance, evaluation, and revision of nursing procedures is a condition that favors the maintenance of a permanent committee. When a permanent committee is organized, provision should be made for the periodic evaluation of its functions, membership, and accomplishments. The need for group participation or judgment may be continuous, but the approach to meeting the need may change with the times. It may be necessary to extend the functions of the committee to cover new situations, or the committee's task may become so involved that in efforts to accomplish the objectives the committee membership has been increased beyond the point of practicality.

The Committee for Patient-centered Care has a membership of fourteen. Were this committee responsible for decision-making, for formulating operational policies, or for revising procedures, its size might impede the attainment of objectives. In fact, some authorities suggest that the probability of accomplishing results decreases markedly when the committee membership exceeds seven. The committee has representatives from five different groups: physicians, nursing personnel, nursing educators, medical educators, and administrators. The more groups represented, the greater the possibility of conflict in goals and of difficulty in reaching a decision that will satisfy the majority of the membership. And yet, because the purpose of this committee is coordination and communication among the major professional groups involved in providing care for patients, it is essential to have sufficient representation to provide a comprehensive picture of situations. This committee does not set policies; other organized groups establish policies in specialized areas. This committee brings problems and issues into the open and discusses them in order to clarify roles and responsibilities. It makes recommendations to standing committees when action is needed.

The membership of the Committee for Patient-centered Care was appointed, not elected. The composition of the original committee was determined by the administrator to assure the major objectives of the committee, communication and coordination. The administrator selected the key persons in each group, individuals who had the authority to make commitments for the groups they represented. The membership of any committee should be selected in terms of the objectives to be accomplished. Representation from certain groups will be important in some instances; in other situations the ability of the individual members will be considered. It is as important that the ability of the member matches the job of the committee as it is that the ability of an employee be equal to the position for which he is employed. This principle negates the practice of electing members to committees unless each person eligible for nomination is equally able to contribute to the objectives of the committee.

Equal importance should be attached to the selection of the chairman, for the "right" chairman is one key to effective committee operation. He should be selected for his ability to stimulate others to contribute and to maintain an impartial role in sharing ideas and responsibilities. Too many committees have failed to serve their true purpose because the chairmen were either too autocratic or too indifferent. The organizational relationship between the chairman and the committee members will have some influence on committee functioning. If the chairman is a department head and the members are subordinates, care must be taken that members do not feel that their jobs are threatened if they choose to support an opinion which is different from that of a chairman who holds a superior position in the organization. If the membership is composed of colleagues and peers, the chairman must not be reluctant to assume the leadership necessary to produce purposeful and efficient group action.

Like any other administrative tool, a committee has a place. Given certain diagnoses, a committee is the treatment of choice. When a wide divergence of information is needed, when an outline of all possible ramifications will facilitate execution, when coordination is needed between several departments or divisions, and when vital issues demand representation from several groups, a committee should be organized. If prompt action is needed, if the task is such that one individual has the information and qualifications to make an adequate decision, if it is a question of execution and not decision, the individual approach should be used.

It was mentioned earlier that one of the chief disadvantages of the use of committees is the cost in man hours. This cost is the time used in attendance, in individual preparation for meetings, in arranging a time when a number of persons can meet together, in informing other members of the organization of the decisions and accomplishments of the committee, and in time lost from some other endeavor. A committee requires time to deliberate if a true exchange of ideas and information is to be accomplished before a decision is reached. An individual can usually reach a decision in less time. It should also be noted that a committee is not automatically a democratic group. It can operate as a power group or a clique with a lack of regard for the organization as a whole. It does, however, function as a group only during meetings. Once the members leave the conference room, each again assumes his individual identification and operates accordingly. On the other hand, this tool is unparalleled for obtaining a meeting of the minds, for furnishing a clearinghouse for mutual problems, and for extending the viewpoints of members.

The Charles Evans Memorial Hospital is not unique in having a Committee for Patient-centered Care. Many hospitals have such committees, modeled after the Joint Commission for the Improvement of the Care of the Patient, which was established in 1947 "to provide a forum for free and open discussion among representatives of the medical profession, the nursing profession and hospital administration." [1]

That the director of nursing, in this case, took the initiative and suggested the formation of such a committee is unique perhaps. Too frequently, nursing has waited for an invitation rather than assert its rightful role in improving care for the patient. This particular committee was organized at the highest level of authority and responsibility. In some hospitals committees with similiar purposes have been organized within specialized clinical areas and on individual wards. The purpose is the same—coordination and communication to improve care for patients. Each committee at the ward level should have representatives of the medical staff, of the educational programs that use the unit for student experiences, and of the nursing staff. Although it would not generally be feasible or necessary for a representative of the hospital administrative staff to attend each ward meeting, provision should be made for such participation when an administrative problem arises. The other constituent groups on the hospital team are the dietary personnel, the physical and occupational therapists, and the social workers

[1] Howard Christian Naffziger, M.D., in Office of Defense Mobilization Health Resources Advisory Committee: *Mobilizing Your Personnel Resources for Better Patient Care,* Washington, D.C., 1954, p. v.

—to name but a few. Communication and coordination are needed with these groups, too. Since the medical and nursing staffs have continuous, direct contacts with and responsibilities for the care of the patient, however, the need for conferences between these two disciplines is great. Representatives of the other professional groups should be invited to attend when problems relate to their specific areas. This will serve to keep the membership of the ward area or the hospital committee small enough to facilitate effective action and yet provide for the participation of other groups as the occasion demands.

The initial resistance to the formation of another committee manifested by the persons involved in the case situation is not surprising. The fact that the committee is in existence and apparently functioning well is a tribute, in part, to the chairman (or perhaps chairmen. Since the report does not reveal names, it is not known whether the same person served as chairman from the inception of the committee). The case data indicate some of the means used to create and maintain an effective group. An agenda was distributed in advance of the meeting. This apprised the members of the subjects to be broached at the meeting and permitted them to assemble pertinent information in advance or to elicit comments and opinions from their colleagues. An agenda also helps in directing the progress of a committee meeting. In arranging the agenda, the chairman may place the most pressing or most important items first. It is his responsibility to guide the deliberations so that each item of business receives the attention commensurate with its relative value to the purpose of the committee. Committee members should be advised to notify the chairman, in advance, of items they wish to place on the agenda. One does need to consider how much advance information should be included in an agenda. Notice that in the case situation, the item on progressive patient care created interest and elicited speculation. Rumors may develop from such an incident prior to the meeting and grow beyond the realm of possibility before the real meaning of the item is disclosed. This agenda was distributed to a group of persons accustomed to considering long-range plans so that it is reasonable to assume that no harm was caused by the speculation in this instance. With other groups, a chairman who wishes to stimulate the committee members by a break in routine may wisely include under new business an item which reads, "To be announced later," or "Time out for brainstorming," or "Fifteen minutes for free wheeling."

The effective functioning of many committees is impeded by the lack of attention to seemingly minor details. Failure to start and finish a meeting on time is one violation of good committee practice. This in reality is a lack of respect for the value of the group's time. Permitting interruptions to answer telephone calls is another violation. The chairman should arrange to have resource material available and to have materials prepared prior to or following a meeting so that valuable time is not consumed in deliberating over minor details. For example, prior to a procedures committee meeting, the members should be advised of the procedures to be formulated or revised. A copy of old procedures or of tentative procedures should be distributed in advance so that members may have time to study the procedures and prepare questions or recommendations to bring to the meeting. This advance preparation may be done by the chairman, by a part-time secretary assigned to assist the committee, by an individual committee member, or by a subcommittee appointed for the task.

The "out-of-orbit," "away from the humdrum" change-of-pace technique may revitalize committee meetings. This is of particular value when the usual business of the committee is concerned with resolving conflicts or untangling problems. The occasional introduction of a subject of no immediate concern to any member of the group will tend to stimulate discussion because no one has a vested interest in the topic. This often gives the members a chance to see one another in a different light.

The chairman who introduces this device will need to maintain a permissive atmosphere. There are universal tendencies toward conformity and practicality. Too often persons tend to say, "That won't work here," or, "But isn't that too idealistic for our institution?" Ideas or thoughts should be contributed freely, but analysis or evaluation should be postponed until the matter is actually being considered for the future plans of the institution. Note that the chairman did not immediately admonish the members for their practical or evaluative comments, but when he noticed that the trend continued in this direction he suggested the broader more philosophical approach.

The subject of progressive patient care was introduced because it was and still is a concept being discussed widely among groups responsible for patient care, not because there were any plans to initiate this approach at the Charles Evans Memorial Hospital. A committee to stimulate innovation for the improvement of care must consider all new trends in patient care.

The concept of progressive patient care is not the first innovation that has been proposed in patient care, but it has been subjected to far more widespread study and experimentation than previous proposals. It is one approach to alleviating some of the difficulties experienced in the traditional arrangement in hospital services: [2]

> The principal objective of this growing concept is to provide better treatment and care by organizing hospital services around the individual patient's medical and nursing needs. Specially planned and organized units are set up to which patients are assigned in accordance with their degree of illness and need for care.

The concept incorporates six elements: intensive care, intermediate care, self-care, long-term care, home care, and outpatient care; and it views the hospital as the center of community health facilities. In order to provide continuity of care for patients, it brings convalescent homes and home-nursing services under the direct guidance and control of the hospital. When the patient's medical and nursing needs change, he is transferred to the area of the medical center which has the facilities, specialized equipment, and trained personnel to meet his needs of the moment. Hospitals have been doing this in part, for many years, by using the recovery room for surgical patients postoperatively. The concept is not offered as the solution to all problems of meeting the needs of the patient, but it has proved effective in many communities where it has been implemented. Many questions still need to be answered, particularly in the area of home-care programs. Many persons question the effect on the patient of several transfers during a single hospital stay. On the other hand, others state that the progressive patient care concept provides better utilization of both medical and nursing personnel.

The future will undoubtedly bring other new concepts to consider. Even when an institution does not find it feasible to adopt a new concept, discussion of the concept may produce ideas that are applicable to existing situations. A glance at the few opinions recorded in this case will indicate that the committee's discussion may well lead to some innovations in patient care at the Charles Evans Memorial Hospital.

There are other ways to vary committee meetings to maintain interest and to rouse the members out of their routinized patterns of thought. A change of meeting place, a guest speaker, occasionally, a tour through

[2] Public Health Service, Division of Hospital and Medical Facilities, *Elements of Progressive Patient Care,* U.S. Department of Health, Education and Welfare, Washington, D.C., 1962, p. 1.

problem areas, a change in the membership, a joint meeting with another committee, or time out to summarize the accomplishments of a committee may aid in keeping a committee productive by enchancing the members' sense of accomplishment and feeling of service.

The use of and participation in committees should not be limited to top level personnel. Staff nurses should be given the opportunity to participate. A committee can serve as a training ground for the skills needed to accomplish things by and with people. It is a way of encouraging administrative leadership at the staff nurse level.

SUPPLEMENTARY READING LIST

Abdellah, Faye G., et al.: *Patient-Centered Approaches to Nursing,* The Macmillan Company, New York, 1960, pp. 39–52.

Abdellah, Faye G., and E. Josephine Strachan: "Progressive Patient Care," *American Journal of Nursing,* vol. 59, pp. 649–655, May, 1959.

Alfano, Genrose: "Administration Means Working with Nurses," *American Journal of Nursing,* vol. 64, pp. 83–85, June, 1964.

Bennett, Addison C.: "Importance of Meetings in Two-way Communication," *Hospital Topics,* vol. 46, pp. 45–47, August, 1968.

Brown, Esther Lucile: *Newer Dimensions of Patient Care, Part II, Improving Staff Motivation and Competence in the General Hospital,* Russell Sage Foundation, New York, 1962, pp. 134–157.

De Armond, Fred: "How to Run a Do-Something Meeting," *Hospital Topics,* vol. 39, pp. 21–22, June, 1961.

Ewell, Charles M., Jr.: "The Joint Planning Committee and Long-range Objectives," *Hospitals, J.A.H.A.,* vol. 42, pp. 51–52, 98, December 16, 1968.

Finer, Herman: *Administration and the Nursing Services,* The Macmillan Company, New York, 1952, pp. 233–237.

Freeman, Lucy: *The Improvement of Long-term Care: A New Responsibility for Community Hospitals,* W. K. Kellogg Foundation, Battle Creek, Michigan, 1967.

Haldeman, Jack C., and Faye G. Abdellah: "Concepts of Progressive Patient Care," *Hospitals, J.A.H.A.,* vol. 33, pp. 38–42, 142, 144, May 16, 1959 (Part I); *Hospitals, J.A.H.A.,* vol. 33, pp. 41–46, June 1, 1959 (Part II).

Health Resources Advisory Committee, Subcommittee on Hospital Service: *Mobilizing Your Personnel for Better Patient Care,* Office of Defense Mobilization, Washington, D.C., 1954.

Kellett, Thomas R.: "Fresh Air for Conferences," *Hospitals, J.A.H.A.,* vol. 35, p. 41, July 16, 1961.

Newman, William H., and Charles E. Summer, Jr.: *The Process of Management: Concepts, Behavior and Practice,* Prentice-Hall, Inc., Englewood Cliffs, N.J., 1961, pp. 103–105, 451–453.

Parkinson, C. Northcote: *Parkinson's Law and Other Studies in Administration,* Houghton Mifflin Company, Boston, 1957, pp. 33–44.

Pearsall, Marion, and M. Sue Kern: "Behavioral Science, Nursing Services, and the Collaborative Process: A Case Study," *Journal of Applied Behavioral Science,* vol. 3, no. 2, pp. 243–266, 1967.

Prince, George M.: "How to Be a Better Meeting Chairman," *Harvard Business Review,* vol. 47, pp. 98–108, January–February, 1969.

Public Health Service, Division of Hospital and Medical Facilities: *Elements of Progressive Patient Care,* U.S. Department of Health, Education, and Welfare, Washington, D.C., 1962.

"Symposium of Progressive Patient Care," *Hospitals, J.A.H.A.,* vol. 33, pp. 42–56, January 16, 1959.

Tillman, Rollie, Jr.: "Problems on Review: Committees on Trial," *Harvard Business Review,* vol. 38, pp. 6–8, 11 ff, May–June, 1960.

Weeks, Lewis E., and John R. Griffith (ed.): *Progressive Patient Care: An Anthology,* The University of Michigan, Ann Arbor, 1964.

case 10

Reorganizing for Nursing Practice

One of the prime responsibilities of the Director of Nursing Service and Nursing Education at the Charles Evans Memorial Hospital is that of making decisions regarding the organization and delivery of nursing services. A nursing audit is one of the tools used by Miss Elliott to provide data for consideration during the application of the *administrative blueprint* to this vital component of her job.

Case Data	*Case Notes*
When the chairman of the Nursing Audit Committee submitted the results of the nursing audit of the last quarter of the year to the Director of Nursing Service and Nursing Education, she requested that Miss Elliott meet with the committee at its next meeting to present her impressions of the work of the committee and to suggest future directions. Miss Elliott read the summary forms prepared by each nursing department and then compared the current reports with the summaries of each department for the previous six quarters. A substantial improvement was noted in both the quantity and the quality of nursing notations on the records of patients on all nursing divisions. The quarterly reports of the Nursing Audit Committee revealed that two chart forms had been revised on the basis of the audit findings and were now in use on all nursing units. Miss Elliott decided that the initial objective of the committee—that the nursing records in patient charts should reflect more completely the nursing care being provided—had been achieved. It was evident, however, that the present method of auditing did not provide data on the attempts of the nursing staff to identify and to meet the needs	

Case Data | *Case Notes*

of patients in special diagnostic categories within the broad clinical classifications such as medicine, surgery, or pediatrics. Miss Elliott presented her findings to the Nursing Audit Committee and explored with the committee the possibility of auditing charts on the basis of diagnostic categories rather than on the basis of patient assignment to a nursing unit. The committee members initially expressed some doubts about this change. Several reasons were given:

1. The nursing audit is now being accepted by all levels of the nursing staff. A change will evoke new reactions to the process.

2. Patients in some of the special diagnostic categories require more attention from the professional nurses than from auxiliary nursing personnel. Singling out charts in these categories may seem to be critical of the care given by professional nurses.

3. Before such a change is instituted, standards would have to be devised against which the nursing records of patients in these special categories could be evaluated. The present standards for the nursing audit are based on "good nursing care" and current medicolegal requirements for any patient regardless of diagnosis.

Following discussion of each of the doubts expressed, the nursing supervisors of the medical and surgical units suggested that standards be developed for the nursing care of patients with cardiovascular problems in order to explore the feasibility of this approach. Recently there had been a significant increase in the number of patients admitted for diagnosis and treatment of such problems on the medical and surgical units. The committee approved the recommendation and set a target date of the end of the second quarter for the first audit of nursing care for patients with cardiovascular problems.

After the meeting Miss Elliott asked the supervisors of the medical and surgical units to meet with her in a few days to discuss the nursing care problems precipitated by this apparent

Case Data *Case Notes*

shift in the composition of the patient census on the units under their supervision. She suggested that they consider whether this might be the time to add a clinical specialist to the nursing staff on one or both of the services, or whether some other pattern of recognition such as the establishment of a research program within the nursing department might lead to a higher quality of nursing care. The medical and surgical nursing supervisors immediately expressed their willingness to discuss these ideas with the director. Miss Elliott emphasized that this would be an exploratory discussion and that any proposals formulated would be presented to the Planning Committee for consideration and recommendations.

DISCUSSION

The ultimate goal of evaluation of nursing practice is to provide more effective nursing care for patients. Every effort must be made to ensure that any tool utilized to assess the quantity and quality of nursing care serves that purpose and does not become an administrative device for limiting creativity or rigidly controlling nursing practice.

The nursing audit was instituted at the Charles Evans Memorial Hospital as one of several tools for evaluating current nursing practice and for identifying means of improving practice. The case data do not reveal whether the proposal for an audit originated with the Director of Nursing Service and Nursing Education, with a member of the nursing staff, with a member of the medical staff, or with one of the hospital administrators. The data do reveal, however, that the audit findings are used by the nursing director and by the nursing staff. The staff had proposed new chart forms to facilitate recording, and Miss Elliott examined the findings for elements of comprehensive nursing care not revealed by the audit process. This was done so that the method could be changed to provide evidence of the presence or absence of any element vital to therapeutically effective care or so that some additional tool could be devised to provide the necessary evidence. In this situation she suggested that the method of audit be revised.

The nursing audit is a structured, standardized, objective, and recorded appraisal of the nursing care provided for patients as revealed by the data recorded in the medical records of hospitalized patients or the records of patients under the care of community health nursing services. The nursing audit is similar to an audit performed by accounting departments in that the appraisal is based on records (not on observation), interviews, or other data collection methods. It differs from a financial audit in that it is conducted by nurses within the agency, not by individuals from external agencies. The nursing audit is similar to the medical audit used by physicians to assess the quality of medical care for patients. It is a process that offers the nursing personnel in a health agency the opportunity to create and enforce standards of nursing care and to examine their own practice in a systematic manner.

The specific details in the conduct of an audit of nursing care will vary among nursing service departments or agencies, but the process is the same:

1. The objectives of a nursing audit are formulated.
2. A group responsible for conducting the audit is established.
3. The standards of nursing care are established or made explicit enough to guide the collection of data from the medical record.
4. A determination is made of the manner in which charts are to be selected for auditing.
5. An audit schedule is established.
6. Decisions as to the disposition of the findings of the audit are made.

The prime objective of a nursing audit is to provide evidence of the quality of nursing services being rendered. The *Standards for Organized Nursing Services,* established by the American Nurses' Association in 1965, states that "The nursing department continuously evaluates its administrative, supervisory, and nursing care practices."[1] Notice that the statement decrees that this is the responsibility of the department as a whole, not of the person or persons holding any one position in the nursing department. The statement of standards further suggests that the results of the appraisal are to be used to measure progress, uncover problems, improve nursing care in existing units, and plan for new services.[2] The nursing department at the University of Illinois Research and Educational Hospitals included an additional aim for a nursing audit. The audit was viewed as an instructional device to promote the

[1] American Nurses' Association, *Standards for Organized Nursing Services,* New York, 1965, p. 7.

[2] *Ibid.,* p. 7.

maintenance of the medical record and to increase the medicolegal protection of the institution.[3] A particular agency or department may establish additional objectives for a nursing audit as long as the basic premise is respected. A nursing audit is an instrument for the evaluation of care rendered by the nursing department. It is *not* a device for the evaluation of the performance of individual members of the nursing staff.

The nursing department must determine who is to conduct the audit. The responsibility may be assigned to an existing committee, such as a committee on nursing practice. Most groups that have utilized a nursing audit suggest that an audit program is implemented more effectively when the supervision is the responsibility of a committee established for the purpose of formulating policies for the program and of receiving the findings of audits conducted by various units within the department. Leadership of the nursing team and supervision of nursing care are the responsibilities of professional nurses. It is advisable, therefore, for all categories of professional nurses to be represented on any committee responsible for establishing and evaluating standards of nursing care.

The specific manner in which charts are selected for auditing and the schedule for auditing is established depend somewhat on the types of services provided by the agency and the classifications of patients served. The Charles Evans Memorial Hospital is a voluntary, non-profit, general hospital. The average length of stay of the majority of patients is less than one week. In the course of a year's time few patients are admitted a second time. The tenure of nursing personnel is not indicated in the description of the nursing department; however, most non-governmental, general hospitals in metropolitan areas report a relatively rapid and constant turnover in nursing personnel. It is undoubtedly for these reasons that the nursing department of the hospital conducts an audit every three months. For nursing departments in similar settings a monthly audit may be indicated. For health agencies that provide services to patients for a prolonged period of time, semi-annual or annual audits may be conducted. Psychiatric hospitals, rehabilitation and chronic disease hospitals, and public health nursing services represent health agencies that provide long-term nursing services to the same patients.

The case data do not reveal the manner by which charts are selected

[3] Helen W. Dunn and Elizabeth M. Morgan, *The Nursing Audit,* The League Exchange No. 84, National League for Nursing, New York, 1968, p. 4.

for auditing, although one can infer from the data that records of patients from each nursing unit are examined. In some agencies the medical record librarian is given criteria to use in selecting charts to be submitted to the audit committee. In other agencies the records of all patients discharged in a specified span of time are selected. Miss Elliott suggested that diagnosis might be the criterion for selection, at least from time to time. The important factor to be considered in the establishment of record selection policies is adequate representation of all aspects of nursing care.

Once the policies and procedures for the audit are formulated and refined through experience, the recording of the audit does not require a substantial investment of time from nursing personnel. The utilization of nursing personnel to record has at times been questioned. The justification for the practice is derived from two principles. Professional persons are obligated to set standards for and to control their own practice. Implicit in this obligation is the responsibility for assessing the quality of the services they render. In addition, objectivity and thoroughness in nursing care "is fostered by staff participation in the auditing process."[4]

If a nursing audit is to contribute to the improvement of nursing care the findings must be examined for clues to deficiencies and inadequacies that inhibit the attainment of established standards of care and to innovations that may promote such accomplishment. If the audit is conducted at the nursing unit level, all nursing personnel on the unit should be advised of the degree to which the nursing care given to patients on the unit matches the standards established for care. The care provided by the nursing personnel on a unit is not to be compared against that provided on another nursing unit; standards, not performance of individuals, serve as the criteria of assessment. If the audit is conducted within clinical nursing services such as maternity, pediatric, and medical, then the findings are presented to all nursing personnel in the particular clinical service. The staff is then encouraged to explore means of increasing the quantity and quality of nursing care for patients on the service.

In the situation described in this case, some responsibilities of the director of nursing in relation to the evaluation of nursing care are revealed. Miss Elliott, in reviewing past and present summaries of the findings of the audit, noted an apparent deficiency in the established procedures. She found no evidence of the adaptation of nursing care to meet the needs of patients with similar diagnoses. There is little doubt that the grouping of patients according to similarity of needs has led to more therapeutically effective care. At present, the patients of Charles Evans Memorial Hospital are assigned to nursing units on the basis of broad medical specialty classifications such as medicine, surgery, and pediatrics rather than on the basis of specific diagnostic categories. This practice does not preclude considering patients with similar diagnoses as a group if nursing personnel are attuned to this approach. Miss Elliott may have been seeking information as to the degree to which nursing staff required guidance in recognizing similarities of needs. That the director was also looking for clues to innovation that may lead to raising the quality of nursing care is revealed by her immediate response to the nursing supervisors who reported changes in the composition of the patient census on their clinical services. It is interesting to speculate as to why Miss Elliott suggested that the supervisors consider the addition of a clinical specialist and the establishment of a nursing research program as means of increasing the effectiveness of care. Did she want to convey to the supervisors her expectation that tentative proposals for problem solution should be included in the supervisors' presentation of the nursing care problems on their units? Was she capitalizing on an expressed interest of one or both of the supervisors? Did she perceive that this was an opportune time to introduce some changes that had been shown to be effective in other nursing settings?

The nursing literature presents many philosophical and experiential discussions of the contributions to nursing care of those functioning as clinical specialists. Yet it is not always clear whether the benefits are derived from a new position in the structure of the nursing department which requires certain qualifications or from the individual skills and qualities of the persons designated as clinical specialists. Just as nursing has frequently clutched at the straw of team nursing without incorporating the rationale on which the concept is based, so also has the title of "clinical specialist in nursing" been ascribed to positions which require technical skill but not the cognitive and decision-making skills that are vital components of the role if it is to meet the expectation of improvement of nursing care.

The nurse is prepared in diploma, associate degree, and baccalaureate programs to function as a generalist in a variety of settings. As a practitioner in a specific setting over a period of time, she increases her knowledge of the requirements of the setting, the needs of the particular kinds of patients cared for in the setting, and of the skills required to provide that care. She is specializing only in the sense of adapting her knowledge and skills to a specific end or use. She is not a specialist in the sense of devoting herself to some special branch of "learning," nor is she "distinguished by some unusual quality." The clinical specialist in nursing is a specialist in the full sense of the word in that she devotes herself to one clinical aspect of nursing and not just to one clinical setting; she develops qualities and skills beyond those of the general practitioner in nursing; and she is committed to expanding the knowledge related to the clinical area in which she specializes. It has been suggested that the title *nurse clinician* be used to designate the generalist who has acquired special skills in a particular setting and that the title of *clinical specialist* or *clinical nurse specialist* be utilized to distinguish the nurse who possesses a depth of knowledge and expertise in a recognized specialty field in nursing. The Michigan Nurses' Association defines a Clinical Nursing Specialist as one who "gives expert nursing care and treatment based on scientific knowledge, clinical acumen, and professional judgment, either in a general or special clinical service, and engages in clinical research or teaching and consultation with colleagues in nursing and medicine.[5] A master's degree with special preparation in a clinical area has been established as the qualification for this position. The California Nurses' Association adds to the above requirement that of "documentary evidence of exceptional expertise in a field of specialized competence."[6] In other words, it is not the possession of an advanced degree that alone qualifies one for the position of clinical nurse specialist. There must also be evidence that the knowledge and skills acquired during the educational experience have been applied to the care of patients.

The clinical specialist is expected to contribute directly and indirectly to the nursing care of patients. She participates directly in giving care to those patients who require her special clinical competencies and to those patients who present nursing care problems which other nursing

[5] Michigan Nurses' Association, *Recommended Qualifications and Employment Standards for Professional Nurse Positions—1967,* The Association, Lansing, Michigan, 1967, p. 7.

[6] California Nurses' Association, *Clinical Nurse Specialist,* The Association, San Francisco, 1967, p. 5, mimeo.

personnel are unable to diagnose. In both instances she concentrates primarily on evolving nursing care plans and procedures which other members of the nursing care team will then implement. The clinical specialist also has a direct responsibility for engaging in research at the bedside (or "grassroots" level), to the end that more effective means of care are found and perhaps even new knowledge discovered. Indirectly the clinical specialist promotes patient care by influencing other members of the nursing care team and by collaborating with colleagues in other health care disciplines.

To a degree these expectations are held for the professional nurse who is functioning in a staff nurse or nurse team leader position in health agencies. How then does the patient care given by the clinical nurse specialist differ from the care given by these general practitioners? Johnson, Wilcox, and Moidel suggest that the practice of the clinical specialist is distinguished by (1) the depth of knowledge and cognitive ability she utilizes in assessing, explaining, prescribing, and evaluating nursing care situations and (2) the greater degree of proficiency demonstrated in decision making.[7] Reiter points out that the team leader in the present system of patient services is concerned primarily with the *amount* of care while "the nurse clinician, by contrast, is concerned with the *kind* of care."[8] Others emphasize that the primary sub-role of the clinical specialist is that of "change agent."[9, 10] The staff nurse and the team leader may, on occasion, identify the need for and initiate change that leads to more effective nursing care; however, the clinical specialist is committed to the role of change agent and has gained the additional knowledge and expertise requisite to the execution of this role.

The staff nurse and the team leader consult with physicians and members of other health care disciplines regarding the care of individual patients for whom they provide nursing care. They seek advice on problems encountered in carrying out medical orders; they convey to others

[7] Dorothy Johnson, Joan Wilcox, and Harriet Moidel, "The Clinical Specialist As a Practitioner," *American Journal of Nursing*, vol. 67, pp. 2298–2303, November, 1967.

[8] Frances Reiter, "The Nurse-Clinician," *American Journal of Nursing*, vol. 66, p. 278, February, 1966.

[9] Marjory Gordon, "The Clinical Specialist As Change Agent," *Nursing Outlook*, vol. 17, pp. 37–39, March, 1969.

[10] Maxine E. Loomis, "The Clinical Specialist As a Change Agent," *Nursing Forum*, vol. 7, no. 2, pp. 136–145, 1968.

who share responsibility for the care of the patient the needs of the patient for service. The clinical specialist goes beyond seeking advice from and referring problems to other disciplines. She works jointly and deliberates with those in health care disciplines who are specialists in areas related to her clinical field of competence. Just as members of other disciplines assume responsibility for representing the discipline as a whole and expect to be held accountable for the contribution of the discipline to the health care of the patient, so, too, in these deliberations does the clinical specialist act as a representative of nursing and is held accountable.

In the case situation, Miss Elliott implied that the addition of a clinical specialist would necessitate reorganization of the nursing department. This suggestion was derived undoubtedly from the experiences of others in attempting to absorb nurses with a depth of clinical nursing knowledge and a high level of competence in nursing practice into the existing line organization of nursing departments. In traditional nursing settings, the supervisor has limited direct contact with patients. Her span of control over patients and personnel is so extensive that the data which she utilizes in decision making comes from second-, third-, or fourth-hand sources, not from direct contact with the patient whose care she is expected to guide personnel in giving. The head nurse often has nominal responsibility for the care given to patients on the nursing unit twenty-four hours a day, seven days a week. Her actual range of authority is frequently limited, however, to the period of time that she is actually present on the division. The assessment of her competence as a head nurse is generally based on patient and personnel "tension indices" rather than on the therapeutic effectiveness of the nursing care given by the personnel on the unit. These factors do not preclude the possibility of effective functioning of clinical nurse specialists in these traditional positions in nursing. They are, however, factors that must be considered seriously in attempting to improve the quality of nursing practice through the introduction of a new position such as that of clinical specialist. Aydelotte proposes that the present view of administration in nursing as "maintaining and protecting a system or meeting the needs of personnel" rather than as serving the needs of patients is one of the obstacles to the functioning of the clinical nurse specialist.[11]

[11] Myrtle K. Aydelotte, "Issues in Professional Nursing: The Need for Clinical Excellence," *Nursing Forum,* vol. 7, no. 1, p. 83, 1968.

The literature seems to indicate that Miss Elliott and the Planning Committee may encounter more difficulty in introducing the concept of clinical specialist than in establishing a program of research in the nursing department. There is a growing recognition among all professional nurse practitioners that health needs, social conditions, and knowledge are advancing and changing so rapidly that change has become one constant in almost every setting and situation. There is also increasing awareness among nurse practitioners that responses to the need for change must be planned, not made on the spur of the moment, and that these responses must emanate from explorations of nursing practice. The clinical specialist in nursing is prepared to conduct these explorations within her area of clinical expertise, but she is not necessarily ready to go beyond this area to examine practice in other clinical areas. A nursing research program, under the direction of a qualified nurse researcher, can foster the necessary spirit of clinical inquiry in all areas of nursing practice within the nursing department, can provide the assistance needed by nurse practitioners in designing and implementing studies, and can assist specialists in various areas to identify the commonalities in nursing care problems and to apply the findings of one area to nursing practice in other clinical areas. Improvements in nursing practice are dependent not only on the provision for nurses with depth of knowledge in the various clinical areas of practice but also on experimentation to identify more therapeutic practices and to develop theories of nursing practice.

The director of the nursing department does not give nursing care to patients personally. She is actively engaged, however, with the nursing staff in designing an organizational structure that enables the nursing personnel to practice nursing in ways that provide patients with therapeutically effective nursing care. The structure of the organization of today may not be adequate for the health care services needed in the future. Each professional nurse has the obligation to be an assessor, evaluator, and innovator in nursing practice. The director of nursing must also be an instigator of necessary changes.

SUPPLEMENTARY READING LIST

Abraham, Gertrude E.: "Promoting Nursing Research in an Organized Nursing Service," *American Journal of Nursing*, vol. 68, pp. 818–821, April, 1968

American Nurses' Association: *Standards for Organized Nursing Services,* The Association, New York, 1965.

American Nurses' Association, Commission on Nursing Services: *The Position, Role and Qualifications of the Administrator of Nursing Services,* The Association, New York, 1969.

Aydelotte, Myrtle K.: "Issues in Professional Nursing: The Need for Clinical Excellence," *Nursing Forum,* vol. 7, no. 1, pp. 72–86, 1968.

Ayers, Rachel, et al.: "Action for Change: An Experiment in Nursing Service Reorganization," *American Journal of Nursing,* vol. 69, pp. 783–786, April, 1969.

Baziak, Anna T.: "Prospects for Change in Nursing," *Nursing Forum,* vol. 6, no. 2, pp. 134–152, 1967.

Davis, K. G.: "Give Nurses a Chance to Explore These Twelve Roads to Better Care," *The Modern Hospital,* vol. 111, pp. 82–85, October, 1968.

Deeken, Sister Mary Helen Louise: *A Guide for the Nursing Service Audit,* Catholic Hospital Association, St. Louis, Missouri, 1960.

Dunn, Helen W., and Elizabeth M. Morgan: *The Nursing Audit,* The League Exchange No. 84, National League for Nursing, New York, 1968.

Ellis, Rosemary: "The Practitioner as Theorist," *American Journal of Nursing,* vol. 69, pp. 1434–1438, July, 1969.

Fagin, Claire M.: "The Clinical Specialist As Supervisor," *Nursing Outlook,* vol. 15, pp. 34–36, January, 1967.

Gordon, Marjory: "The Clinical Specialist As Change Agent," *Nursing Outlook,* vol. 17, pp. 37–39, March, 1969.

Johnson, Dorothy, Joan Wilcox, and Harriet Moidel: "The Clinical Specialist As a Practitioner," *American Journal of Nursing,* vol. 67, pp. 2298–2303, November, 1967.

Johnson, Everett A.: "Nursing Reorganization Strengthens Head Nurse Role, Provides Special Nursing Consultants," *Hospitals, J.A.H.A.,* vol. 42, pp. 85–90, June 16, 1968.

Little, Dolores: "The Nurse Specialist," *American Journal of Nursing,* vol. 67, pp. 552–556, March, 1967.

Loomis, Maxine E.: "The Clinical Specialist As a Change Agent," *Nursing Forum,* vol. 7, no. 2, pp. 136–145, 1968.

McGuire, Rita L.: "Bedside Nursing Audit," *American Journal of Nursing,* vol. 68, pp. 2146–2148, October, 1968.

Paynich, Mary L., et al.: "Is There a Role for the Nurse Clinician in Public Health?" *Nursing Outlook,* vol. 17, pp. 32–36, July, 1969.

Phaneuf, Marie C.: "Analysis of a Nursing Audit," *Nursing Outlook,* vol. 16, pp. 57–60, January, 1968.

Phaneuf, Marie C.: "A Nursing Audit Method," *Nursing Outlook,* vol. 12, pp. 42–45, May, 1964.

Phaneuf, Marie C.: "The Nursing Audit for Evaluation of Patient Care," *Nursing Outlook,* vol. 14, pp. 51–54, June, 1966.

Ramphal, Marjorie: "Clinical Nursing Supervision," *American Journal of Nursing,* vol. 68, pp. 1900–1902, September, 1968.
Reiter, Frances: "The Nurse-Clinician," *American Journal of Nursing,* vol. 66, pp. 274–280, February, 1966.
Thomas, Lauraine A.: "Action for Change: A Rationale for Nursing Administration," *American Journal of Nursing,* vol. 69, pp. 774–776, April, 1969.
Young, Lucie S.: "The Modern Nurse Administrator," *Journal of Nursing Education,* vol. 8, pp. 13–17, 20–24, August, 1969.

case **11**

Planning for the Future

The Planning Committee of the Nursing Department meets monthly. Its primary purpose is to coordinate the activities of the various nursing divisions and to serve as a clearing house for proposals of changes in nursing practice. Proposed changes are referred to standing committees or to special work committees for investigation. These committees then submit their recommendations to the Planning Committee for action. The membership is composed of the director of nursing, the assistant directors, the nursing supervisors, and representatives from the head nurse group. The Director of Nursing Service and Nursing Education serves as chairman of the committee.

Case Data | *Case Notes*

As the Planning Committee assembled for the March meeting, Miss Helen Robertson, Supervisor of Specialty Services, commented to one of the other supervisors, "Miss Elliott looks as though she is about to 'burst' with news of some kind."

As the meeting progressed several other members commented to one another on Miss Elliott's exhilaration and speculated on which item on the agenda may have generated this intense interest. Finally Miss Elliott announced, "You know how many times we have said, 'If only the nursing department could have been in on the original planning things would have been different!' Our chance to do so has come! It is anticipated that when the new facilities for the research laboratories are constructed an additional patient unit will be built on the top floor of the new addition. There are, as yet, no plans on paper for this unit. This time nursing will have a chance to contribute to the planning from the start."

The expressions on the faces of the members of the Planning Committee seemed to reflect Miss

Case Data *Case Notes*

Elliott's enthusiasm. Questions were raised quickly.

"Where do we start?"

"How much time do we have?"

"What kind of patients will be admitted?"

For some of these questions Miss Elliott had answers. The division was to have a capacity for twenty-four medical patients referred from the outpatient department. The tentative plans suggested two- and four-bed rooms. The forecast called for the unit to be ready for occupancy in eighteen months.

One of the head nurses suggested that the new unit may be an ideal place to experiment with the unit manager pattern of organization. Someone questioned whether it was wise to try a new scheme when a new unit was being opened. At that point Miss Elliott suggested that instead of discussing the relative merits of each proposal the group spend the remaining time in listing questions and suggestions to consider in planning the new unit. The following were voiced by the group:

Would a new head nurse take over the unit or would one be transferred from an existing division?

Would it be possible to purchase new equipment for the unit? If so, what would be the budget allotment?

Could an audiovisual system be installed from the patients' rooms to the nurses station?

The nurses station might be located in the center instead of at one end of the division.

A combination day-dining and visitors room should be planned for the unit.

Tub and shower facilities should be provided.

Would the same ratio of professional-to-nonprofessional personnel be used as was now being used on most of the divisions?

Would this division use the team or functional method of assignment?

Which supervisor would be responsible for the division?

Case Data *Case Notes*

Shouldn't the dietary and housekeeping departments be included in the planning?

As the meeting drew to a close Miss Elliott suggested that the following subcommittees be formed to participate in developing plans for the new unit:

1. A liaison committee to work with the Planning Committee of the Medical Staff.
2. A staffing subcommittee.
3. An equipment and supplies subcommittee.
4. A physical facilities subcommittee.

She asked members to tell which subcommittee assignment they preferred and to suggest additional personnel who might contribute to the planning. She then announced that as soon as the liaison committee clarified with the medical staff planning committee some of the major questions, the other subcommittees would be activated. At the close of the meeting she said, "In the meantime, you are welcome to view the architect's plans for the clinical research laboratory facilities. These will give you some indication of the space that will be available."

DISCUSSION

The first case report in this series considered the responsibility of the staff nurse in formulating a plan of care for an individual patient. It seems fitting that the final case be concerned with the responsibility of the entire nursing service department in planning the facilities for the care of patients in the future. The case reports were arranged in this order to allow the reader to move from the relatively simple to the more complex situations and to emphasize the crucial role that planning plays in the administrative process. Planning, including thinking, is the foundation upon which the rest of the process depends.

Throughout the discussions of the preceding cases, evidence of planning is noted. Every organization has structured plans and informal traditions that provide a framework within which specific decisions are made. The vacation policy mentioned in Case 6 is one such plan. The visiting-hour policy mentioned in Case 5 is another plan. These are examples of standing plans. The same decision is used to guide action over and over again.

A fire drill routine is a standing plan. A standardized order form is another type of standing plan. All these are decisions made to serve as guides to action in recurring situations. In contrast, this last case involves the formulation of a "single-use plan," a plan devised to deal with a particular problem or to guide action for a specific time period.

In an earlier case discussion the decision-making process was applied to an emergency situation and to the formulation of a standing plan, a visiting-hour policy. The same steps may be used to evolve the recommendations of the nursing service department for the arrangement of the new patient division:

1. Recognize the problem. What is the purpose or goal to consider? What are the limitations to consider?
2. Outline alternative solutions.
3. Collect the data.
4. Analyze and compare the possible solutions.
5. Select the preferred solution.

These recommendations, along with the proposals of the other departments involved with inpatient units—i.e., the medical staff, the dietary department, the housekeeping department—will be subjected to the same five steps by the person or committee appointed to reach a final decision and to consult with the architect and contractor. Once the working drawings have been approved, the sixth step in the formulation of a single-use plan will be taken: the decision may be programmed. The principal steps for achieving the objective of opening a new unit for patients will be outlined, an approximate time may be designated for the completion of each step, and the person or persons who are to take each step may be indicated. It is to be hoped that the nursing department will have an opportunity to offer recommendations regarding its role in the program for the project. The forwarding of well-defined recommendations for the new unit may enhance this possibility.

The easiest way to plan is to perpetuate current practice. Indications of such a tendency are revealed in the case data. The first few questions raised by members of the Planning Committee sought specific information about the extent of the new project. Subsequent questions, for the most part, reflected inclinations to transplant present facilities and practices to a new setting. One exception is noted in the suggestion to introduce a unit manager pattern of organization on the new patient unit as an experiment. The head nurse who proposed this may have been trying to introduce a more dynamic note.

One aspect of the first step in the planning process is to consider the limitations specified or inherent in the project. These are the only decisions about the new unit disclosed by Miss Elliott:

1. This was to be an inpatient unit with beds for twenty-four medical patients.

2. Two- and four-bed rooms were suggested.

3. The patients would be referred for admission by the outpatient clinic; in other words, their medical care would be provided by interns and residents under the guidance of the faculty of the school of medicine.

4. The location of the unit was predetermined—the top floor of an addition being built to house the clinical research laboratories.

5. A tentative opening date had already been set.

To these stated facts or decisions may be added several implied restrictions. The actual space available for the unit was limited to no more than that already planned for the research laboratory on the floor or floors below. Since the architect's plans for those areas were available, it may be presumed that the patient unit was an afterthought. One may also assume that access to the ward was already determined since the addition would undoubtedly connect to an existing building. These restrictions, both explicit and implicit, are relatively few in number. Of all of them, the time factor is perhaps the most limiting. It does take time to propose alternative solutions and to subject them to careful analysis. However, there is a wide range of possible suggestions open to the nursing staff.

Miss Elliott's excitement over this first opportunity to contribute to the plans is understandable. The case data do not indicate why the suggestions of the nursing department are being sought. This is of no great importance to the case at hand. It is important, however, that the department accept the responsibility now, not so much for the prestige or satisfaction of the nursing staff as for the benefit of the patients. No other group has more sustained contact with patients. No other group has greater potential for contributing to the planning of the environment for the patient.

The approach of the nursing director to the presentation of the problem seemed to be designed to stimulate the interest of the group. It is assumed that the reference to the slights in the past was intended to challenge the staff to "pick up the gauntlet." This negative approach may have the effect of dampening the enthusiasm of the group for the entire project, or it may encourage them to play safe by using a traditional instead of a creative approach to the problem. One wonders what responses would have been evoked by an invitation to "think big" and to make all suggestions, no matter how remote they may be from current practice. It seems evident that Miss Elliott was conscious of the need to maintain a permissive atmosphere so that each member would feel free to propose ideas. When one of the staff started to question the proposal of another, the director suggested a moratorium on analysis and evaluation.

Miss Elliott also recognized that the task may be accomplished more expeditiously by several small groups than by one large group. In this way, staff members would have the opportunity to explore areas of special interest and special talents, and more members of the nursing staff would be involved in the planning process while keeping committees to a manageable size.

Although undoubtedly suggested as a means of capitalizing on individual interests, the "volunteer" method of forming committees may not be the most suitable for a liaison committee that will have responsibility, in part, for determining the purpose or goal of a new unit for medical patients. Suppose that none of the representatives from the medical nursing units elected to serve on the liaison committee? In a situation such as this, where special data or experience may be required, individuals that meet the requirements should be requested to serve to provide necessary information. This would not prohibit other interested persons from volunteering to fill out the membership of a committee.

There seems to be another drawback to the procedure outlined by the Director of Nursing. At the close of the initial meeting it had been announced that the planning committees for physical facilities, equipment and supplies, and staffing would be activated *after* the liaison committee had met with the medical planning committee to clarify some of the major questions. What major questions? None of the questions recorded in the case data can be considered consequential at this stage of planning. They are seeds for thought, but they are not yet guides for action. Before a group begins to study the placement of the nurses station, the need for a visual intercommunication system, the selection of a head nurse, or the method of assignment, the purpose of the plan must be established. It is to be a plan for a unit for twenty-four medical patients, but need it be a traditional hospital unit for medical patients? May it be used as an intensive care unit; an adolescent unit; a rehabilitation unit; a research unit; a convalescent unit; or a diagnostic unit? It is assumed that a need has been identified for increasing the number of beds for clinic patients on the medical service by twenty-four. Since no other qualification has been declared by the persons making the initial decision, one must assume that they did not identify any outstanding need for specialized care. This does not mean that the need does not exist. It is possible that the persons who made the decision know only that there is a long list of clinic patients waiting for admission. If a division were opened to meet some of the special needs of twenty-four patients presently accommodated on existing medical divisions, the same net increase in available beds may result and, most likely, the care of patients may be improved and extended immeasurably. Nursing cannot assume a passive role in such situations. It must consider the situation, collect the facts, analyze them carefully, and formulate a rational recommendation. In the case situation this vital first step seems to have been bypassed, unless Miss Elliott is assuming that the liaison committee will draw up a recommendation regarding the purpose or goal for the unit before meeting with the medical planning committee. If this is so, the majority of the membership of the Planning Committee is being denied the opportunity to participate fully in the planning. The greater the number of persons included in the phase of clarifying the problem, the greater the possibility of obtaining a wide selection of alternative solutions.

The time limitation undoubtedly influenced the approach to this situation. At times such as these the director and her staff need to evaluate the importance of the project. Is it worth sacrificing or delaying other plans temporarily to devote time to this one? This decision has to be made in light of the importance of other plans to patient care. It may be possible, for example, to suspend the work of the procedures committee temporarily and to elicit the concentrated assistance of this group in some of the fact finding. It may be possible to rearrange the responsibilities of the assistant directors to free one of them to serve as coordinator for the planning period. It may save time in the long run if such a coordinator would interview key persons on the nursing staff to elicit ideas or problem situations, to group the suggestions for trends and issues, then present them to the entire Planning Committee for consideration in clarifying the real problem. Once the group has made a recommendation regarding the goal for the unit, the more detailed planning can be done in the areas of equipment and supplies, physical facilities, and staffing.

In making recommendations regarding physical layout and equipment, an idea that has not been used before, or inability of the staff to conceptualize how the idea could be transformed into reality, should not deter suggestions. The staff is not expected to have the technical knowledge necessary for drafting architectural drawings. They are expected to be able to present their ideas clearly and objectively, and to substantiate the reasons for a proposal.

When the board of trustees approves the preliminary plan for an addition or a new venture, some limitation is placed on the expenditures for the project. In the initial planning phase, it is expected that the needs of the patients and the staff will be considered before cost. Suppose, for example, that an intensive care unit is being planned. In order to ensure the maximum supervision of patients by conservation of nursing time, a locker room and a rest room for the nursing staff should be provided, even though these facilities are not provided for the staff on other divisions. Before submitting any proposals the planning groups should identify the advantages and disadvantages of a specific choice. Their plan should provide for the desirable maximum, but they should be prepared to substantiate the minimum acceptable for effective functioning. Once the final plans for the project have been accepted and the final budget set, the nursing department should expect to operate within the allocated budget. The cost of equipment for a new unit should be included in the project budget, but not the operating expenditures for supplies and staffing. The director of nursing will have to prepare a request for an additional allocation to cover these costs for the remainder of the fiscal year if the budget for the year has already been determined. In this instance sufficient time would seem to be available for the Director of Nursing to include the costs of staffing and supplying the unit in the annual budget request of the nursing department.

As the plans progress, some of the questions first raised by the staff will be answered relatively easily. Other questions will require intensive study. The suggestion regarding the use of the unit manager concept on the new nursing division is one that can only be answered after exploration and discussion with several other departments within the organization. The unit or services manager system is designed to bring the hospital administration to the patient unit in order to free the head nurse and her staff from administrative tasks not directly related to nursing. The unit manager assumes the responsibility for directing and coordinating all the services for the patient except nursing functions. He supervises the general housekeeping and maintenance on the unit, arranges for the transportation of patients within the hospital, and keeps supplies in stock and equipment in repair. In other words, he is responsible for all the services that support the medical treatment and nursing care needed by patients.

The inauguration of a system such as this would necessitate a reorganization of the administrative structure. In some hospitals the unit manager system has been incorporated within the nursing department. In other hospitals or health agencies a department distinct from and independent of the nursing department has been established. The latter form of organization provides for a sharper distinction between patient care and patient service functions. Under this system the nursing department is not required to compensate for absences or deficiencies within the unit manager department. The unit manager coordinator is responsible and accountable for the services required by the patient.

If the analysis of the situation at the Charles Evans Memorial Hospital reveals that the unit manager system is feasible and desirable, the organization chart of the hospital (page 145) may be revised to clarify lines of communication and responsibility. The chart shown in Figure 9 represents one possible form of organization. Because the unit managers would be coordinating the activities of personnel in several departments, distinct channels of communication would need to be established. These paths are suggested by dotted lines in the chart. The assistant directors responsible for the separate departments would have to establish specific procedures to accomplish the desired objectives. These are some of the ramifications of the application of the *administrative blueprint* to one suggestion put forth spontaneously in the discussion of the addition of a new unit within an established organization. The proposal may have no direct bearing on the physical design of the new unit, but it does have implications for the functioning of the unit. It must, therefore, be considered in the design process.

Once the architect's plans have been drawn and the contractors have started to work, activation of the plans will continue. Arrangements would have to be made for staffing the unit. The respective merits of transferring a head nurse or appointing a new head nurse will have to be decided in light of the personnel available. It is to be hoped that the leadership training program has identified and trained staff to assume vacancies when they occur. If not, there is sufficient time to prepare

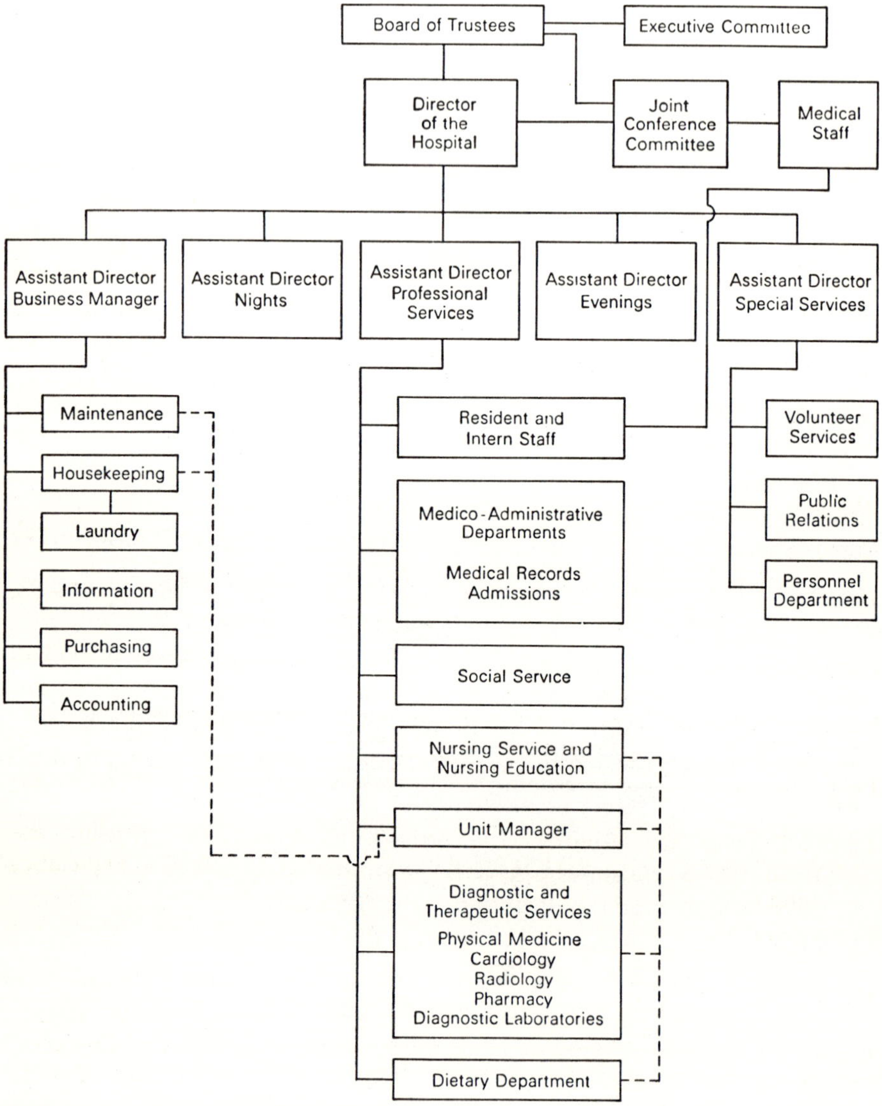

FIGURE 9. Proposed revision of the organization chart, Charles Evans Memorial Hospital

a nurse to assume the direction of the ward. Plans should be made for the head nurse to be available on the unit as the equipment is placed and the division is stocked with supplies. The staff should be appointed and available prior to the arrival of patients on the unit. If the decision is made to use this unit to meet the special needs of patients, the entire staff should be available in advance to plan the procedures and policies to be used in providing this care for patients.

Nurses must take a dynamic part in planning patient care and the environment for patient care. The use of the administrative process is vital to planning and accomplishing this goal. It is also vital in selling this plan to others. The demonstration that a careful analysis has been done, and the conviction that the selections can be explained, will contribute to the acceptance of the plan. With this will come increasing respect for the ability of nurses to provide and implement comprehensive care for patients.

SUPPLEMENTARY READING LIST

American Journal of Nursing, "Illinois Research Tries Unit Managers," vol. 63, p. 47, December, 1963.

American Journal of Nursing, "The Realities of Staffing," vol. 62, pp. 56–63, November, 1962.

American Journal of Nursing, "Unit Manager System Tried at One More Hospital," vol. 64, p. 42, August, 1964.

Bennett, Addison C.: "Importance of Meetings in Two-way Communication," *Hospital Topics,* vol. 46, pp. 45–47, August, 1968.

Bennett, Addison C.: "Organization Analysis," *Hospital Topics,* vol. 46, pp. 43–46, March, 1968.

Brodt, Dagmar E.: "The Service Manager: Innovation for Nursing and Health Organization," *Hospital Progress,* vol. 47, pp. 69–74, September, 1966.

Editorial: "The Lonely Room at the Top," *American Journal of Nursing,* vol. 62, p. 55, November, 1962.

Egolf, Marion G.: "Unit Management Program Provides More Effective Use of Personnel," *Hospitals, J.A.H.A.,* vol. 43, pp. 77–82, July 16, 1969.

Gaulin, Richard P.: "Nursery Planning: Considerations of the Engineer," *Hospital Topics,* vol. 43, pp. 108–109, August, 1965. (See also the articles by Daniel A. Lagozzino and Louise A. Murray.)

Henderson, Cynthia: "Freeing the Nurse to Nurse," *American Journal of Nursing,* vol. 64, pp. 72–77, March, 1964.

Katz, Geneva: "A Nurse Administrator and New Design Concepts," *Nursing Outlook,* vol. 15, pp. 50–52, July, 1967.

Lagozzino, Daniel A.: "Nursery Planning: Medical Guidelines for the Designer," *Hospital Topics*, vol. 43, pp. 107–109, August, 1965.

Lambertsen, Eleanor C.: "Reorganize Nursing to Re-emphasize Care," *The Modern Hospital*, vol. 108, pp. 68–71, 138, January, 1967.

McBeth, Max A., and Douglas C. Carpenter: "Seven-year Appraisal of a Ward Manager System," *Hospitals, J.A.H.A.*, vol. 40, pp. 79–80, 82, 84, 86, March 16, 1966.

Murray, B. Louise: "Nursery Planning: Contribution of the Nurse to Design," *Hospital Topics*, vol. 43, pp. 110–116, August, 1965.

Nellis, W. L.: "Unit Managers Cut Patients' Complaints 50 Percent," *Hospitals, J.A.H.A.*, vol. 46, pp. 42–45, June, 1968.

Newman, William H., and Charles E. Summer, Jr.: *The Process of Management: Concepts, Behavior and Practice*, Prentice-Hall, Inc., Englewood Cliffs, N.J., 1961, pp. 359–389, 598–601.

Pitel, Martha: "A Nurse's View: Hospital Design Should Focus on Patient's Needs," *Hospitals, J.A.H.A.*, vol. 43, pp. 67–68, May 16, 1969.

Purdy, Frances: "The Nursing Service Department in the Hospital," in Edythe Alexander et al., *Nursing Service Administration*, The C. V. Mosby Company, St. Louis, 1962, pp. 81–139.

Rinehart, Elma L.: *Management of Nursing Care*, The Macmillan Company, New York, 1969.

Rourke, Anthony J. J.: "In Nursing Unit Planning . . . Design Follows Function," *Hospitals, J.A.H.A.*, vol. 39, pp. 42–47, August 1, 1965.

Scott, Jessie M.: "Seeing Nursing Activities As They Are," *American Journal of Nursing*, vol. 62, pp. 70–71, November, 1962.

Smith, Dorothy M.: "Nursing Practice Within a Hospital Nursing Service," in National League for Nursing, Department of Hospital Nursing, *Blueprint for Progress in Hospital Nursing*, National League for Nursing, New York, 1963.

Stull, Richard J.: "Personal Advantages To a Budget," *Hospitals, J.A.H.A.*, vol. 33, p. 50, February 16, 1959.

Stull, Richard J.: "Planning: Vital Function of Administrative Nurses," *Hospital Topics*, vol. 43, pp. 46–49, February, 1965.

Wheeler, Dorothy V.: "A New Direction for Directors?" *American Journal of Nursing*, vol. 62, pp. 64–66, November, 1962.

Zimmerman, James P.: "Initiating a Unit Management System," *Hospital Progress*, vol. 49, pp. 64–66, 72, February, 1968.

15

Predictions

by Evelyn M. Hamil

In the foregoing pages an attempt has been made to describe nursing service administration as it presently exists and to present some new thinking as to what it may become in the future. A firm commitment to the triumvirate approach to administration is evidenced throughout the text—the belief that the ultimate success achieved in a position of administration is directly related to and equally dependent upon the characteristics of the person occupying the position, the extent to which this person is familiar with the place in which he is an administrator, and his knowledge of the administrative process. Directly deriving from this belief is the prediction that nursing service administration will move forward at a rate that parallels the rate with which less and less attention is given to the minutia of the job—the isolated techniques or tools of the job—and more and more attention is given to the person, the place, and the process. But the real significance of this prediction rests with the *kind* of attention that is given to these three elements of administration. Sound experimentation conducted by members of the nursing profession is the attention that will serve to carry nursing administration forward.

If the desired influence of this text is achieved, much that has been written will be subjected to a critical evaluation by way of structured investigations. Most certainly the effects of a liberal education on the person, as herein stated, will be studied in an effort to scientifically validate or reject the statements. Can effects that have been identified only through empirical observations, despite the experience of the observer, be accepted without question?

The assumption that administration is administration in any setting will surely be tested by many nurse researchers. Too long the belief has been held by too many that the hospital setting is unique. And, as a part of the same question, additional explorations will be made in an effort to understand better the effects of the hospital as a social organization on the individuals in the organization. In the institutional hierarchy, does each employee tend to rise to his level of incompetence, as has been suggested by Dr. Laurence J. Peter, professor of education at the University of Southern California? Does the system develop, perpetuate, and reward incompetence?

But the forecast that is the most plainly visible one is undoubtedly the further substantiation that will be sought in the area of the process of administration. Nursing will assume its rightful role in researching administrative theories—the ones that have been proposed and the hypotheses that have not yet been postulated. The proposition that all nurses perform some functions that are administrative in nature, the practicality of the *administrative blueprint*, and the effectiveness of case analysis as a method of teaching and learning the administrative process should stir the imagination of the inquiring mind and promote the concept of administrative relevance.

If these predictions materialize, the future of nursing will be brighter. The outcomes of these investigations are not the consequential consideration here, but rather the fact that thinking nurses equipped to assume the role of principal investigators have elected to make a contribution to this field of knowledge—to add to the developing science of administration.

Index

Index